Animal Virology

Animal Virology

Editor: Henry Robinson

R CALLISTO
REFERENCE

www.callistoreference.com

Callisto Reference,
118-35 Queens Blvd., Suite 400,
Forest Hills, NY 11375, USA

Visit us on the World Wide Web at:
www.callistoreference.com

ISBN: 978-1-64116-252-4 (Hardback)

Cataloging-in-Publication Data

Animal virology / edited by Henry Robinson.
    p. cm.
Includes bibliographical references and index.
ISBN 978-1-64116-252-4
1. Veterinary virology. 2. Virology. 3. Animals. 4. Virus diseases. I. Robinson, Henry.
SF780.4 .A55 2020
636.089 601 94--dc23

Table of Contents

Permissions

List of Contributors

Index

Preface

This book has been an outcome of determined endeavour from a group of educationists in the field. The primary objective was to involve a broad spectrum of professionals from diverse cultural background involved in the field for developing new researches. The book not only targets students but also scholars pursuing higher research for further enhancement of the theoretical and practical applications of the subject.

Animal virology is the science concerned with the study of viruses in animals. It is a sub-field of veterinary medicine. Several families of viruses are of particular interest in the study of animal virology, such as rhabdoviruses, pestiviruses, arteriviruses, toroviruses, coronaviruses, circoviruses, etc. Rhabdoviruses are a family of single stranded RNA viruses which can infect insects, fish and mammals. Notable examples of rhabdoviruses are rabies virus and vesicular stomatitis virus. Foot-and-mouth disease virus is a cause of foot-and-mouth disease in cattle, pigs, sheep and goats. Pestiviruses cause bovine viral diarrhea and classical swine fever. RNA viruses of the family orthomyxoviridae cause influenza in birds and mammals. This book includes some of the vital pieces of work being conducted across the world, on various topics related to animal virology. It studies, analyzes and upholds the pillars of animal virology and its utmost significance in modern times. It includes contributions of experts and scientists which will provide innovative insights into this field.

It was an honour to edit such a profound book and also a challenging task to compile and examine all the relevant data for accuracy and originality. I wish to acknowledge the efforts of the contributors for submitting such brilliant and diverse chapters in the field and for endlessly working for the completion of the book. Last, but not the least; I thank my family for being a constant source of support in all my research endeavours.

Editor

The Antiviral Effect of High-Molecular Weight Poly-Gamma-Glutamate against Newcastle Disease Virus on Murine Macrophage Cells

Melbourne Talactac,[1,2] Jong-Soo Lee,[2] Hojin Moon,[2] Mohammed Y. E. Chowdhury,[2,3] and Chul Joong Kim[2]

[1]College of Veterinary Medicine and Biomedical Sciences, Cavite State University, 4122 Cavite, Philippines
[2]College of Veterinary Medicine, Chungnam National University, Daejeon 305-764, Republic of Korea
[3]Chittagong Veterinary and Animal Sciences University, Chittagong 4202, Bangladesh

Correspondence should be addressed to Chul Joong Kim; cjkim@cnu.ac.kr

Academic Editor: Subhash Verma

This study demonstrates the capacity of HM-γ-PGA treatment to significantly protect murine macrophage cells (RAW 264.7 cells) against NDV infection. Such protection can be explained by the induction of antiviral state of HM-γ-PGA in RAW 264.7 cells via TLR4-mediated IRF-3, IRF-7, IFN-β, and IFN-related gene induction as shown in time-dependent changes in mRNA expression confirmed by polymerase chain reaction (PCR). Moreover, the present research also showed that HM-γ-PGA can induce proinflammatory cytokine secretion in RAW 264.7 as measured by enzyme-linked immunosorbent assay (ELISA). Therefore, our findings suggest that HM-γ-PGA can be a potential antiviral substance that can inhibit NDV infection through its stimulation of antiviral state on RAW 264.7 cells. These results have been consistent with the previous studies showing that HM-γ-PGA can protect RAW 264.7 cells and mice against influenza infection. However, it should be noted that although murine macrophage cells are susceptible to NDV, they are not the natural host cells of the virus; thus further in vivo and in vitro studies involving chicken and chicken immune cells are needed to fully assess the efficacy and applicability of HM-γ-PGA in the poultry industry.

1. Introduction

Newcastle disease virus (NDV) is a member of the Paramyxoviridae family under the genus *Avulavirus* [1, 2] and is currently designated as avian paramyxovirus virus serotype 1 (APMV-1) [3]. According to the Office International des Epizooties (OIE) in 2009, NDV strains can be classified into five pathotypes according to the clinical signs shown by the affected chickens, namely, viscerotropic velogenic (high mortality and hemorrhagic intestinal lesions), neurotropic velogenic (high mortality, respiratory, and nervous signs), mesogenic (low mortality, respiratory signs with occasional nervous signs), lentogenic (subclinical or mild infection), and asymptomatic enteric (subclinical enteric infection) ones [4].

Newcastle disease remains prevalent worldwide, though a number of live and inactivated NDV vaccines are available to control the disease [5, 6]. However, the currently available commercial vaccines have their limitations and one of them is the absence of genetic markers for serological differentiation between vaccinated and naturally infected birds. There are also reports suggesting that the types of NDV strains that have been identified circulating in poultry already showed major antigenic drift. Thus, there is a need for better NDV vaccines which can solve such problems, wherein viral vector vaccines prove to be a good alternative [7], as exemplified by the first licensed commercial recombinant vaccine, a recombinant Newcastle disease virus vaccine, using fowl pox virus as the vector to express immunogenic proteins from the NDV [8]. However, recombinant vaccines are not widely used by the poultry industry due to their inability for use in population-based mass application procedures and high cost [5].

In addition, currently available vaccines cannot provide adequate immunity in poultry even with the use of multiple vaccinations and live vaccines do not completely prevent infection or virus shedding [7–9]; thus natural substances with the ability to inhibit or prevent NDV infections might provide much needed additional protection against the disease. One of the natural substances which is widely studied for its various biological functions and applications is the high-molecular-weight poly-γ-glutamate (HM-γ-PGA) (>3000 kDa), a natural, edible, and biodegradable polymer derived from *Bacillus subtilis* subsp. *chungkookjang* [10–12]. Recently, the antiviral function of HM-γ-PGA against influenza virus through stimulation of Type I interferon (IFN) and Mx1 proteins both *in vitro* and *in vivo* was demonstrated [13]. Additionally, several studies have shown that HM-γ-PGA is functionally better than low molecular weight poly-γ-glutamate (LM-γ-PGA) (10–1,000 kDa) when it comes to antitumor activity and immune stimulation and when used as an adjuvant [14, 15].

In this study, the antiviral effect of HM-γ-PGA against NDV was evaluated on murine macrophage cell line (RAW 264.7). Based on the results, this study has shown that HM-γ-PGA protects murine macrophage cells from NDV infection through Type I interferon induction.

2. Methodology

2.1. Preparation of HM-γ-PGA.

Endotoxin-free poly-γ-glutamate (γ-PGA) produced from *Bacillus subtilis* subsp. *chungkookjang* was prepared and provided by BioLeaders Corporation (Daejeon, Korea) in 0.85% sterile NaCl solution. Briefly, the culture broth of *B. subtilis* subsp. *chungkookjang* was collected and mixed with 3 times volume of ethanol. The precipitate was lyophilized and reconstituted in 10 mM Tris-HCl buffer (pH 7.5), treated with proteinase K, and dialyzed in distilled water. Next, the γ-PGA was purified by anion-exchange chromatography and dialyzed using Sep-Pak Plus Waters Accell Plus QMA cartridge (Millipore, USA) equilibrated with distilled water. Next, the cartridge column charged with γ-PGA was stepwise developed with NaCl solutions from 0.1 to 1.0 M. By estimating the concentration of glutamate in hydrolyzed γ-PGA using an amino acid analyzer, the content of γ-PGA was calculated by the following formula: content of γ-PGA (%) = (amount of glutamate/amount of sample) × $(A/B) \times 100$. $A = 129$ (molecular mass of γ-glutamyl residue in γ-PGA); $B = 147$ (molecular mass of glutamate). The number and weight-average molecular masses (Mn and Mw, resp.) along with the polydispersity (Mw/Mn) of γ-PGA molecules were measured by gel permeation chromatography using a GMPWXL column (Viscotek, USA) and a LR125 Laser Refractometer (Viscotek, USA). Polyacrylamide standards (American Polymer Standard, USA) were used to construct a calibration curve and polydispersity of high-molecular weight γ-PGA was measured. The content of high-molecular mass γ-PGA was increased to >99%, and polydispersity was decreased after anion-exchange chromatography. To thoroughly get solubilized γ-PGA, the pH was adjusted to 7.0 by adding 5N sodium hydroxide (NaOH) solution to the acid

form of PGA. Only purified HM-γ-PGA was used in this study [16].

2.2. Cell Culture and Virus.

RAW 264.7 cells (ATCC TIB-71) were maintained in Dulbecco's Modified Eagles Minimum essential medium (DMEM) (Invitrogen, USA) containing 10% fetal bovine serum (FBS) (Gibco, USA) and 1% antibiotic/antimycotic (Gibco, USA) at 37°C with 5% CO_2 until use.

The NDV-green fluorescence protein (NDV-GFP) was kindly provided by Dr. J. Jung of University of Southern California. The virus was amplified in 9- to 10-day-old embryonated eggs. Collected allantoic fluid was ultracentrifuged at 20,000 ×g for 2.5 hours at 8°C in 20% sucrose solution for viral concentration. Viral pellet was resuspended in PBS and 500 ul aliquots were kept at −70°C until use.

2.3. Antiviral Assay.

To evaluate the antiviral effect of HM-γ-PGA against NDV infection, the inhibition of virus replication was examined. Briefly, RAW 264.7 cells were cultured with a suitable number (8×10^5 cells/well) onto 12-well tissue culture (TC) plates (Nunc, Denmark) for 12 hours. Then, the medium was substituted with DMEM (for w/o treatment and medium treated cells) and DMEM with 1 mg/mL HM-γ-PGA. DMEM with 1000 units of recombinant mouse interferon-β (Sigma, USA) served as the positive control. After 12 hours of incubation, cells were infected with 1 multiplicity of infection (MOI) of NDV-GFP virus. The GFP expression was observed at 200x magnification 12 hours after infection (hpi) [13].

Cell viability was carried out via trypan blue exclusion test as described elsewhere. Briefly, RAW 264.7 cells were treated with 1 mg/mL of HM-γ-PGA, recombinant mouse interferon-β, or DMEM only (NC and medium treated cells) for 12 hours. After incubation, the cells were infected with NDV-GFP virus and cell viability was determined by trypan blue exclusion test at 30 hpi. Clarified cells from each group were mixed with 0.4% trypan blue stain (Invitrogen, USA) at 1 : 1 ratio. After staining, 10 μL of the mixture was applied to a hemocytometer, wherein to get the percentage of viable cells, the total number of viable/live cells per mL of aliquot was divided by the total number of cells/mL of aliquot multiplied by 100. Cell counting was done thrice.

Lastly, following the instructions of the manufacturer, the GFP expression levels of medium only, 1 mg/mL HM-γ-PGA, and IFN-β treated cells 12 h before NDV-GFP infection were measured 24 hpi using Glomax multidetection system (Promega, USA). Briefly, the cells from each treatment group as described above were collected separately and centrifuged at 1200 rpm for 3 minutes. The resulting cell pellet was diluted in PBS and transferred to 96-well black plate for GFP detection. The test was done in triplicate [17].

2.4. NDV-GFP mRNA Expression on RAW 264.7 Cells.

Total mRNA from RAW 264.7 cells was extracted and amplified in order to estimate the NDV-GFP mRNA expression [18]. Briefly, cells (8×10^5/well) were cultured on 12-well TC plates (Nunc, Denmark) for 12 hours. Then, the medium was replaced with DMEM (for w/o treatment and medium treated cells) and DMEM with 1 mg/mL HM-γ-PGA. After

TABLE 1: Primer sets used to quantify viral RNA expression.

Genes	Primers	
	Forward	Reverse
APMV-1 M gene	5′-AGTGATGTGCTCGGACCTTC-3′	5′-CCTGAGGAGAGGCATTTGCTA-3′
Murine GAPDH	5′-TGACCACAGTCCATGCCATC-3′	5′-GACGGACACATTGGGGGTAG-3′

TABLE 2: Primer sets used to quantify antiviral gene mRNA expression.

Genes	Primers	
	Forward	Reverse
GAPDH	5′-TGACCACAGTCCATGCCATC-3′	5′-GACGGACACATTGGGGGTAG-3′
IFN-β	5′-TCCAAGAAAGGACGAACATTCG-3′	5′-TGCGGACATCTCCCACGTCAA-3′
Mx1	5′-GATCCGACTTCACTTCCAGATGG-3′	5′-CATCTCAGTGGTAGTCAACCC-3′
IRF-3	5′-GTGCCTCTCCTGACACCAAT-3′	5′-CCAAGATCAGGCCATCAAAT-3′
IRF-7	5′-AAGCTGGAGCCATGGGTATG-3′	5′-GACCCAGGTCCATGAGGAAG-3′
ISG15	5′-CAATGGCCTGGGACCTAAA-3′	5′-CTTCTTCAGTTCTGACACCGTCAT-3′
GBP1	5′-AAAAACTTCGGGGACAGCTT-3′	5′-CTGAGTCACCTCATAAGCCAAA-3′

12 hours of incubation, cells were infected with 1 MOI of NDV-GFP virus. Cells were collected at 0, 6, 12, and 24 hours after infection. Total mRNA was extracted from RAW 264.7 cells using the RNeasy Mini Kit (Qiagen, USA). Reverse transcription of the total mRNA was carried out using M-MLV Reverse Transcriptase (Enzynomics, Korea), oligo (dT) 16-primers, and dNTP (0.5 μM). M-MLV Reverse Transcriptase was incubated at 72°C for 5 minutes and 37°C for 60 minutes and terminally inactivated by heating at 72°C for 15 minutes. The polymerase chain reactions (PCR) using specific primers for Matrix gene of APMV-1 [19] and murine glyceraldehyde 3-phosphate dehydrogenase (GAPDH) housekeeping gene (internal control) [20] were carried out using emerald PCR master mix (Takara, USA) with 1 pM of each primer set (Table 1). The cDNA was amplified for 30 cycles with optimized annealing temperature for each primer set. Final extension was performed at 72°C for 5 minutes. Equal amounts of PCR products were run on 1.5% ethidium bromide impregnated agarose gels and visualized using GelDoc Imaging System (Bio-Rad, USA). On the other hand, relative band intensity (RBI) of the Matrix gene and GAPDH mRNA expression was determined using GelDoc Imaging System Band Quantification Software (Bio-Rad, USA).

2.5. Stimulation of an Antiviral State by HM-γ-PGA Treatment. To confirm the upregulation in mRNA expression level of antiviral related genes on RAW 264.7 cells, the method of Moon et al. [13] was used with some modifications. Briefly, the RAW 264.7 cells were seeded to each well of a 6-well TC plate (Nunc, Denmark) and cultured for 12 hours. Separately, the cells were treated with 1 mg/mL of HM-γ-PGA in DMEM with 1% FBS, 100 ng/mL LPS in DMEM as the positive control, and DMEM with 1% FBS only as the negative control. The treated cells were harvested at 0, 3, 6, 12, and 24 hours posttreatment. Afterward, preparation of total RNA and RT-PCR was performed using the same method above. The specific primers for PCR are listed in Table 2 [13, 20, 21].

2.6. Detection of Proinflammatory Cytokines Induced by HM-γ-PGA on RAW 264.7 Cells by ELISA. The proinflammatory cytokine inducing effect of HM-γ-PGA on RAW 264.7 cells was examined using commercial ELISA kits for murine interleukin-6 (IL-6), interleukin-12 (IL-12), tumor necrosis factor-alpha (TNF-α) (BD Bioscience, USA), and murine interferon-β (IFN-β) (PBL Interferon Source, USA) [13, 22, 23]. Briefly, a suitable number (2×10^6/well) of RAW 264.7 cells were seeded to each well of a 6-well TC plate (Nunc, Denmark) and cultured. Twelve hours later, the culture medium was removed and the cell monolayer was washed once with PBS. The cells were then treated with 100 ng/mL of lipopolysaccharide (LPS) derived from *E. coli* O111:B4 (Sigma-Aldrich, USA) or 1 mg/mL of HM-γ-PGA in DMEM with 1% FBS and incubated at 37°C with 5% CO_2. Cells treated with DMEM with 1% FBS only served as negative control. Supernatant from each treatment group was harvested at 0, 6, 12, 24, and 36 hours posttreatment and clarified by centrifugation at 2500 ×g for 10 minutes at 4°C. Clarified supernatant was dispensed into the murine IFN-β ELISA plate for the measurement of secreted murine IFN-β, while 10-fold diluted supernatant was dispensed into the mouse TNF-α, IL-6, and IL-12 capture antibody coated ELISA plate. The test was performed in triplicate.

2.7. Statistical Analysis. Differences between groups were analyzed by Student's t-test. P values less than 0.05 were regarded as significant and those less than 0.01 were regarded as highly significant.

3. Results

3.1. Inhibition of Virus Replication by HM-γ-PGA on RAW 264.7 Cells. Previous studies revealed that HM-γ-PGA has beneficial functions to immune responses [12, 14, 16]. Recent studies also confirmed the role of γ-PGA in inducing cytokines involved in antiviral states in cells, leading to inhibition of virus replication [13].

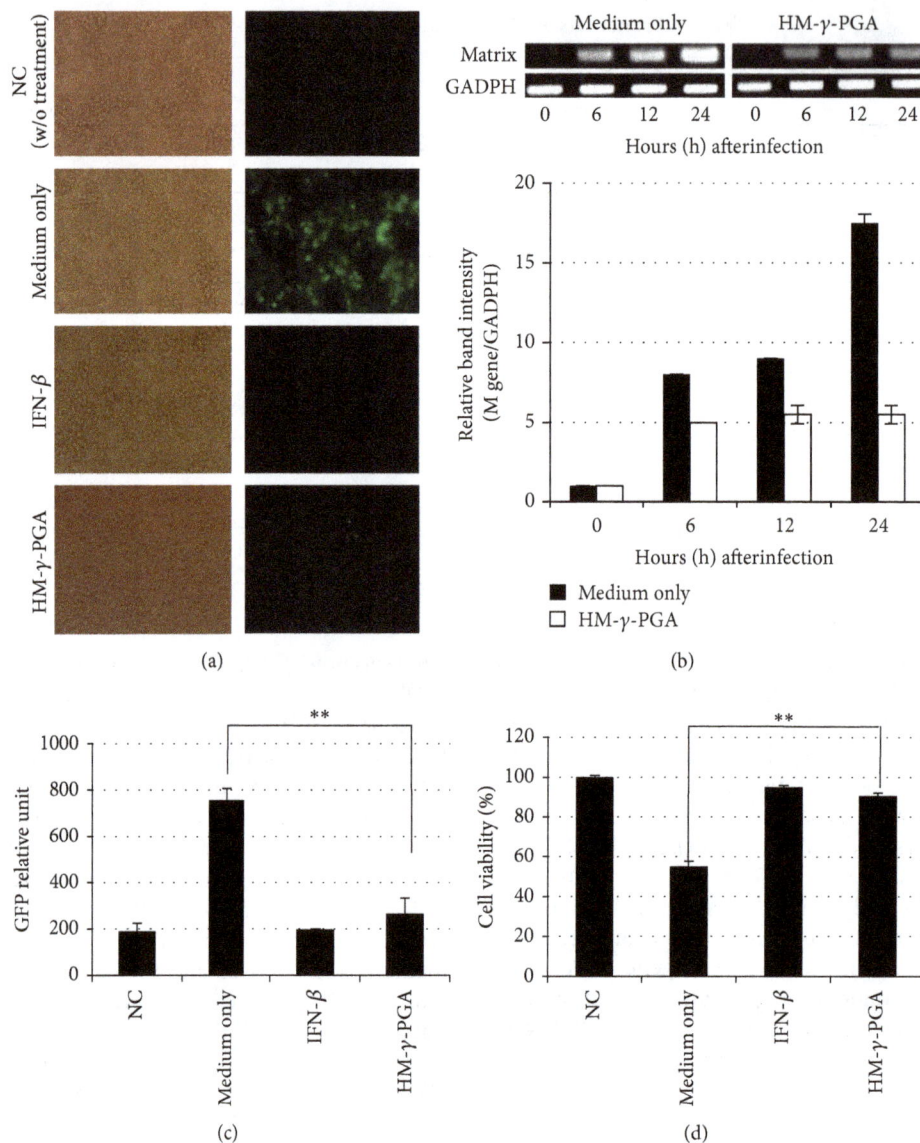

(a)

(b)

(c)

(d)

FIGURE 1: Antiviral function of HM-γ-PGA in murine macrophage cell line. (a) GFP expression images of medium only, 1 mg/mL HM-γ-PGA, and 1000 units/mL recombinant mouse IFN-β treated cells 12 h before NDV-GFP infection. Images taken 12 hpi (200x magnification). (b1) Viral mRNA expression level of Matrix gene of NDV-gfp over time in each treatment group was confirmed by specific RT-PCR primers which are shown in Table 1. Equal amounts of PCR products were run on 1.5% ethidium bromide impregnated agarose gels and visualized using GelDoc Imaging System. All samples were normalized using their respective GAPDH gene expression. (b2) Relative band intensity (RBI) of the Matrix gene mRNA expression of (b1). RBI was determined (Gene/GAPDH) using GelDoc Imaging System Band Quantification Software. Error bars indicate the range of values obtained from two independent experiments. (c) GFP expression level of media treated, 1 mg/mL HM-γ-PGA, and IFN-β treated cells 12 h before NDV-GFP (La Sota strain) infection. GFP expression was measured 24 hpi using Glomax multidetection system. (d) Cell viability was determined by trypan blue exclusion test at 30 hpi. The results are presented as a percentage of the control (cells without treatment). Error bars on Figures (c) and (d) indicate the range of values obtained from triplicate counting ($^{**}P < 0.001$, highly significant difference).

In this study, HM-γ-PGA treated RAW 264.7 cells showed markedly reduced virus replication while the medium treated cells demonstrated high level of GFP expression (Figures 1(a) and 1(c)). HM-γ-PGA treated cells showed a significant twofold reduction of GFP expression compared to medium treated cells.

Likewise, after virus infection, HM-γ-PGA treated cells showed less than 10% cell death while medium treated cells showed more than 50% cell death at 30 hpi (Figure 1(d)). Additionally, with the failure of the NDV-GFP virus to bud successfully from RAW 264.7 cells, we opted to measure the mRNA expression of the Matrix gene of the virus via RT-PCR to estimate virus replication (Figure 1(b)). As expected, the M gene expression of the HM-γ-PGA treated cells is relatively lower than the medium treated cells from 6 to 24 hours after infection. The medium treated cells also showed continuous expression of the M gene up to 24 hours after infection while HM-γ-PGA treated cells demonstrated nonincreasing pattern beginning after 12 hours.

3.2. Induction of Antiviral Genes and Proinflammatory Cytokines by HM-γ-PGA in RAW 264.7 Cells. To determine the mechanism by which HM-γ-PGA induces antiviral state in RAW 264.7 cells, the antiviral related gene expression and secreted proinflammatory cytokines from the murine macrophage cells were confirmed after HM-γ-PGA stimulation. RAW 264.7 cells were treated with 1 mg/mL of HM-γ-PGA and compared with 100 ng/mL of LPS treated cells.

HM-γ-PGA treated RAW 264.7 cells showed increased mRNA expression of interferon regulatory transcription factors 3 (IRF-3) and 7 (IRF-7) and IFN-stimulated genes such as myxovirus resistance protein 1 (Mx1) and interferon-induced guanylate-binding protein 1 (GBP1) almost comparable with the level induced by LPS beginning 3 hours posttreatment (Figure 2). However, IFN-β as well as interferon stimulated gene-15 (ISG-15) mRNA expression levels was not as high as compared to LPS treated cells, though still evidently higher in contrast to the negative control. Since mRNA expression does not necessarily correlate with the secreted protein levels, proinflammatory cytokine secretion was also measured after HM-γ-PGA stimulation via murine cytokine ELISA kits (Figure 3). The present research showed that HM-γ-PGA can induce cytokine secretion in RAW 264.7 cells comparable with the LPS treated cells.

4. Discussion

The capacity of NDV to cause a highly contagious infection resulting in high mortality and reduced farm efficiency remains to threaten the global poultry industry. Currently available vaccines cannot provide adequate immunity in poultry even with the use of multiple vaccinations [9]; hence natural substances which have antiviral activity are of great importance. One of the natural substances widely studied for its various biological functions and applications is the HM-γ-PGA, a natural, edible, and biodegradable polymer derived from *Bacillus subtilis* subsp. *chungkookjang* [10–12]. HM-γ-PGA is secreted from γ-PGA synthetase ABC complex on the wall of *Bacillus subtilis* subsp. *chungkookjang* [11]. This naturally secreted HM-γ-PGA is a safe and edible polymer which contains negligible toxins which do not interfere with its beneficial effects/applications such as satisfactory adjuvant function, antitumor effect, and innate immunity inducible role [14, 16]. Among its biological functions, its capacity to initiate immune responses in mice via TLR4 signaling just like LPS makes HM-γ-PGA a potent immunomodulator with a big potential as a therapeutic agent [12]. Briefly, TLRs are considered to be a major component of the pattern recognition system which detects invading pathogens by recognizing pathogen associated molecular patterns (PAMPs). And one of the well-studied TLRs is TLR4. Mammalian (mouse) TLR4 signaling pathway starts by the transfer of LPS-binding protein (LBP) of the detected LPS to the cluster of differentiation 14 (CD14) on the surface of inflammatory cells. This reaction eventually leads to the transfer of LPS to TLR-4 via

myeloid differentiation-2 (MD-2) [24]. Successful activation of TLR4 initiates intracellular activation of myeloid differentiation primary response protein-88 (MyD88-) dependent and MyD88-independent pathways. MyD88-dependent pathway utilizes MyD88 and Toll-interleukin 1 receptor (TIR) domain-containing adapter protein (TIRAP) to successfully export nuclear factor-Kβ (NF-Kβ) to the nucleus to initiate transcription of proinflammatory cytokine genes, while MyD88-independent pathway makes use of Toll/interleukin-1 receptor-domain-containing adapter-inducing interferon-β (TRIF) and TRIF-related adapter molecule (TRAM) to effectively activate transcription factor IRF-3 and subsequent production of IFN-β [25]. Though proinflammatory cytokines such as TNF-α, IL-6, and IL-12 are important for a successful inflammatory response, induction of Type I interferon is much more considered to be indispensible for antiviral resistance. Nonetheless, TLR4 is considered to be unique among the TLR family in the fact that LPS recognition results in activation of both MyD88-dependent and the TRAM/TRIF-dependent signaling pathways [26].

In this study, HM-γ-PGA has been tested through several experiments to evaluate its application to control Newcastle disease virus replication on murine macrophage cells (RAW 264.7). Since the immune-stimulating effect of HM-γ-PGA has been well established in mice and murine macrophage cells [11–13, 16] and previous studies have already elucidated the interaction between NDV and murine macrophages [21, 27], we decided to use murine macrophages to evaluate the antiviral effect of HM-γ-PGA against NDV.

In the pretreatment antiviral assay, HM-γ-PGA treatment was able to reduce viral replication on NDV-GFP infected RAW 264.7 cells as shown by lower NDV M gene and GFP expressions and higher cell survivability after infection (Figure 1). However, coincubation of the virus with HM-γ-PGA and postinfection treatment with HM-γ-PGA did not reduce the gfp expression of the virus.

Based on these findings, HM-γ-PGA has been hypothesized to be involved with the antiviral state in cells via induction of Type I interferons. The previous study showed that the expression of antiviral effector molecules protein kinase R (PKR), 2'-5'-ologoadenylate synthetase (OAS), and Mx, as induced by Type 1 interferons, correlates with the susceptibility to NDV infection in both primary macrophages and macrophage-derived tumor cells (e.g., RAW cells) as these molecules inhibit critical steps during RNA translation and/or assembly of virus particles in viral replication [21]. In addition, ISG-15 protein, a ubiquitin-like modifier, greatly expressed after Type I interferon stimulation has been shown to mediate protection in a number of different viral infection models [28].

Likewise, the same paper also demonstrated that RAW cells have delayed IFN secretion after NDV infection thus making them susceptible to the said virus [21]. However, as compared to chicken cells, mammalian cells have innate resistance with the V protein of NDV which can block production of IFN [29]. On the other hand, Moon et al. showed that HM-γ-PGA can induce a significant amount

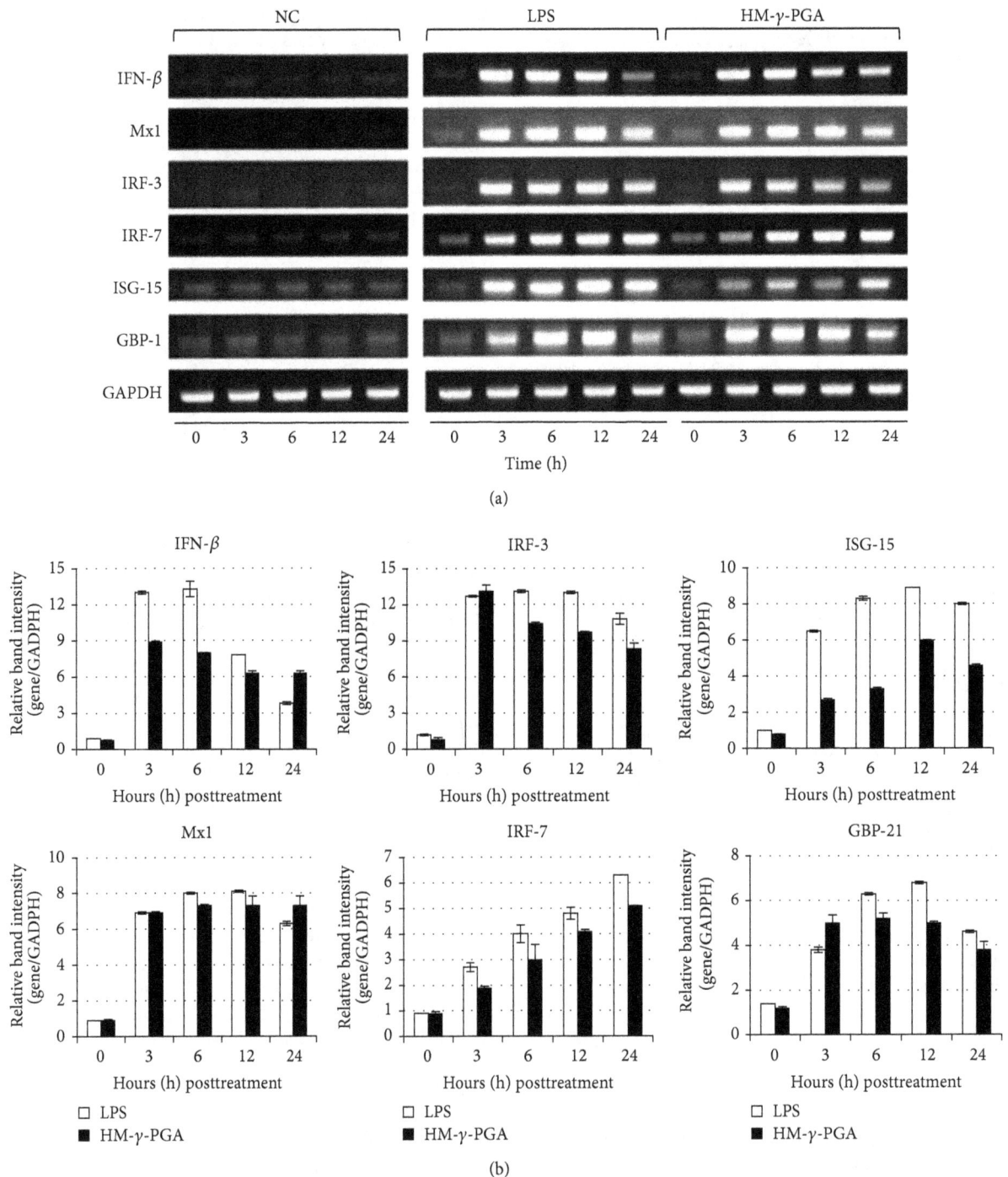

FIGURE 2: Induction of antiviral genes and proinflammatory cytokines by HM-γ-PGA in RAW 264.7 cells. (a) Cells were treated with medium only, HM-γ-PGA (1 mg/mL), and 100 ng/mL of LPS. The time-dependent changes in mRNA expression after treatment were confirmed by PCR. All samples were normalized using GAPDH wherein equal amounts PCR products were run on 1.5% ethidium bromide impregnated agarose gels and visualized using GelDoc Imaging System. (b) RBI (Gene/GAPDH) of the IFN-β, IRF-3, IRF-7, and IFN-related genes of Figure (a). RBI was determined using GelDoc Imaging System Band Quantification Software. Error bars indicate the range of values obtained from two independent experiments.

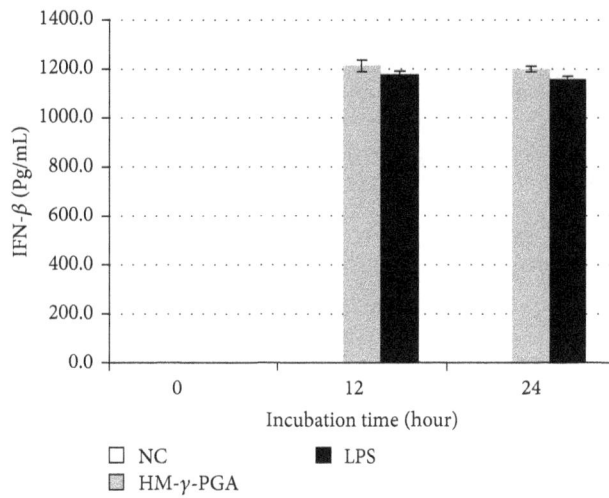

(a)

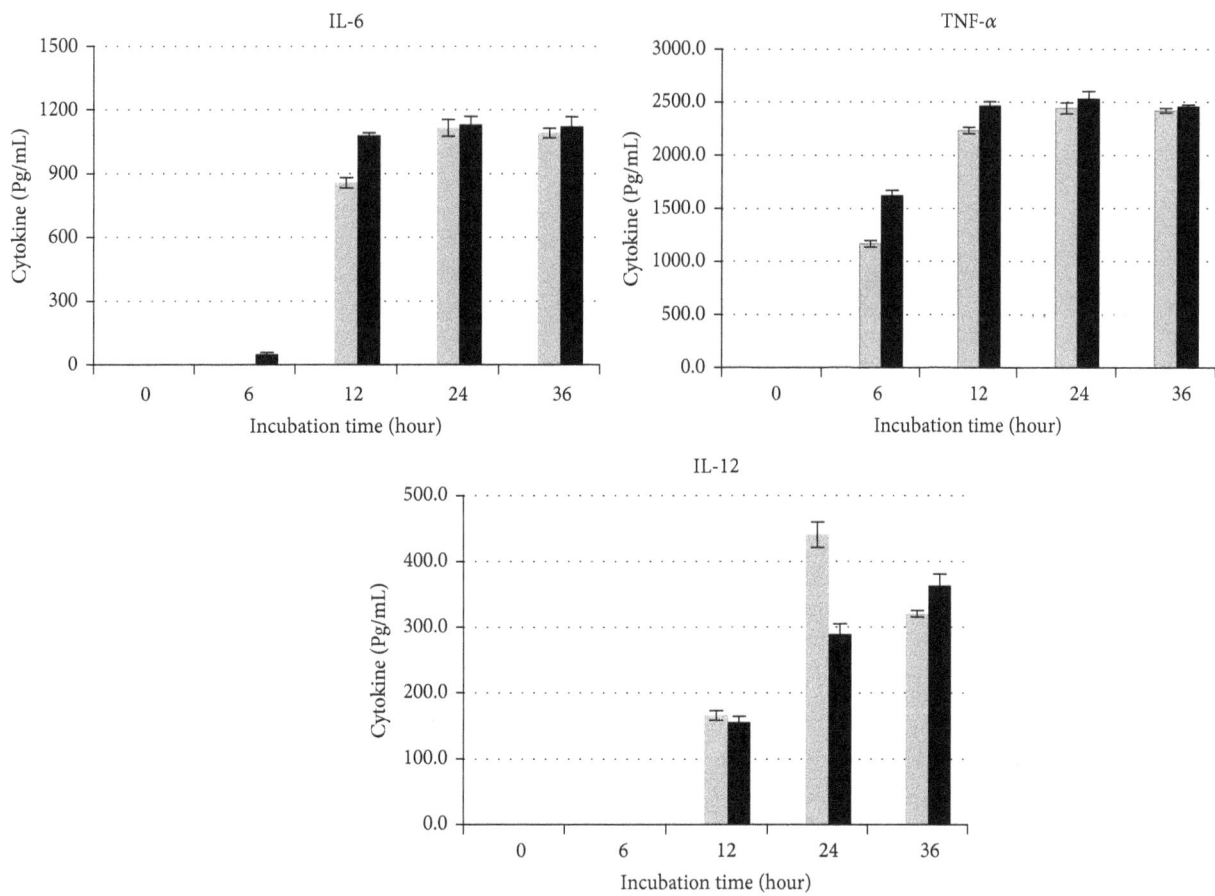

(b)

FIGURE 3: Ability of HM-γ-PGA to induce proinflammatory cytokine secretion in murine macrophage cell line. Cells were treated with medium only, HM-γ-PGA (1 mg/mL), and 100 ng/mL of LPS. The time-dependent changes in cytokine secretion after treatment were determined by ELISA (a) IFN-β; (b) proinflammatory cytokines. The data show representative means ± SD of each murine cytokine measured over time from three independent assays.

of IFN-β in RAW 264.7 cells comparable with LPS induced IFN-β secretion as measured by murine cytokine ELISA [13]. With this in mind, the researchers hypothesized that the early induction of Type I interferon can also protect RAW 264.7 cells against NDV infection. In the present study, HM-γ-PGA treated Raw 264.7 cells showed increased mRNA expression of transcriptional factors IRF-3, IRF-7, and IFN-stimulated genes such as Mx1 and GBP1 almost comparable with the level induced by LPS beginning 3 hours posttreatment. However, IFN-B as well as ISG-15 mRNA expression levels was not as high as compared to LPS treated cells, though still evidently higher in contrast to the negative control. Such observations are in accordance with the findings of group of Wilden in 2009 that strong expression of antiviral genes IRF-3, IRF-7, and IFN-β and retinoic acid-inducible gene 1 (RIG-I) can provide protection against NDV infection [21]. Although RIG-1 was not measured in this study, the strong expression of IRF-3 and IRF-7 alone can strongly suggest that antiviral state has been achieved in HM-γ-PGA treated RAW 264.7 cells since these transcriptional factors are indispensable for the induction of Type I IFNs [30].

However, since mRNA expression does not necessarily correlate with the secreted protein levels, proinflammatory cytokine secretion was also measured. Using commercial murine cytokine ELISA kits for detection of IL-6, IL-12, TNF-α, and IFN-β, the present research showed that HM-γ-PGA can induce cytokine secretion in RAW 264.7 cells comparable with the LPS treated cells. Nevertheless, overstimulation of the innate immunity can possibly lead to excessive cytokine release which can be detrimental to the cells. This study is no exception with the possibility of a cytokine storm after treatment of an immune-stimulating agent, HM-γ-PGA, and infection of NDV, a virus known to aberrantly affect cytokine responses. Based on the limited results of the study, pretreatment of murine macrophage cells prior to NDV infection only resulted in less than 10% cell death in contrast to more than 50% of the medium treated cells. Assuming that excessive cytokine release indeed occurred in cells pretreated with HM-γ-PGA, the results still suggest that the upregulation of cytokines in this study did not adversely affect the treated cells as compared to medium treated cells. Thus we can observe that pretreatment of HM-γ-PGA at the appropriate time prior to NDV infection provided protection rather than death to the susceptible cells.

Moreover, since we did not test the protein expression levels of the interferon stimulated antiviral proteins Mx, OAS, PKR, and ISG 15, we could only speculate that these proteins have been sufficiently expressed and successfully inhibited virus replication; thus pathogen recognition receptors (PRRs) were not maximally stimulated, preventing a possible cytokine storm. Therefore, our findings suggest that HM-γ-PGA, if given at the appropriate time prior to NDV-GFP infection, can be a significant antiviral substance which can inhibit NDV infection through its stimulation of antiviral state on RAW 264.7 cells.

Though the experiments were done on cells not normally infected by NDV, the promising results of the present study serve as justification for conducting tests on the applicability of HM-γ-PGA in chicken immune cells. Nonetheless, our lab has already started the evaluation of the anti-NDV activity of HM-γ-PGA in both chicken and chicken immune cells, to fully assess the applicability of HM-γ-PGA in the poultry industry.

Acknowledgments

The authors would like to thank the BioLeaders Corporation for providing the HM-γ-PGA. The study was supported by the research fund of the Chungnam National University.

References

[1] M. A. Mayo, "Virus taxonomy," *Archives of Virology*, vol. 147, pp. 1071–1076, 2002.

[2] M. A. Mayo, "A summary of taxonomic changes recently approved by ICTV," *Archives of Virology*, vol. 147, no. 8, pp. 1655–1663, 2002.

[3] D. J. Alexander, "Newcastle disease and other avian paramyxoviruses," *Revue Scientifique et Technique*, vol. 19, no. 2, pp. 443–462, 2000.

[4] Office International des Epizooties, "Manual of Diagnostic Tests and Vacc ines for Terrestrial Animals," 2012, http://web.oie.int/eng/normes/MMANUAL/A_Index.htm.

[5] B. S. Seal, D. J. King, and H. S. Sellers, "The avian response to Newcastle disease virus," *Developmental and Comparative Immunology*, vol. 24, no. 2-3, pp. 257–268, 2000.

[6] Y.-J. Lee, H.-W. Sung, J.-G. Choi et al., "Protection of chickens from Newcastle disease with a recombinant baculovirus subunit vaccine expressing the fusion and hemagglutinin-neuraminidase proteins," *Journal of Veterinary Science*, vol. 9, no. 3, pp. 301–308, 2008.

[7] S. Kumar, B. Nayak, P. L. Collins, and S. K. Samal, "Evaluation of the newcastle disease virus f and hn proteins in protective immunity by using a recombinant avian paramyxovirus type 3 vector in chickens," *Journal of Virology*, vol. 85, no. 13, pp. 6521–6534, 2011.

[8] K. Yamanouchi, T. Barrett, and C. Ka, "New approaches to the development of virus vaccines for veterinary use," *Revue scientifique et technique*, vol. 17, no. 3, pp. 641–653, 1998.

[9] D. J. Alexander, "Newcastle disease," *British Poultry Science*, vol. 42, no. 1, pp. 5–22, 2001.

[10] S.-R. Bae, C. Park, J.-C. Choi, H. Poo, C.-J. Kim, and M.-H. Sung, "Effects of ultra high molecular weight poly-γ-glutamic acid from *Bacillus subtilis* (chungkookjang) on corneal wound healing," *Journal of Microbiology and Biotechnology*, vol. 20, no. 4, pp. 803–808, 2010.

[11] M.-H. Sung, C. Park, C.-J. Kim, H. Poo, K. Soda, and M. Ashiuchi, "Natural and edible biopolymer poly-γ-glutamic acid: synthesis, production, and applications," *Chemical Record*, vol. 5, no. 6, pp. 352–366, 2005.

[12] H. Poo, C. Park, M.-S. Kwak et al., "New biological functions and applications of high-molecular-mass poly-γ-glutamic acid," *Chemistry and Biodiversity*, vol. 7, no. 6, pp. 1555–1562, 2010.

[13] H.-J. Moon, J.-S. Lee, Y.-K. Choi et al., "Induction of type I interferon by high-molecular poly-γ-glutamate protects B6.A2G-*Mx1* mice against influenza A virus," *Antiviral Research*, vol. 94, no. 1, pp. 98–102, 2012.

[14] T.-Y. Lee, Y.-H. Kim, S.-W. Yoon et al., "Oral administration of poly-gamma-glutamate induces TLR4- and dendritic cell-dependent antitumor effect," *Cancer Immunology, Immunotherapy*, vol. 58, no. 11, pp. 1781–1794, 2009.

[15] T. Yoshikawa, N. Okada, A. Oda et al., "Nanoparticles built by self-assembly of amphiphilic γ-PGA can deliver antigens to antigen-presenting cells with high efficiency: a new tumor-vaccine carrier for eliciting effector T cells," *Vaccine*, vol. 26, no. 10, pp. 1303–1313, 2008.

[16] W. K. Tae, Y. L. Tae, C. B. Hyun et al., "Oral administration of high molecular mass poly-γ-glutamate induces NK cell-mediated antitumor immunity," *The Journal of Immunology*, vol. 179, no. 2, pp. 775–780, 2007.

[17] C. Puig-Saus, A. Gros, R. Alemany, and M. Cascalló, "Adenovirus i-leader truncation bioselected against cancer-associated fibroblasts to overcome tumor stromal barriers," *Molecular Therapy*, vol. 20, no. 1, pp. 54–62, 2012.

[18] S. M. Shin, J. H. Kwon, S. Lee et al., "Immunostimulatory effects of *Cordyceps militaris* on macrophages through enhanced production of cytokines via the activation of NFκB," *Immune Network*, vol. 10, no. 2, pp. 55–63, 2010.

[19] M. G. Wise, D. L. Suarez, B. S. Seal et al., "Development of a real-time reverse-transcription PCR for detection of Newcastle disease virus RNA in clinical samples," *Journal of Clinical Microbiology*, vol. 42, no. 1, pp. 329–338, 2004.

[20] J. R. Reed, R. P. Leon, M. K. Hall, and K. L. Schwertfeger, "Interleukin-1beta and fibroblast growth factor receptor 1 cooperate to induce cyclooxygenase-2 during early mammary tumourigenesis," *Breast Cancer Research*, vol. 11, no. 2, article R21, 2009.

[21] H. Wilden, P. Fournier, R. Zawatzky, and V. Schirrmacher, "Expression of RIG-I, IRF3, IFN-β and IRF7 determines resistance or susceptibility of cells to infection by Newcastle Disease Virus," *International Journal of Oncology*, vol. 34, no. 4, pp. 971–982, 2009.

[22] T. L. Wadsworth and D. R. Koop, "Effects of the wine polyphenolics quercetin and resveratrol on pro-inflammatory cytokine expression in RAW 264.7 macrophages," *Biochemical Pharmacology*, vol. 57, no. 8, pp. 941–949, 1999.

[23] K. von Maltzan and S. B. Pruett, "ELISA assays and alcohol: Increasing carbon chain length can interfere with detection of cytokines," *Alcohol*, vol. 45, no. 1, pp. 1–9, 2011.

[24] E. M. Pålsson-McDermott and L. A. J. O'Neill, "Signal transduction by the lipopolysaccharide receptor, Toll-like receptor-4," *Immunology*, vol. 113, no. 2, pp. 153–162, 2004.

[25] M. Yamamoto, S. Sato, H. Hemmi et al., "TRAM is specifically involved in the Toll-like receptor 4-mediated MyD88-independent signaling pathway," *Nature Immunology*, vol. 4, no. 11, pp. 1144–1150, 2003.

[26] A. Marijke Keestra and J. P. M. van Putten, "Unique properties of the chicken TLR4/MD-2 complex: selective lipopolysaccharide activation of the MyD88-dependent pathway," *The Journal of Immunology*, vol. 181, no. 6, pp. 4354–4362, 2008.

[27] H. Wilden, V. Schirrmacher, and P. Fournier, "Important role of interferon regulatory factor (IRF)-3 in the interferon response of mouse macrophages upon infection by Newcastle disease virus," *International Journal of Oncology*, vol. 39, no. 2, pp. 493–504, 2011.

[28] D. J. Morales and D. J. Lenschow, "The antiviral activities of ISG15," *Journal of Molecular Biology*, vol. 425, no. 24, pp. 4995–5008, 2013.

[29] M.-S. Park, A. García-Sastre, J. F. Cros, C. F. Basler, and P. Palese, "Newcastle disease virus V protein is a determinant of host range restriction," *Journal of Virology*, vol. 77, no. 17, pp. 9522–9532, 2003.

[30] M. Sato, H. Suemori, N. Hata et al., "Distinct and essential roles of transcription factors IRF-3 and IRF-7 in response to viruses for IFN-α/β gene induction," *Immunity*, vol. 13, no. 4, pp. 539–548, 2000.

Molecular Detection of Torque Teno Sus Virus and Coinfection with African Swine Fever Virus in Blood Samples of Pigs from Some Slaughterhouses in Nigeria

Pam D. Luka,[1,2] Joseph Erume,[1] Bitrus Yakubu,[2] Olajide A. Owolodun,[2] David Shamaki,[3] and Frank N. Mwiine[1]

[1]Department of Biomolecular Resources and Biolab Sciences, College of Veterinary Medicine, Animal Resources and Biosecurity, Makerere University, Kampala, Uganda
[2]Biotechnology Division, National Veterinary Research Institute, Vom, Plateau State, Nigeria
[3]Virology Division, National Veterinary Research Institute, Vom, Plateau State, Nigeria

Correspondence should be addressed to Frank N. Mwiine; fmwiine@gmail.com

Academic Editor: Alessandra Lo Presti

Torque teno sus virus 1 (TTSuV1a/TTSuV1b) infection is present in pig herds worldwide. This study investigated the prevalence of TTSuV1a/TTSuV1b infections in domestic pigs from some slaughterhouses in Nigeria as well as coinfection with African swine fever virus (ASFV) and described the phylogeny in relation to global strains. One hundred and eighty-one (181) blood samples from four slaughterhouses were used for the study and viral nucleic acid detection was carried out by PCR. Comparative sequence analysis was carried out to infer phylogeny. The overall prevalence of TTSuV1a/b was 17.7%. Prevalence of individual genotypes was 10.5% and 7.2% for TTSuV1a and TTSuV1b, respectively. Coinfection of ASFV/TTSuV1a/b was 7.7% while that of TTSuV1a and TTSuV1b was 1.7%. ASFV alone was detected in 11.91% of the total samples. The Nigerian TTSuV1a and TTSuV1b shared a sequence identity of 91–100% and 95–100%, respectively, among each other. The ASFV sequences were 100% identical to members of genotype 1. This is the first report on the presence of TTSuV1a/b in domestic pigs in Nigeria and coinfection with ASFV. Although the prevalence of TTSuV1a/b in Nigeria was low, we recommend further studies to establish the trend and possible role in the pathogenesis of ASFV.

1. Introduction

Torque teno virus (TTV) is a small icosahedral and nonenveloped, single-stranded DNA (ssDNA) virus. It is circular with a negative genome that was first reported in a human with posttransfusion hepatitis in Japan [1]. The virus has also been reported to infect domestic animals such as pigs and boars [2, 3]. TTV are classified into the family Anelloviridae including 9 different genera among which is the genus *Iotatorquevirus*. Genetic analysis has shown that two genotypes of the genus *Iotatorquevirus* [torque teno sus virus 1 (TTSuV1) and torque teno sus virus 2 (TTSuV2)] and the newly grouped genotype TTSuVk2 of the genus *Kappatorquevirus* exist in pigs [4].

Torque teno viruses have been reported to be distributed globally with human TTV being ubiquitous while several other reports of swine TTSuV infection have been reported in Spain, Italy, Russia, China, and very recently Uganda in Africa [5–8]. TTSuV has been reported in coinfection with other pathogens but its evidence as a pathogen of pigs and its involvement in causality is yet to be elucidated [6].

The disease caused by TTSuV has not yet been defined even though it is widely spread and species specific. However, TTSuV2 (now TTSuV1b) has been reported in domestic reared pigs with other pathogens such as porcine circovirus 2 (PCV-2), hepatitis E virus (HEV), postweaning multisystemic wasting syndrome (PMWS), porcine endogenous retrovirus, and Ndumu virus [9–13]. On the other hand,

TTSuV1a has been suggested to trigger PMWS development in gnotobiotic pigs coinfected with PCV-2 [14]. Furthermore, coinfection of TTSuV1a and *porcine reproductive and respiratory syndrome virus* (PRRSV) [15] has also been reported; Blomström et al. [12] have also reported a novel variant of porcine parvovirus 4 (PPV4) from bushpig (*Potamochoerus larvatus*) coinfecting with TTSuV1a and TTSuV1b. Therefore, the potential association of swine TTSuV with other disease occurrence in pigs is of scientific interest.

The rising demand for livestock products in Nigeria has resulted in government agricultural intervention leading to increased pig production [16]. However, with the advent of African swine fever in 1997, the prospect of the pig industry has continued to dwindle [17, 18]. Some regions in Nigeria preferred pig to other food animals due to its relative rapid growth rate, short cycle, and large litter size. Given the extensive/semi-intensive farming system common in Nigeria and the rising contact between pigs and humans in addition to poor farm practices, any potential risk from TTSuV or coinfection with other pathogens could lead to public health consequences in terms of the pig's capacity to serve as reservoir and/or transmitter of several emerging and reemerging diseases. As part of ASF surveillance in Nigeria, blood samples from selected slaughterhouses were analyzed to determine the presence of TTSuV1. The main objective of this study was to determine the presence of swine TTSuV1a and TTSuV1b genotypes in association with ASFVs in Nigeria.

2. Materials and Methods

2.1. Study Area and Sample Collection. Blood samples from 181 domestic pigs were collected from four slaughterhouses from four localities in Nigeria: Jos, Makurdi and Ibadan abattoirs, and Kafanchan pig market slaughter slab (Figure 1). Sampling was carried out between January and March 2014 as part of a research project on the epidemiology of African swine fever in some pig producing states of Nigeria. This project was with the mandate of National Veterinary Research Institute (NVRI), Vom, and the Federal Department of Veterinary and Pest Control Services of the Federal Ministry of Agriculture, Abuja. Apparently healthy pigs presented to the slaughterhouses were sampled.

2.2. Sample Processing and DNA Extraction. Blood samples (n = 181) were collected in sterile sample bottles with ethylenediaminetetraacetic acid (EDTA) anticoagulant and kept at +4°C to +8°C until used for DNA extraction. The DNA extraction was carried out using a DNeasy blood and tissue kit (Qiagen, Hilden Germany) following the manufacturer's guidelines. Extracted DNA was kept at −20°C pending PCR.

2.3. Confirmation of ASFV by PCR. ASFV was confirmed using the primer pair ASF-1 and ASF-2 according to the Manual of Diagnostic Tests and Vaccines [19]. ASF specific primers targeting the major capsid protein (VP72 gene) 278-bp fragment within the conserved region were amplified as described by the OIE manual. A 478-bp C-terminus of the

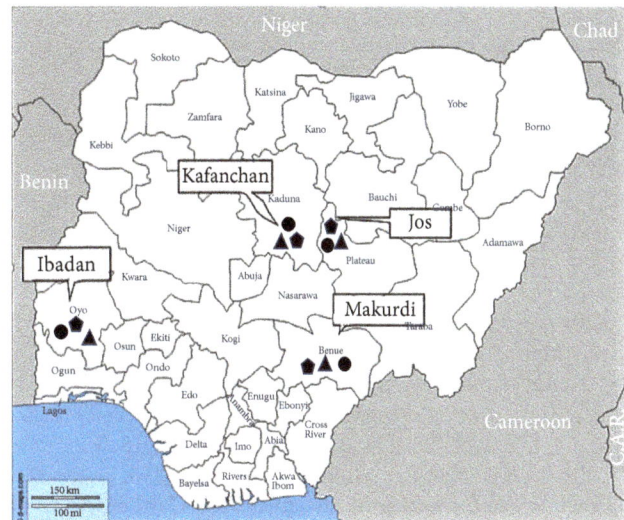

Presence of virus
▲ TTSuV1
● TTSuV
⬟ ASFV

FIGURE 1: Map of Nigeria showing the 4 locations of slaughterhouses where samples were collected.

p72 gene was also amplified for genotyping as described by Bastos et al. [20].

2.4. TTSuV1 and TTSuV2 Detection and Partial Sequencing. The sample extracted DNA was used for the detection of TTSuV1a and TTSuV1b. Assessment of TTSuV genotypes 1a and 1b from the collected samples was analyzed by amplifying an untranslated region (UTR) of the TTSuV1 viral genome using species specific primers as reported by Segalés et al. [5]. The amplification was performed on a GeneAmp® PCR System 9700 machine (Applied BioSystems, USA).

The PCR amplicons were resolved on 1.8% agarose in Tris-borate-EDTA- (TBE-) buffered gels stained with ethidium bromide. Ten microlitres of the PCR product from each of the tubes was mixed with 1 μL of 6x buffer and electrophoresed along with a 50-bp DNA molecular weight marker (GeneRuler, MBI Fermentas) at a constant voltage of 100 V for 45 min in 1x TBE buffer. Amplified products were viewed using a Bio-Rad Gel Doc™ XR system. The PCR positive products were purified using Wizard® SV Gel and PCR clean-up system (Promega Corporation, Madison, WI, USA) according to the manufacturers' instructions and eluted in 30 μL EB. The purified products were sequenced by Inqaba Biotec®, South Africa.

2.5. Statistical Analyses of TTSuV Genotype Prevalence. The prevalence data generated with the screening of TTSuV and ASFV DNA in apparently healthy population was analyzed with statistical tests carried out in SPSS, version 17.0. Student's *t*-test, Pearson's correlation, and chi-square/Fisher's exact test were applied wherever relevant. *P* value <0.05 was considered significant.

Table 1: Prevalence of swine TTSuV1a and TTSuV1b species in some pig slaughterhouses in Nigeria.

Location	TTSuV1a	TTSuV1b	Overall	Coinfected TTSuV1a/TTSuV1b	Coinfected TTSuV1/ASF
Jos	12/77 (15.6%)	2/77 (2.6%)	14/77 (18.2%)	0/77 (0%)	4/77 (5.2%)
Kafanchan	3/24 (12.5%)	5/24 (20.8%)	8/24 (33.3%)	2/24 (8.3%)	6/24 (25.0%)
Makurdi	1/38 (2.6%)	2/38 (5.3%)	3/38 (7.9%)	1/38 (2.6%)	0/38 (0%)
Ibadan	3/42 (7.1%)	4/42 (9.5%)	7/42 (16.7%)	0/42 (0%)	4/42 (9.5%)
Total positives	**19/181 (10.5%)**	**13/181 (7.2%)**	**32/181 (17.7%)**	**3/181 (1.7%)**	**14/181 (7.7%)**

2.6. Phylogenetic Analysis. The chromatograms were edited in SeqMan (Lasergene 9, DNASTAR Inc., Madison, USA). The edited sequences were subsequently aligned by ClustalW in BioEdit http://www.mbio.ncsu.edu/bioedit/bioedit.html. The phylogenetic relationship among the TTSuV1a and TTSuV1b sequences from this study was compared to previously published sequences available from GenBank http://www.ncbi.nlm.nih.gov/genbank using Mega 6.0 [21] for the construction of a phylogenetic tree using the Maximum-Likelihood algorithm with the Tamura 3-parameter model substitution with a bootstrap value of 1000.

3. Results

3.1. Detection of ASFV from Blood. Of the 181 samples collected from the four slaughterhouses, overall blood positivity rate for the pig populations was 12.71% (23/181). Location-wise, 77, 24, 42, and 38 blood samples were collected from Jos, Kafanchan, Ibadan, and Makurdi, respectively. A total of 9 (11.69%), 7 (29.17%), 5 (11.91%), and 2 (5.26%) were positive for ASFV from Jos, Kafanchan, Ibadan, and Makurdi, respectively (Table 1). Our result showed that Kafanchan had the highest number of pigs positive for ASFV and Makurdi was with the lowest number of ASFV positives.

3.2. Detection of TTSuV Genotypes from Blood. A total of 181 suspected samples collected from four slaughterhouses, Jos, Makurdi, Ibadan, and Kafanchan, were screened for ASFV and TTSuV1 genome, respectively. Of these samples 32 were positive for TTSuV1 genotypes 1a and 1b by TTSuV1F/R and TTSuV2F/R primer amplification from all the slaughterhouses. TTSuV1a and TTSuV1b infections were found in all the slaughterhouses in the four cities (Table 1). There was no statistically significant difference (p = 0.075) between the prevalence of genotype 1a infection alone (10.5%, 19/181) and 1b alone (7.2%, 13/181) for the four different locations. Nevertheless, there was a statistically significant (p = 0.011) difference between the genotypes with coinfection (1.7%, 3/181) and also between the overall TTSuV1 infections (17.7%, 32/181) with coinfection (p = 0.005) with ASFV (7.7%, 14/181). No coinfection of the genotype (TTSuV1a/TTSuV1b) was detected in Jos and Ibadan. Similarly, coinfection of TTSuV1/ASFV was detected in all the slaughterhouses with the exception of Makurdi (Table 1). TTSuV1a was more prevalent than TTSuV1b (Table 1).

3.3. Phylogenetic Relationships between TTSuV1 Genotypes. A total of 8 TTSuV1 sequences generated from PCR products and those from the GenBank were used to infer phylogeny.

All the sequences obtained from this study were deposited in the GenBank with accession number KT160265-72.

The TTSuV1a sequences from our study revealed a sequence similarity of 91–100% to one another and 91%–97% to other sequences from the GenBank. The phylogenetic analysis of Nigerian TTSuV1a revealed no unique clustering with other global sequences from the GenBank (Figure 2).

Equally the Nigerian TTSuV1b sequences displayed a similarity of 95–100% among each other and 85%–97% when compared with 16 sequences from the GenBank. However, no clear geographical grouping was observed phylogenetically (Figure 2).

4. Discussion

To the best of our knowledge, this is the first study in Nigeria to investigate the presence of TTSuV1 in domestic pigs. Our present study confirms that the infection is prevalent (17.7%) in Nigerian domestic pigs infected with either of the 2 TTSuV1 genotypes. It is not clear whether sample number or sampling season played a role in the prevalence rate but our finding is in agreement with Brink et al. [8] in Uganda who reported 51.6% positivity from 95 samples collected during ASF studies. TTSuV1 was detected in all the 4 slaughterhouses but the prevalence was low compared to reports from China and Uganda [7, 8].

Interestingly the genotype TTSuV1b was found in fewer pigs when compared to TTSuV1a and only a few pigs (3/181, 1.7%) were coinfected with both genotype. This is in agreement with previous reports by Brinks et al. [8] in Uganda and Mei et al. [7] in China.

In addition, we also observed coinfection of TTSuV1 with ASFV in domestic pigs in Nigeria. Interestingly, TTSuV1 and ASFV coinfection was higher than TTSuV1a/b but overall coinfection with either of the genotypes (32/181, 17.7%) was higher than with ASFV (14/181, 7.7%). From the total number of samples analyzed, ASFV detection was 11.6%. ASFV has been reported to be endemic in Nigeria [17]; however the potential role of TTSuV1 in the infection and epidemiology of ASFV still needs to be explored. TTSuV1 coinfection has been reported with other diseases of pigs such as porcine circovirus associated diseases [14, 15]. In humans, TTV coinfection with other viruses has been described to enhance the pathogenic potential of the coinfecting viral agent and thereby worsen clinical manifestation [22–24].

Genetically, the similarity of Nigerian TTSuV1 UTR regions is higher for TTSuV1b (95–100%) than TTSuV1 (91–100%). Similarly, the sequence identity with other TTSuV1 globally revealed a related pattern (TTSuV1a: 91–97%;

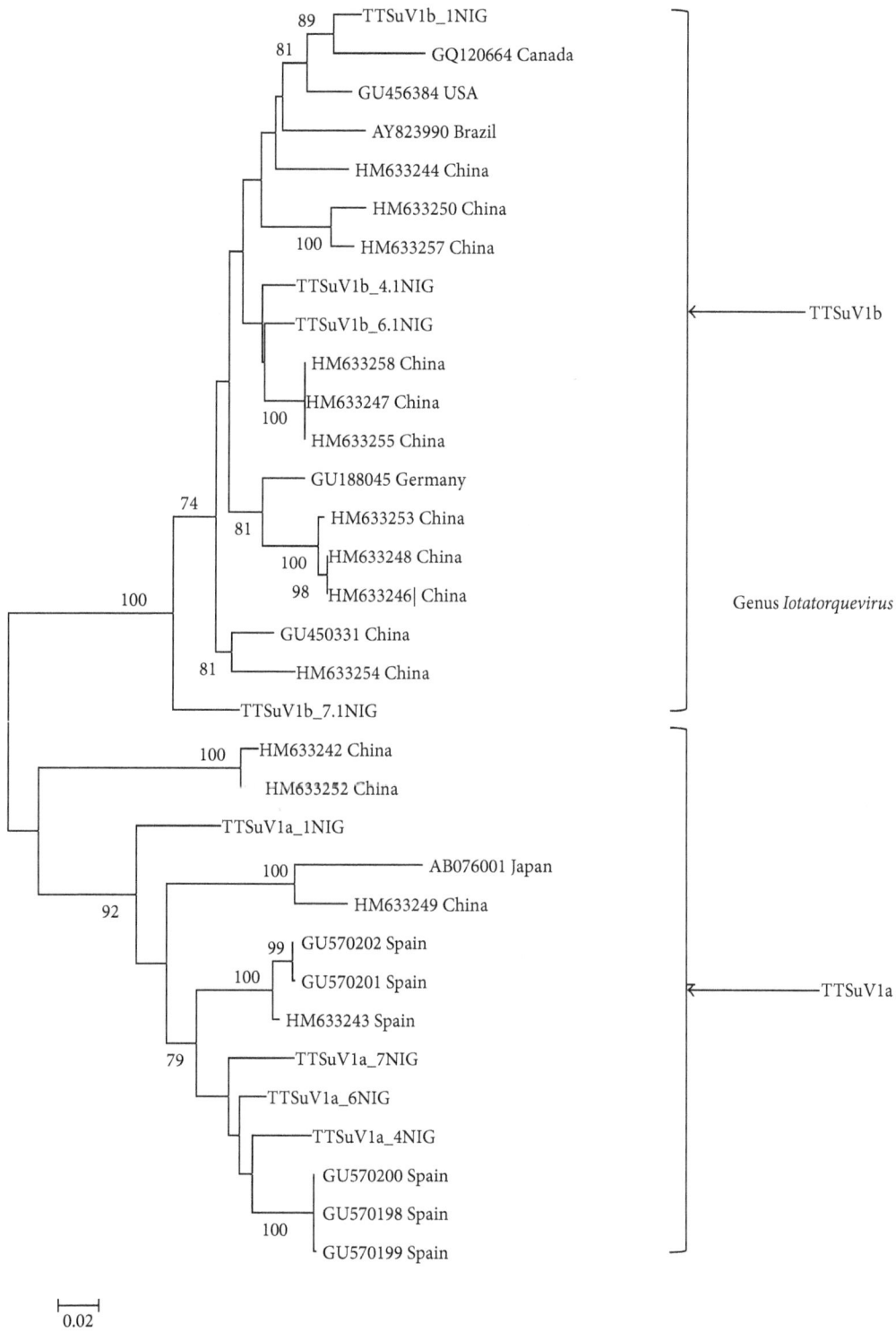

FIGURE 2: Molecular phylogenetic analysis of TTSuV1a and TTSuV1b sequences of the UTR region using Maximum-Likelihood method based on the Tamura 3-parameter model. A discrete gamma distribution was used to model evolutionary rate differences among sites (5 categories (+G, parameter = 0.3029)). Only bootstrap values above 70% are shown and sequences from this study are bold and highlighted (red).

TTSuV1b: 85–97%). However, previous studies using the UTR region did not reveal distinct geographical clustering. The phylogenetic analysis of the Nigerian sequences showed TTSuV1a and TTSuV1b distribution among other sequences globally as described by ICVT (2011) new classification. However, sequences from our study revealed a similar pattern to TTSuV1 reports from Spain and Uganda [5, 8].

In contrast, other studies had suggested the use of ORF1 capsid gene as a marker for better resolution and molecular epidemiology because the gene is under selection pressure [5]. A complete genome sequencing has also been advocated for a better understanding of the virus dynamics [4, 25, 26].

ASFV sequences obtained from our study showed 100% sequence identity of the p72 gene to all other members of genotype 1 included in the analysis and phylogenetically clustered together (data not shown).

The capacity of TTSuV1 on its own to cause disease or influence ASF is yet to be fully elucidated, but it has been reported to be involved directly or indirectly in the development of other diseases such as PMWS and PCV-2. Its association with PCV-2 has been reported especially in diseased animals [12, 14]. From the total number of samples analyzed, 14 were positive for ASFV from apparently healthy pigs suggesting state of nonclinical manifestation of disease. Phylogenetically, the viruses were similar to those previously reported to be circulating in Nigeria. It is however possible that the pigs positive for ASFV brought to the slaughterhouse could be ASFV carriers without developing the disease or could have been brought into the slaughterhouse prior to visible signs or part of emergency sale.

5. Conclusion

We reported the circulation of TTSuV1 in Nigeria coinfecting with ASFV and like other parts of the world TTSuV1a/b infection is not very common among domestic pigs in Nigeria. However, having detected TTSuV1 coinfecting with ASFV and given the lethal nature of ASFV, we hypothesize that TTSuV1 may play an exacerbating role in the pathogenesis of ASF in domestic pigs in Nigeria. Further investigation needs to be carried out to establish if the trend is rising. The role of TTSuV in the infection and epidemiology of ASFV needs to be explored.

References

[1] T. Nishizawa, H. Okamoto, K. Konishi, H. Yoshizawa, Y. Miyakawa, and M. Mayumi, "A novel DNA virus (TTV) associated with elevated transaminase levels in posttransfusion hepatitis of unknown etiology," *Biochemical and Biophysical Research Communications*, vol. 241, no. 1, pp. 92–97, 1997.

[2] L. Martínez, T. Kekarainen, M. Sibila et al., "Torque teno virus (TTV) is highly prevalent in the European wild boar (*Sus scrofa*)," *Veterinary Microbiology*, vol. 118, no. 3-4, pp. 223–229, 2006.

[3] H. Okamoto, M. Takahashi, T. Nishizawa et al., "Genomic characterization of TT viruses (TTVs) in pigs, cats and dogs and their relatedness with species-specific TTVs in primates and tupaias," *Journal of General Virology*, vol. 83, no. 6, pp. 1291–1297, 2002.

[4] ICTV, *Virus Taxonomy, Ninth Report of the International Committee on Taxonomy of Viruses*, ICTV, 2012.

[5] J. Segalés, L. Martínez-Guinó, M. Cortey et al., "Retrospective study on swine Torque teno virus genogroups 1 and 2 infection from 1985 to 2005 in Spain," *Veterinary Microbiology*, vol. 134, no. 3-4, pp. 199–207, 2009.

[6] S. Hino and H. Miyata, "Torque teno virus (TTV): current status," *Reviews in Medical Virology*, vol. 17, no. 1, pp. 45–57, 2007.

[7] M. Mei, L. Zhu, Z. Xu et al., "Molecular investigation of *Torque teno sus virus* in geographically distinct porcine breeding herds of Sichuan, China," *Virology Journal*, vol. 10, article 161, 2013.

[8] M. Brink, K. Ståhl, C. Masembe, A. Okurut, M. Berg, and A.-L. Blomström, "First time molecular detection and phylogenetic relationships of torque teno sus virus 1 and 2 in domestic pigs in Uganda: further evidence for a global distribution," *Virology Journal*, vol. 9, article 39, 2012.

[9] T. Kekarainen, M. Sibila, and J. Segalés, "Prevalence of swine *Torque teno virus* in post-weaning multisystemic wasting syndrome (PMWS)-affected and non-PMWS-affected pigs in Spain," *Journal of General Virology*, vol. 87, no. 4, pp. 833–837, 2006.

[10] T. Kekarainen and J. Segalés, "Torque teno Sus virus in pigs: an emerging pathogen?" *Transboundary and Emerging Diseases*, vol. 59, no. 1, pp. 103–108, 2012.

[11] B. Savic, V. Milicevic, J. Bojkovski, B. Kureljusic, V. Ivetic, and I. Pavlovic, "Detection rates of the swine torque teno viruses (TTVs), porcine circovirus type 2 (PCV2) and hepatitis E virus (HEV) in the livers of pigs with hepatitis," *Veterinary Research Communications*, vol. 34, no. 7, pp. 641–648, 2010.

[12] A.-L. Blomström, S. Belák, C. Fossum, L. Fuxler, P. Wallgren, and M. Berg, "Studies of porcine circovirus type 2, porcine boca-like virus and torque teno virus indicate the presence of multiple viral infections in postweaning multisystemic wasting syndrome pigs," *Virus Research*, vol. 152, no. 1-2, pp. 59–64, 2010.

[13] C. Masembe, G. Michuki, M. Onyango et al., "Viral metagenomics demonstrates that domestic pigs are a potential reservoir for Ndumu virus," *Virology Journal*, vol. 9, article 218, 2012.

[14] J. A. Ellis, G. Allan, and S. Krakowka, "Effect of coinfection with genogroup 1 porcine torque teno virus on porcine circovirus type 2-associated postweaning multisystemic wasting syndrome in gnotobiotic pigs," *American Journal of Veterinary Research*, vol. 69, no. 12, pp. 1608–1614, 2008.

[15] S. Krakowka and J. A. Ellis, "Evaluation of the effects of porcine genogroup 1 torque teno virus in gnotobiotic swine," *American Journal of Veterinary Research*, vol. 69, no. 12, pp. 1623–1629, 2008.

[16] K. El-Hicheri, "Emergency assistance on control and eradication of an outbreak of African swine fever in Western Nigeria," Report of the FAO Consultancy Mission to Nigeria TCP/NIR/7822(E), FAO, Rome, Italy, 1998.

[17] O. A. Owolodun, B. Yakubu, J. F. Antiabong et al., "Temporal dynamics of African swine fever outbreaks in Nigeria, 2002–2007," *Transboundary and Emerging Diseases*, vol. 57, no. 5, pp. 330–339, 2010.

[18] O. O. Babalobi, B. O. Olugasa, D. O. Oluwayelu, I. F. Ijagbone, G. O. Ayoade, and S. A. Agbede, "Analysis and evaluation

of mortality losses of the 2001 African swine fever outbreak, Ibadan, Nigeria," *Tropical Animal Health and Production*, vol. 39, no. 7, pp. 533–542, 2007.

[19] OIE Office International des Epizooties, "African swine fever," in *Manual of Diagnostic Tests and Vaccines for Terrestrial Animals*, OIE, Paris, France, 6th edition, 2008.

[20] A. D. S. Bastos, M.-L. Penrith, C. Crucière et al., "Genotyping field strains of African swine fever virus by partial p72 gene characterisation," *Archives of Virology*, vol. 148, no. 4, pp. 693–706, 2003.

[21] K. Tamura, G. Stecher, D. Peterson, A. Filipski, and S. Kumar, "MEGA6: molecular evolutionary genetics analysis version 6.0," *Molecular Biology and Evolution*, vol. 30, no. 12, pp. 2725–2729, 2013.

[22] D. Bhavnani, J. E. Goldstick, W. Cevallos, G. Trueba, and J. N. S. Eisenberg, "Synergistic effects between rotavirus and coinfecting pathogens on diarrheal disease: evidence from a community-based study in northwestern Ecuador," *American Journal of Epidemiology*, vol. 176, no. 5, pp. 387–395, 2012.

[23] M.-B. Tang, C.-P. Yu, S.-C. Chen, and C.-H. Chen, "Coinfection of adenovirus, norovirus and torque teno virus in stools of patients with acute gastroenteritis," *Southeast Asian Journal of Tropical Medicine and Public Health*, vol. 45, no. 6, pp. 1326–1336, 2014.

[24] C. Liu, L. Grillner, K. Jonsson et al., "Identification of viral agents associated with diarrhea in young children during a winter season in Beijing, China," *Journal of Clinical Virology*, vol. 35, no. 1, pp. 69–72, 2006.

[25] M. Cortey, L. Macera, J. Segalés, and T. Kekarainen, "Genetic variability and phylogeny of *Torque teno sus virus 1* (TTSuV1) and 2 (TTSuV2) based on complete genomes," *Veterinary Microbiology*, vol. 148, no. 2–4, pp. 125–131, 2011.

[26] Y. W. Huang, Y. Y. Ni, B. A. Dryman, and X. J. Meng, "Multiple infection of porcine Torque teno virus in a single pig and characterization of the full-length genomic sequences of four U.S. prototype PTTV strains: implication for genotyping of PTTV," *Virology*, vol. 396, no. 2, pp. 289–297, 2010.

3

Evaluation of NxTAG Respiratory Pathogen Panel and Comparison with xTAG Respiratory Viral Panel Fast v2 and Film Array Respiratory Panel for Detecting Respiratory Pathogens in Nasopharyngeal Aspirates and Swine/Avian-Origin Influenza A Subtypes in Culture Isolates

K. H. Chan,[1] K. K. W. To,[1,2,3] P. T. W. Li,[1] T. L. Wong,[1] R. Zhang,[1] K. K. H. Chik,[1] G. Chan,[1] C. C. Y. Yip,[4] H. L. Chen,[1,2,3] I. F. N. Hung,[5] J. F. W. Chan,[1,2,3] and K. Y. Yuen[1,2,3,6]

[1]*Department of Microbiology, The University of Hong Kong, Pokfulam, Hong Kong*
[2]*State Key Laboratory for Emerging Infectious Diseases, The University of Hong Kong, Pokfulam, Hong Kong*
[3]*Carol Yu Centre for Infection, The University of Hong Kong, Pokfulam, Hong Kong*
[4]*Department of Microbiology, Queen Mary Hospital, Pokfulam, Hong Kong*
[5]*Department of Medicine, The University of Hong Kong, Pokfulam, Hong Kong*
[6]*The Collaborative Innovation Center for Diagnosis and Treatment of Infectious Diseases,*
 The University of Hong Kong, Pokfulam, Hong Kong

Correspondence should be addressed to K. H. Chan; chankh2@hkucc.hku.hk and K. Y. Yuen; kyyuen@hkucc.hku.hk

Academic Editor: Subhash C. Verma

This study evaluated a new multiplex kit, Luminex NxTAG Respiratory Pathogen Panel, for respiratory pathogens and compared it with xTAG RVP Fast v2 and FilmArray Respiratory Panel using nasopharyngeal aspirate specimens and culture isolates of different swine/avian-origin influenza A subtypes (H2N2, H5N1, H7N9, H5N6, and H9N2). NxTAG RPP gave sensitivity of 95.2%, specificity of 99.6%, PPV of 93.5%, and NPV of 99.7%. NxTAG RPP, xTAG RVP, and FilmArray RP had highly concordant performance among each other for the detection of respiratory pathogens. The mean analytic sensitivity (TCID50/ml) of NxTAG RPP, xTAG RVP, and FilmArray RP for detection of swine/avian-origin influenza A subtype isolates was 0.7, 41.8, and 0.8, respectively. All three multiplex assays correctly typed and genotyped the influenza viruses, except for NxTAG RRP that could not distinguish H3N2 from H3N2v. Further investigation should be performed if H3N2v is suspected to be the cause of disease. Sensitive and specific laboratory diagnosis of all influenza A viruses subtypes is especially essential in certain epidemic regions, such as Southeast Asia. The results of this study should help clinical laboratory professionals to be aware of the different performances of commercially available molecular multiplex RT-PCR assays that are commonly adopted in many clinical diagnostic laboratories.

1. Introduction

Respiratory tract infections (RTIs) are caused by various pathogens that are often indistinguishable from one another by clinical diagnosis. RTIs are a major cause of mortality, morbidity, and hospitalization, especially in children aged below five years, and pose significant economic burden [1–6].

Most RTIs are caused by viruses. Common respiratory viruses include influenza virus, adenovirus, parainfluenza virus, respiratory syncytial virus (RSV), human coronaviruses, human metapneumovirus (hMPV), and rhinovirus [7, 8].

Rapid and accurate identification of the causative pathogens of RTIs can help guide treatment decisions, possibly reducing the length of hospital stays and associated healthcare costs. Moreover, it aids in epidemiologic tracking of local outbreaks or epidemics by implementing proper infection control measures and administering effective antimicrobial therapy. Rapid laboratory identification of RTI pathogens has been associated with up to 50% reduction in hospital stays, 30% reduction in the inappropriate use of antibiotics, and 20% reduction in unnecessary diagnostic tests and procedures [9]. Multiplexed molecular assays that can concurrently detect multiple pathogens from the same sample in a single reaction have been increasingly adopted in clinical microbiology laboratories in the recent years [10]. Several studies have shown that these molecular tests have superior diagnostic capacity and cost-effectiveness of molecular tests when compared to conventional and other diagnostic methods [11, 12].

For influenza viruses, rapid molecular tests based on polymerase chain reaction (PCR) using primers that target the relatively conserved matrix (M) gene are frequently used for achieving rapid and accurate laboratory diagnosis. However, variations in the gene and amino acid sequences in different influenza virus subtypes due to rapid mutations of the viral RNA polymerase may affect the results of these tests. With the emergence of human infections due to the swine-origin influenza A H3N2 variant (H3N2v) virus in North America in 2010 and more recently the avian-origin influenza A H7N9 and H5N6 in China [13–15], it would be important to ascertain the analytical sensitivities of these rapid tests for the novel influenza viruses [16, 17]. In a previous study, we have demonstrated that xTAG RVP has lower sensitivity for detection of H7N9 in patient samples and culture isolates [16, 17].

NxTAG Respiratory Pathogen Panel (RPP), CE-IVD (Luminex Molecular Diagnostics, Toronto, Canada), is a recent new qualitative multiplex molecular test for the detection of nucleic acids from multiple respiratory viruses and bacteria extracted from respiratory specimens. It detects 22 viral and bacterial targets including influenza A virus, influenza A virus subtype seasonal H1, influenza A virus subtype seasonal H3, influenza A virus subtype swine-origin H1N1pdm09, influenza B virus, RSV A and B, parainfluenza viruses types 1 to 4, adenovirus, hMPV, rhinovirus/enterovirus, human coronavirus- (HCoV-) 229E, HCoV-OC43, HCoV-NL63, HCoV-HKU1, human bocavirus, *Chlamydophila pneumoniae*, *Mycoplasma pneumoniae*, and *Legionella pneumophila* (Table 1). Although there were several studies about the performance of NxTAG RPP using RUO (research use only) assay, the performance of the NxTAG RPP, CV-IVD, for detection of respiratory viruses, particularly the sensitivity and specificity of influenza A subtypes, remains unclear [18–20]. The purpose of this study is to evaluate the NxTAG RPP, CE-IVD, and compare it with Luminex xTAG Respiratory Viral Panel (RVP) Fast v2 (Luminex Molecular Diagnostics, Toronto, Canada) and FilmArray Respiratory Panel (RP) (bioMérieux, Marcy l'Étoile, France), using nasopharyngeal aspirate (NPA) samples obtained from patients with RTIs and culture isolates of different swine and avian-origin influenza A subtypes (H2N2, H3N2v, H5N1, H5N6, H7N9, and H9N2).

2. Materials and Methods

2.1. Clinical Specimens. The 133 NPA specimens selectively collected from patients with symptoms and signs of RTIs who were managed in Queen Mary Hospital, Hong Kong, and with clinical PCR results were used in this study. These NPA samples were collected into a viral transport medium as described previously [21] and were tested by direct immunofluorescence (DFA) (D^3® Ultra 8™ DFA Respiratory Virus Screening and Identification Kit, Diagnostic Hybrids, Inc. (Quidel), USA) for influenza A virus, influenza B virus, parainfluenza viruses types 1 to 4, respiratory syncytial virus, human metapneumovirus, and adenovirus, and an aliquot of each NPA was sent to Hong Kong Government Virus Laboratory, the Department of Health, for further testing by RT-PCR for detection of influenza A virus, influenza B virus, parainfluenza viruses types 1 to 4, respiratory syncytial virus, adenovirus, and rhinovirus/enterovirus, as part of the routine clinical diagnostic protocol. Single RT-PCR for detection of human metapneumovirus, human coronavirus- (HCoV-) 229E, HCoV-OC43, HCoV-NL63, HCoV-HKU1, human bocavirus, *Chlamydophila pneumoniae*, *Mycoplasma pneumoniae*, and *Legionella pneumophila* was used as described previously [22–27]. All these PCR results were used as positive reference. The remaining samples were then recruited for NxTAG RVP evaluation. A sufficient quantity of the samples was used for further testing with xTAG RVP and FilmArray RP.

2.2. Influenza Isolates. Two swine-origin and four avian-origin influenza A human isolates, namely, H1N1pdm09 (A/415742/09/H1N1), H3N2v (A/Wisconsin/12/2010), H2N2 (A/Asia/57/3), H5N1 (A/Vietnam/3028/04), H7N9 (A/Anhui/1/2013), and H9N2 (A/HK/1073/99), were used in this study. Additionally, an H5N6 avian isolate [H5N6 (A/Great Egret/H5N6/HK/2016)] was also included. The viruses were cultured for 2 days in Madin-Darby Canine Kidney (MDCK) cells with tosyl sulfonyl phenylalanyl chloromethyl ketone- (TPCK-) treated trypsin (2 μg/ml) (Sigma, St. Louis, MO) as previously described [28]. Aliquots of culture supernatant were frozen at −80°C until use. Serial tenfold dilutions of the virus stock with serum-free minimal essential medium (MEM) (Gibco BRL, Grand Island, NY) were tested in NxTAG RPP, xTAG RVP, and FilmArray RP. The viral M gene genome copy numbers per ml of each virus dilution were determined by real-time, quantitative RT-PCR (q-PCR) as previously described with modification [29, 30]. Briefly, 5 μL purified RNA was amplified in a 25 μL reaction containing 0.5 μL Superscript III Reverse Transcriptase/Platinum Taq DNA polymerase (Invitrogen, Carlsbad, California, USA), 0.05 μL ROX reference dye (25 mM), 12.5 μL of 2x reaction buffer, 800 nmol/L forward primer (5'-GACCRA-TCCTGTCACCTCTGAC-3'), 800 nmol/L reverse primer (5'-AGGGCATTYTGGACAAAKCGTCTA-3'), and probe 200 nmol/L (FAM-5'-TGCAGTCCTCGCTCACTGGGC-ACG-3'-BHQ1). The thermal cycling conditions were 30 minutes at 50°C for reverse transcription and then 2 min at 95°C for RT inactivation/initial denaturation, followed by 50 cycles of 15 s at 95°C and 30 s at 55°C. All reactions

TABLE 1: Detectable pathogens and targets.

Viruses	NxTAG RPP	xTAG RVP Fast v2	FilmArray RP
Influenza A virus	√	√	√
Subtype (H1, H1pdm09, H3)	√	(H1, H3)	√
Influenza B virus	√	√	√
Respiratory syncytial virus	(A, B)	(A, B)	√
Human coronavirus (229E, OC43, NL63, HKU1)	√	√	√
Parainfluenza viruses 1–4	√	√	√
Human metapneumovirus	√	√	√
Adenovirus	√	√	√
Human bocavirus	√	√	
Human rhinovirus/Enterovirus	√	√	√
Chlamydophila pneumoniae	√		√
Legionella pneumophila	√		
Mycoplasma pneumoniae	√		√
Bordetella pertussis			√
Total targets	22	18	20

were performed using StepOnePlus Real-Time PCR System (Applied Biosystems, Foster City). For quantitative assay, a reference standard plasmid was prepared by cloning the target M gene amplicon into pCRII-TOPO vector (TOPO™ TA Cloning™ Kit, Invitrogen, San Diego, CA) according to the manufacturer's instructions. The copy number of the standard plasmid was determined based on molar concentration of the plasmid (1 molar is equivalent to about 6.0221415×10^{23} copies numbers). A series of 6 log10 dilutions, equivalent to 1×10^{1} to 1×10^{6} copies per reaction, were then prepared from the reference standard plasmid to generate calibration curves and run in parallel with the test samples. The limit of detection of the M gene qRT-PCR is 10 copies per reaction at 95% confidence level. The same virus dilutions were inoculated onto MDCK cells to determine the 50% tissue culture infective dose (TCID50) using the Reed-Muench method as previously described [28].

2.3. Nucleic Acid Extraction. Nucleic acid was detected using easyMAG extraction platform (bioMérieux, Marcy l'Étoile, France) and extracted for NxTAG RPP and xTAG RVP from the specimens as previously described [31]. Total nucleic acid extraction was isolated by using the NucliSENS easyMAG instrument (bioMérieux). Briefly, 10 μl of MS2 internal control was first added to 200 μl of sample. The mixture was added to 2 ml of lysis buffer and was incubated for 10 minutes at room temperature. The lysed sample was then transferred to the well of a plastic vessel with 100 μl of silica. This was followed by automatic magnetic separation. Nucleic acid was recovered in 110 μl elution buffer. By using a parallel specimen (300 μl), nucleic acid extraction, PCR, and detection were performed in FilmArray according to the manufacturer's instructions. The NxTAG RPP incorporates multiplex Reverse Transcriptase-Polymerase Chain Reaction (RT-PCR) with the Luminex proprietary universal tag sorting system on the Luminex platform for detecting respiratory pathogen targets according to the manufacturer's instructions. Briefly, the extracted total nucleic acid is added to

preplated Lyophilized Bead Reagents (LBRs) and mixed to resuspend the reaction reagents. The reaction is amplified via RT-PCR and the reaction product undergoes bead hybridization within the sealed reaction well. The hybridized, tagged beads are then sorted and read on the MAGPIX instrument, and the signals are analyzed using the NxTAG Respiratory Pathogen Panel Assay File for SYNCT™ Software (Luminex, Austin, Texas, USA).

2.4. Statistical Analysis. Diagnostic sensitivity, specificity, PPV, and NPV of the assays against the positive references and agreement between the assays were calculated by VassarStats: Website for Statistical Computation (http://vassarstats.net).

3. Results

3.1. Clinical Samples and Performance of NxTAG RPP. A total of 133 NPA specimens were tested in this study. The specimens were collected from 75 males and 58 females with a mean age of 32.5 years (range: 2 months to 99 years of age). Of 133 specimens, 75 positives were detected by DFA and 151 positives were detected by PCR [influenza A virus = 16 (H3 = 12, H1pdm09 = 3, H7 = 1), influenza B virus = 10, parainfluenza virus 1 = 10, parainfluenza virus 2 = 10, parainfluenza virus 3 = 10, parainfluenza virus 4 = 11, RSV = 11, hMPV = 11, adenovirus = 4, rhinovirus/enterovirus = 28, human coronavirus- (HCoV-) 229E = 3, HCoV-OC43 = 6, HCoV-NL63 = 1, HCoV-HKU1 = 5, human bocavirus = 9, *Chlamydophila pneumoniae* = 1, *Mycoplasma pneumoniae* = 4, and *Legionella pneumophila* = 1]. All 133 specimens were evaluated by NxTAG RPP. Overall, 153 pathogens were identified by NxTAG RPP. Ten positives (H1pdm09 × 1, RSV A × 1, PIF1 × 1, adenovirus × 1, EV/rhinovirus × 4, and bocavirus × 2) were considered as false positives when compared with positive reference. The sensitivity, specificity, positive predictive value, and negative predictive value of NxTAG RPP for detection of respiratory viruses were 95.2% [95% confidence level (Cl): 90.4–97.7], 99.6% (95% Cl: 99.3–99.8), 93.5% (95% Cl: 88.4–96.5), and 99.7% (95% Cl: 99.4–99.9), respectively (Table 2).

3.2. Performance and Concordance of xTAG RVP and FilmArray RP.

Of 133 tested samples, 71 had enough quantity to be used for further testing with xTAG RVP and FilmArray RP. The results of these 71 samples tested by the three assays were then compared. Out of these 71 specimens, 66 were positive and 5 were negative by NxTAG RPP. Both the xTAG RVP and FilmArray RP detected respiratory pathogens in 63 (88.7%) specimens with 96 and 83 pathogens, respectively. The sensitivity, specificity, positive predictive value, and negative predictive value of xTAG RVP and FilmArray RP were 96.9%, 99.9%, 99.0%, and 99.7% and 85.3%, 99.9%, 98.8%, and 98.9%, respectively. When NxTAG RPP was compared with xTAG RVP and FilmArray RP, the Kappa value was 0.97 with 95% CI of 0.95–0.99 and 0.93 with 95% CI of 0.89–0.97, respectively. When xTAG RVP was compared with FilmArray RP, the Kappa value was 0.95 with 95% CI of 0.91–0.98. These results suggested that the three assays were highly concordant as a Kappa value higher than 0.80 indicated concordance.

We have previously shown that xTAG RVP has low sensitivity for detecting H7N9 [16, 17]. In this study, one of the patient specimens with confirmed H7N9 influenza A infection was also not detected by xTAG RVP influenza A but was detected by NxTAG RPP and FilmArray RP influenza A. xTAG RVP has a 1000 and 10 times higher limit of detection for H7N9 than NxTAG RPP and FilmArray RP, respectively (Table 3). These findings show that NxTAG RRP has greatly improved the sensitivity for detecting H7N9 over the xTAG RVP. Besides, NxTAG RPP has also improved sensitivity for detecting other respiratory viruses over xTAG RVP (1 adenovirus and 2 bocavirus). These findings corroborate another recent report on the partial comparison between the NxTAG Respiratory Pathogen Panel Assay and the Luminex xTAG Respiratory Panel Fast Assay v2 [32]. NxTAG RPP detected 12 more pathogens than FilmArray RP in our study, with 50% (6/12) being enterovirus/rhinovirus. The other additional positives detected by NxTAG RPP were adenovirus (2), parainfluenza virus 4b (1), hMPV (1), H1N1pdm (1), and *M. pneumoniae* (1). Overall, 8 positives, hMPV (1), P2 (1), P4 (3), enterovirus/rhinovirus (2), and *M. pneumoniae* (1), were not detected by NxTAG RPP. All these positives indeed had high Ct value (≥35) that may be lower than the limit of detection by NxTAG RPP. Further study should be required if the primers that are suspected do not detect epidemic strains.

Furthermore, the results of 5 samples (4 H1N1pdm 2009 and 1 H7N9) were reported to be "equivocal" by FilmArray RP (Flu A-pan-1 positive, Flu A-pan-2 negative). These 5 specimens were, in fact, true positive as confirmed by other testing methods. These findings indicated that M gene (Flu A-pan-1) was more sensitive than NS1 gene (Flu A-pan-2) for detection of H1N1pdm 2009.

3.3. Analytical Sensitivity of Influenza A Culture Isolates.

When influenza A virus subtype isolates were tested, the mean (range) analytic sensitivities (viral load log10 copies/ml and TCID$_{50}$/ml) of NxTAG RPP, xTAG RVP, and FilmArray RP were 3.0 (1.8–4.2) and 0.7 (0.0056–3.2); 4.3 (3.0–6.4) and 41.8 (0.56–178); and 3.4 (2.7–4.4) and 0.8 (0.1–1.78), respectively (Table 3). All avian- and swine-origin influenza A strains were detected by M gene in NxTAG RPP, xTAG RVP, and FilmArray RP. The swine-origin H1N1pdm09 was correctly genotyped by NxTAG RPP and FilmArray RP. However, H3N2v and seasonal H3N2 could not be differentiated by NxTAG RPP.

4. Discussion

In the recent years, the availability of molecular diagnostic tests has revolutionized the diagnosis and surveillance of infectious diseases and treatment of RTIs. Multiplexed molecular assays simultaneously detect multiple pathogens from the same sample in a single reaction vessel, providing a more comprehensive picture of infection. In this study, the clinical performance of the Luminex NxTAG RPP (CV-IVD) in NPA specimens was found to have high sensitivity (95.2%) and specificity (99.6%) for detection of respiratory viruses. These findings are similar to those reported in recent evaluation studies using NxTAG RPP (RUO) kit by other groups [18–20]. The performances of the NxTAG RPP, xTAG RVP, and FilmArray RP were also compared. Their results were highly concordant, with the highest concordance reported between NxTAG RRP and xTAG RVP [Kappa value = 0.97 (95% Cl: 0.95–0.99)].

According to the manufacturer, M gene (Flu A-pan-1) and NS1 gene (Flu A-pan-2) are used for influenza A typing by FilmArray RP. The result is only interpreted as positive when both genes are positive. The result will be interpreted as "equivocal" when only Flu A-pan-1 is positive, and the system will suggest the users to repeat testing by the same assay or other assays. In this study, the results showed that an "equivocal" result by FilmArray RP is most likely to be a true positive. The correct interpretation of these results should be considered to avoid delay in diagnosis and treatment particularly in patients with severe influenza A virus infection.

In general, the analytical sensitivities of the NxTAG RPP and FilmArray RP for the swine- and avian-origin influenza viruses were comparable, but xTAG RVP had more than one log lower analytical sensitivity than NxTAG RPP and FilmArray RP (Table 3). NxTAG RPP also had higher analytical sensitivity for detecting H5N6 than the xTAG RVP but the same sensitivity as FilmArray RP and higher analytical sensitivity for detecting H3N2v than xTAG RVP and FilmArray RP. All three multiplex assays accurately typed and genotyped the influenza viruses, except for NxTAG RRP that does not distinguish subtyped H3N2 from H3N2v. This finding was further confirmed by testing another H3N2v strain, A/Indiana/08/2011, with 500TCID$_{50}$. A recent study also showed that NxTAG RPP (RUO) only correctly genotyped 95.5% of influenza A virus H1N1pdm09 strains [19].

Rapid multiplex RT-PCR assays for respiratory pathogens detection are important for establishing diagnosis to facilitate the implementation of appropriate treatment and infection control measures. Sensitive and specific laboratory diagnosis

TABLE 2: Performance of NxTAG RRP for detecting respiratory viruses in nasopharyngeal aspirates.

Viruses	NxTAG Pos/Ref Pos	NxTAG Neg/Ref Pos	NxTAG Pos/Ref Neg	NxTAG Neg/Ref Neg	Sensitivity % (95% CI)	Specificity % (95% CI)	PPV % (95% CI)	NPV % (95% CI)
Influenza A	16	0	1	116	100 (75.9–100)	99.1 (94.6–100)	94.1 (69.2–99.7)	100 (96.0–100)
H3	12	0	0	121	100 (69.9–100)	100 (96.2–100)	100 (69.9–100)	100 (96.2–100)
H1pdm09	3	0	1	129	100 (31.0–100)	99.2 (95.1–100)	75 (21.9–98.7)	100 (96.4–100)
H1	0	0	0	133	NA	NA	NA	NA
Influenza B	10	0	0	123	100 (65.5–100)	100 (96.2–100)	100 (65.5–100)	100 (95.5–100)
RSV A	9	0	1	123	100 (62.9–100)	99.2 (94.9–100)	90 (54.1–99.5)	100 (96.2–100)
RSV B	2	0	0	131	100 (19.8–100)	100 (96.4–100)	100 (19.8–100)	100 (96.4–100)
PIF1	10	0	1	122	100 (65.5–100)	99.2 (94.9–100)	99.9 (57.1–99.5)	100 (96.2–100)
PIF2	9	1	0	123	90.0 (54.1–99.4)	100 (96.2–100)	100 (62.9–100)	99.2 (94.9–100)
PIF3	10	0	0	123	100 (65.5–100)	100 (96.2–100)	100 (65.5–100)	100 (96.2–100)
PIF4	8	3	0	122	72.7 (39.0–92.6)	100 (96.2–100)	100 (59.8–100)	97.6 (92.6–99)
Adenovirus	4	0	1	128	100 (39.6–100)	99.2 (95.1–100)	80.0 (29.9–98.9)	100 (96.4–100)
hMPV	10	1	0	122	90.9 (57.1–99.5)	100 (96.2–100)	100 (66.5–100)	99.2 (94.9–100)
HCoV-229E	3	0	0	130	100 (31.0–100)	100 (96.4–100)	100 (31.0–100)	100 (96.4–100)
HCoV-OC43	6	0	0	127	100 (51.7–100)	100 (96.3–100)	100 (51.7–100)	100 (96.3–100)
HCoV-NL63	1	0	0	132	100 (5.5–100)	100 (96.5–100)	100 (5.5–100)	100 (96.5–100)
HCoV-HKU1	5	0	0	128	100 (46.3–100)	100 (96.4–100)	100 (46.3–100)	100 (96.4–100)
EV/rhinovirus	26	2	4	101	92.9 (75.0–98.8)	96.2 (90.0–98.8)	86.7 (68.4–95.6)	98.1 (92.4–100)
Bocavirus	9	0	2	122	100 (62.9–100)	98.4 (93.7–99.7)	81.8 (47.8–96.8)	100 (96.2–100)
C. pneumoniae	1	0	0	132	100 (5.5–100)	100 (96.5–100)	100 (5.5–100)	100 (96.5–100)
M. pneumoniae	3	1	0	129	75.0 (21.9–98.7)	100 (96.3–100)	100 (31.0–100)	99.2 (95.2–100)
L. pneumophila	1	0	0	132	100 (5.5–100)	100 (96.5–100)	100 (5.5–100)	100 (96.5–100)
B. pertussis	0	0	0	133	NA	NA	NA	NA
Total	158	8	11[#]	2882	95.2 (90.4–97.7)	99.6 (99.3–99.8)	93.5 (88.4–96.5)	99.7 (99.4–99.9)

EV, enterovirus; HCoV, human coronavirus; hMPV, human metapneumovirus; PIF, parainfluenza virus; PPV, positive predictive value; NPV, negative predictive value; RSV, respiratory syncytial virus; NA, not applicable; Ref, reference; Pos, positive; Neg, negative. [#]Overall total number of false positives is 10 because influenza A and subtyping were tested for a sample simultaneously.

TABLE 3: Analytical sensitivity of NxTAG RPP, xTAG RVP, and FilmArray RP for detecting influenza A, avian- or swine-origin subtypes.

| Influenza A | | Limit of detection [viral load (log10 copies/ml); log10 TCID50/ml] of influenza A subtype | | | | | |
| | | NxTAG RPP | | xTAG RVP | | FilmArray RP | |
Subtype	Strains	Viral load	TCID$_{50}$	Viral load	TCID$_{50}$	Viral load	TCID$_{50}$
H1N1pdm09	A/HK/415742/09/H1N1	3.0	0.1	3.0	0.1	3.0	0.1
H2N2	A/Asia/57/3	3.7	3.2	3.7	3.2	2.7	0.32
H3N2v	A/Wisconsin/12/2010	2.0	0.1	4.0	10	3.0	1
H5N1	A/Vietnam/3028/04	4.2	0.56	4.2	0.56	4.2	0.56
H5N6	A/H5N6/HK/2016	3.0	1	5.0	100	3.0	1
H7N9	A/Anhui/1/2013	3.4	0.178	6.4	178	4.4	1.78
H9N2	A/HK/1073/99	1.8	0.0056	3.8	0.56	3.8	0.56
Mean		3.0	0.7	4.3	41.8	3.4	0.8

of all influenza A virus subtypes is especially essential in certain epidemic regions, such as Southeast Asia. The correct interpretation of these results is also important and would avoid delay in patient management and infection control, especially in patients with severe seasonal influenza A or avian/swine-origin influenza A virus subtype infection. Clinical microbiologists, infectious disease specialists, and laboratory managers should be aware of and understand the different clinical performances of these commercially available molecular multiplex RT-PCR assays that are commonly adopted in many clinical microbiology laboratories. The sensitivity and specificity of these molecular multiplex assays must be predetermined and be able to confidently detect most of the important avian or swine influenza A subtype infection including H5N1 and H7N9 and this capability is particularly important for use in Southeast Asia.

A limitation of this study is that some target numbers are small. This is due to low prevalent disease and may require a longer period in order to collect a higher number of positives. High cost for these multiplex assays is another limitation for us to study more samples.

5. Conclusion

In this study, the results showed that NxTAG RPP, xTAG RVP, and FilmArray RP assays had high sensitivity and specificity for diagnosis of respiratory diseases. They are suitable for use in clinical diagnostic laboratories for detection of respiratory pathogens in patients with RTIs. However, awareness should be raised that H3N2 could not be distinguished from H3N2v by NxTAG RPP. Further investigation should be performed if H3N2v is suspected to be the cause of disease.

Acknowledgments

The authors would like to thank the staff of the Department of Microbiology, Queen Mary Hospital, for the facilitation of this project. This work was partly supported by the donations of Larry Chi-Kin Yung and Hui Hoy and Chow Sin Lan Charity Fund Limited; the authors also obtained funding from the Consultancy Service for Enhancing Laboratory Surveillance of Emerging Infectious Diseases, the Department of Health, Hong Kong Special Administrative Region; the University Development Fund and the Committee for Research and Conference Grant; the University of Hong Kong; the Collaborative Innovation Center for Diagnosis and Treatment of Infectious Diseases, the Ministry of Education of China; and the Commissioned Research on Control of Infectious Diseases (Phase III) of the Health and Medical Research Fund (HKM-15-M-04) of the Food and Health Bureau of the HKSAR Government.

References

[1] W. Olszewska, M. Zambon, and P. J. M. Openshaw, "Development of vaccines against common colds," *British Medical Bulletin*, vol. 62, no. 1, pp. 99–111, 2002.

[2] World Health Organization, *Burden of Disease Project*, World Health Organization, Geneva, Switzerland, 2005.

[3] B. Ehlken, G. Ihorst, B. Lippert et al., "Economic impact of community-acquired and nosocomial lower respiratory tract infections in young children in Germany," *European Journal of Pediatrics*, vol. 164, no. 10, pp. 607–615, 2005.

[4] M. M. Massin, J. Montesanti, P. Gérard, and P. Lepage, "Spectrum and frequency of illness presenting to a pediatric emergency department," *Acta Clinica Belgica*, vol. 61, no. 4, pp. 161–165, 2006.

[5] K. G. Nicholson, T. McNally, M. Silverman, P. Simons, J. D. Stockton, and M. C. Zambon, "Rates of hospitalisation for influenza, respiratory syncytial virus and human metapneumovirus among infants and young children," *Vaccine*, vol. 24, no. 1, pp. 102–108, 2006.

[6] A. Sauro, F. Barone, G. Blasio, L. Russo, and L. Santillo, "Do influenza and acute respiratory infective diseases weigh heavily on general practitioners' daily practice?" *European Journal of General Practice*, vol. 12, no. 1, pp. 34–36, 2006.

[7] J. S. Tregoning and J. Schwarze, "Respiratory viral infections in infants: causes, clinical symptoms, virology, and immunology," *Clinical Microbiology Reviews*, vol. 23, no. 1, pp. 74–98, 2010.

[8] S. S. Chiu, P.-L. Ho, M. J. S. Peiris, K. H. Chan, and E. L. Y. Chan, "Population-based hospitalization incidence of respiratory viruses in community-acquired pneumonia in children younger than 5 years of age," *Influenza and other Respiratory Viruses*, vol. 8, no. 6, pp. 626-627, 2014.

[9] K. J. Henrickson, "Cost-effective use of rapid diagnostic techniques in the treatment and prevention of viral respiratory infections," *Pediatric Annals*, vol. 34, no. 1, pp. 24–31, 2005.

[10] E. B. Popowitch, S. S. O'Neill, and M. B. Miller, "Comparison of the biofire filmarray RP, Genmark eSensor RVP, Luminex xTAG RVPv1, and Luminex xTAG RVP fast multiplex assays for detection of respiratory viruses," *Journal of Clinical Microbiology*, vol. 51, no. 5, pp. 1528–1533, 2013.

[11] J. B. Mahony, "Detection of respiratory viruses by molecular methods," *Clinical Microbiology Reviews*, vol. 21, no. 4, pp. 716–747, 2008.

[12] J. B. Mahony, A. Petrich, and M. Smieja, "Molecular diagnosis of respiratory virus infections," *Critical Reviews in Clinical Laboratory Sciences*, vol. 48, no. 5-6, pp. 217–249, 2011.

[13] Centers for Disease Control and Prevention, *Swine-Origin Influenza A (H3N2) Virus Infection in Two Children — Indiana and Pennsylvania, July–August MMWR*, 2011.

[14] Y. Chen, W. Liang, S. Yang et al., "Human infections with the emerging avian influenza A H7N9 virus from wet market poultry: clinical analysis and characterisation of viral genome," *Lancet*, vol. 381, pp. 1916–1925, 2013.

[15] Z.-F. Yang, C. K. P. Mok, J. S. M. Peiris, and N.-S. Zhong, "Human infection with a novel avian influenza A(H5N6) virus," *New England Journal of Medicine*, vol. 373, no. 5, pp. 487–489, 2015.

[16] K.-H. Chan, K. K. W. To, J. F. W. Chan, C. P. Y. Li, H. Chen, and K.-Y. Yuen, "Analytical sensitivity of seven point-of-care influenza virus detection tests and two molecular tests for detection of avian origin H7N9 and swine origin H3N2 variant influenza a viruses," *Journal of Clinical Microbiology*, vol. 51, no. 9, pp. 3160-3161, 2013.

[17] K.-H. Chan, K. K. W. To, J. F. W. Chan et al., "Assessment of antigen and molecular tests with serial specimens from a patient with influenza A(H7N9) infection," *Journal of Clinical Microbiology*, vol. 52, no. 6, pp. 2272–2274, 2014.

[18] J. H. K. Chen, H.-Y. Lam, C. C. Y. Yip et al., "Clinical evaluation of the new high-throughput luminex nxtag respiratory pathogen panel assay for multiplex respiratory pathogen detection," *Journal of Clinical Microbiology*, vol. 54, no. 7, pp. 1820–1825, 2016.

[19] Y.-W. Tang, S. Gonsalves, J. Y. Sun et al., "Clinical evaluation of the luminex nxtag respiratory pathogen panel," *Journal of Clinical Microbiology*, vol. 54, no. 7, pp. 1912–1914, 2016.

[20] C. Beckmann and H. H. Hirsch, "Comparing Luminex NxTAG-Respiratory Pathogen Panel and RespiFinder-22 for multiplex detection of respiratory pathogens," *Journal of Medical Virology*, vol. 88, no. 8, pp. 1319–1324, 2016.

[21] I. Hung, V. Cheng, A. Wu et al., "Viral Loads in Clinical Specimens and SARS Manifestations," *Emerging Infectious Diseases*, vol. 10, no. 9, pp. 1550–1557, 2004.

[22] M. Welti, K. Jaton, M. Altwegg, R. Sahli, A. Wenger, and J. Bille, "Development of a multiplex real-time quantitative PCR assay to detect Chlamydia pneumoniae, Legionella pneumophila and Mycoplasma pneumoniae in respiratory tract secretions," *Diagnostic Microbiology and Infectious Disease*, vol. 45, no. 2, pp. 85–95, 2003.

[23] L. J. R. Van Elden, A. M. Van Loon, F. Van Alphen et al., "Frequent Detection of Human Coronaviruses in Clinical Specimens from Patients with Respiratory Tract Infection by Use of a Novel Real-Time Reverse-Transciptase Polymerase Chain Reaction," *Journal of Infectious Diseases*, vol. 189, no. 4, pp. 652–657, 2004.

[24] P. C. Y. Woo, S. K. P. Lau, C.-M. Chu et al., "Characterization and complete genome sequence of a novel coronavirus, coronavirus HKU1, from patients with pneumonia," *Journal of Virology*, vol. 79, no. 2, pp. 884–895, 2005.

[25] S. S. Chiu, K. H. Chan, K. W. Chu et al., "Human coronavirus NL63 infection and other coronavirus infections in children hospitalized with acute respiratory disease in Hong Kong, China," *Clinical Infectious Diseases*, vol. 40, no. 12, pp. 1721–1729, 2005.

[26] J. Kuypers, N. Wright, L. Corey, and R. Morrow, "Detection and quantification of human metapneumovirus in pediatric specimens by real-time RT-PCR," *Journal of Clinical Virology*, vol. 33, no. 4, pp. 299–305, 2005.

[27] S. K. P. Lau, C. C. Y. Yip, T.-L. Que et al., "Clinical and molecular epidemiology of human bocavirus in respiratory and fecal samples from children in Hong Kong," *Journal of Infectious Diseases*, vol. 196, no. 7, pp. 986–993, 2007.

[28] K. H. Chan, S. Y. Lam, P. Puthavathana et al., "Comparative analytical sensitivities of six rapid influenza A antigen detection test kits for detection of influenza A subtypes H1N1, H3N2 and H5N1," *Journal of Clinical Virology*, vol. 38, no. 2, pp. 169–171, 2007.

[29] I. F. Hung, K. K. To, J. F. Chan et al., "Efficacy of Clarithromycin-Naproxen-Oseltamivir Combination in the Treatment of Patients Hospitalized for Influenza A(H3N2) Infection," *Chest*, vol. 151, no. 5, pp. 1069–1080, 2017.

[30] Centers for Disease Control and Prevention, *CDC protocol of realtime RTPCR for influenza A (H1N1)*, Revision 2. Centers for Disease Control and Prevention, Atlanta, GA, 2009.

[31] K. H. Chan, W. C. Yam, C. M. Pang et al., "Comparison of the NucliSens easyMAG and Qiagen BioRobot 9604 nucleic acid extraction systems for detection of RNA and DNA respiratory viruses in nasopharyngeal aspirate samples," *Journal of Clinical Microbiology*, vol. 46, no. 7, pp. 2195–2199, 2008.

[32] S. Esposito, A. Scala, S. Bianchini et al., "Partial comparison of the NxTAG Respiratory Pathogen Panel Assay with the Luminex xTAG Respiratory Panel Fast Assay V2 and singleplex real-time polymerase chain reaction for detection of respiratory pathogens," *Diagnostic Microbiology and Infectious Disease*, vol. 86, no. 1, pp. 53–57, 2016.

4

The Study of Viral RNA Diversity in Bird Samples using De Novo Designed Multiplex Genus-Specific Primer Panels

Andrey A. Ayginin (iD),[1,2] Ekaterina V. Pimkina,[1]
Alina D. Matsvay (iD),[1,2] Anna S. Speranskaya (iD),[1,3] Marina V. Safonova,[1]
Ekaterina A. Blinova,[1] Ilya V. Artyushin (iD),[3] Vladimir G. Dedkov (iD),[1,4]
German A. Shipulin,[1] and Kamil Khafizov (iD)[1,2]

[1]Central Research Institute of Epidemiology, Moscow 111123, Russia
[2]Moscow Institute of Physics and Technology, Dolgoprudny 141700, Russia
[3]Lomonosov Moscow State University, Moscow 119991, Russia
[4]Saint-Petersburg Pasteur Institute, Saint Petersburg 197101, Russia

Correspondence should be addressed to Kamil Khafizov; kkhafizov@gmail.com

Academic Editor: Gary S. Hayward

Advances in the next generation sequencing (NGS) technologies have significantly increased our ability to detect new viral pathogens and systematically determine the spectrum of viruses prevalent in various biological samples. In addition, this approach has also helped in establishing the associations of viromes with many diseases. However, unlike the metagenomic studies using *16S* rRNA for the detection of bacteria, it is impossible to create universal oligonucleotides to target all known and novel viruses, owing to their genomic diversity and variability. On the other hand, sequencing the entire genome is still expensive and has relatively low sensitivity for such applications. The existing approaches for the design of oligonucleotides for targeted enrichment are usually involved in the development of primers for the PCR-based detection of particular viral species or genera, but not for families or higher taxonomic orders. In this study, we have developed a computational pipeline for designing the oligonucleotides capable of covering a significant number of known viruses within various taxonomic orders, as well as their novel variants. We have subsequently designed a genus-specific oligonucleotide panel for targeted enrichment of viral nucleic acids in biological material and demonstrated the possibility of its application for virus detection in bird samples. We have tested our panel using a number of collected samples and have observed superior efficiency in the detection and identification of viral pathogens. Since a reliable, bioinformatics-based analytical method for the rapid identification of the sequences was crucial, an NGS-based data analysis module was developed in this study, and its functionality in the detection of novel viruses and analysis of virome diversity was demonstrated.

1. Introduction

An increase in globalization, climate change, and interaction with livestock animals has resulted in the emergence of novel viral pathogens or zoonoses [1], which pose a serious health problem for birds and animals and ultimately for humans. The natural reservoirs of pathogens, such as birds, bats, rodents, and bloodsucking arthropods play a significant role in the sustenance and transmission of zoonotic infections. Migratory birds warrant special attention, as their rich diversity and migratory behavior contribute to the spread of infections to considerable distances. Such migrations are strongly associated with the emergence of the epidemic and enzootic outbreaks as well as the formation and activation of natural sources of viral infections. Wild birds are widely acknowledged to be reservoirs and transmitters of pathogens responsible for emerging infectious diseases such as severe acute respiratory syndrome virus (SARSV), avian influenza virus A (H10N7), and West Nile virus (WNV), to domestic animals and humans [2, 3]. The rich biodiversity of the wild bird population may increase the risk of spread of pathogens to domesticated poultry. Understanding the viral diversity is critical for predicting future risks of transmission or possible outbreaks of viral diseases. However, identifying and monitoring the transmission of novel viruses are one of the vital requisites for responding to outbreaks. The asymptomatic carriage of viruses, which could be attributed to certain characteristics of bird metabolism and the adaptive capabilities of their immune system, provides ideal conditions for coevolution, leading to the emergence of mutant and recombinant strains of viruses. Hence, the majority of widely used molecular diagnostic methods, such as those employing polymerase chain reaction (PCR), are not sufficiently suitable for the identification of a wide variety of viruses, as the techniques are usually designed for the detection of highly conserved regions in the genomes, which limits the search to a restricted group of viral agents and prevents the identification of new viruses or viral variants. In addition, the Sanger sequencing technique, which has been a standard diagnostic tool for the detection and identification of various pathogens, provides limited sequence information at a higher cost per nucleotide base and can only be used to identify pathogens with a high titer. Moreover, a preliminary evidence of the presence of the certain viruses is required for performing the PCR, in the absence of which the process of pathogen identification could take a significant amount of time, which can be a major obstacle in the prevention and control of the infection.

DNA barcoding is a method which uses a short part of organism's genome (so-called barcode) to identify whether it belongs to a particular family, genera, or even species, by using extensive parallel sequencing technologies (or more commonly NGS [Next Generation Sequencing]). This method was initially developed for studying bacterial communities (e.g., studies on gut microbiota), but today it is widely employed for various tasks, including detection of food adulteration [4], the study of the diets of marine communities [5], and biofuel analysis [6]. Unlike other taxa, viruses lack a universally shared phylogenetic marker (such as *16S* for bacteria, *Cytochrome C oxidase* for birds and mammals, *rbcL* and *matK* for plants, and Internal Transcribed Spacer (*ITS*) for fungi or plants), which makes it impossible to design a universal primer pair to amplify and differentiate diverse viral sequences. Furthermore, the viral taxonomy gives a better indication of the signs of diseases caused, rather than genetic similarity. This fact complicates the barcode (a short, standardized nucleotide sequence of an organism's DNA) selection, even for one genus (for example, mammarenavirus can be serologically, phylogenetically, and geographically divided into two major complexes: the Old World complex prevalent in Africa, Europe, and Asia, and the New World complex found in North and South America [7]), let alone higher taxa. However, metagenomics still allows the detection of different viral pathogens using shotgun sequencing [8]. Despite the constant reduction in the cost of DNA sequencing, this approach is still considerably expensive and is not feasible for screening a large number of samples. Also, metagenomic NGS data-sets are usually predominantly composed of host-derived sequences with only a minor fraction of pathogen sequences. Often, even an approximate fraction of pathogen content is initially unknown, making it practically impossible to estimate how many sequencing reads are needed per sample, in order to detect the pathogen in the final sequencing data file. Another common problem for most NGS-based tests is that complex multistep workflows may pose challenges in the reproducibility of results. Recently, Briese et al. [9] had developed a virome capture sequencing platform for vertebrate viruses (VirCapSeq-VERT), which consisted of ~2 million biotinylated DNA-probes for target enrichment of viral nucleic acids to increase the sensitivity of sequence-based detection and characterization of viruses. The described method allowed the identification (and possibly even sequencing the whole genome assembly of detected viruses) of a large number of viruses including the novel ones. However, the overall cost of sequencing per sample remained considerably high.

Other methods of enrichment are based on the targeted amplification of cDNA region using genus-specific primer pairs in PCR. This approach has been known for a long time [10] and has been used successfully by various researchers, both in the studies of the representatives of individual viral genera and in the analyses of the diversity of viruses in different types of biological material [11–13]. Till recently, a large number of such primers have been described [14–16]. However, most of them were designed for the detection of certain species of viruses. Moreover, it was impossible to use them in multiplex reactions due to primer-specific annealing temperatures, nonspecific amplification, and potential self-complementarity. Thus, in order to analyze one sample, it is necessary to carry out a number of PCR experiments corresponding to the number of primer pairs. The effectiveness of the study could be significantly increased by combining genus-specific PCR and NGS. In this approach, the products of different PCR assays for each sample would be pooled in one tube, purified, eluted in a minimal volume, and prepared for NGS [17]. However, this approach does not exempt the requirement of many PCRs per sample, which is a problem when a large number of samples are studied simultaneously. In addition, there are restrictions on the use of different protocols for the library preparation, particularly when the protocol includes the emulsion PCR stage, which strictly requires PCR products of the same length.

In this study, we have introduced a method for designing oligonucleotide panels for targeted enrichment of viral nucleic acids, where the main objective is to use a minimum number of primer oligonucleotides to cover the maximum number of diverse viral taxa within a single PCR reaction. We have applied this approach to design genus-specific primer pairs for targeted enrichment of cDNA from zoonotic RNA viruses and have evaluated it using several samples from birds. We have also demonstrated a considerable increase in the viral genome coverage.

2. Materials and Methods

2.1. Design of the Genus-Specific Primers Panel. This section contains the technical details of the algorithm for the design of genus-specific primer panels. To enable us to process the enrichment PCR reaction in a single tube, a number of restriction parameters were applied to the positions and structures of oligonucleotides. The availability of validated reference viral nucleic acid sequences is crucial for efficient usage of the algorithm. Although several viral reference sequence databases are publicly available [18], the medically relevant and model organisms are largely overrepresented in most of them, and the genomic diversity of circulating strains is often underrepresented. One such source is the open-source database "The Virus Pathogen Database and Analysis Resource (ViPR)" [19], which was developed back in 2011. The most important advantage of this database is the authenticity of nucleic acid sequences, as the data are curated and managed by experts in virology and bioinformatics. This source was used to retrieve the sequences of the polymerase genes of target viral genera (or other genes in cases where the sequences of polymerase genes were not available). The sequences were filtered by length (≥400 bp), quality, and intrageneric similarity and were combined to the corresponding FASTA files.

In order to create consensus sequences, nucleotide sequences within each FASTA file specific to a genus were aligned using ClustalW [20]. If a minimum of two consensus subsequences with lengths of 20 bp and a maximum of four ambiguous positions with minor nucleotide frequency ≥ 10% were not identified, the original FASTA file was iteratively clustered using CD-HIT [21], with decreasing threshold. The clusters obtained at each step were aligned independently using ClustalW to identify consensus subsequence(s) for all the subsets, which must collectively represent at least 90% of different species within the genus. Finally, at least one aligned FASTA file was obtained for every genus.

For extracting the common subsequences from multiple sequence alignments, a "sliding window" was used within a specified range of lengths. This window "slides" from the 5'- to 3'-end of the alignment with a step of one nucleotide and identifies all subsequences fulfilling the following criteria:

(i) proportion of ambiguous positions (P_{AMB}) ≤ 20%;

(ii) proportion of unique species, which share the subsequence and do not contain gaps (P_{SH}) ≥ 50%;

(iii) GC content of the consensus sequence (P_{GC}) within 35–65% interval;

(iv) absence of self-complementary regions;

(v) absence of formation of homodimers;

(vi) absence of formation of heterodimers with previously selected oligonucleotides.

An amplicon length between two subsequences (primers) was then adjusted between 200 and 400 bp to make the panel compatible with the most popular sequencing platforms (for example, Illumina MiSeq or Ion S5 from Thermo Fisher Scientific). Two subsequences were considered to be a pair if they together covered at least 90% of species related to a target genus or cluster and shared over 90% of the species. The pairs were then filtered according to their annealing temperature (50°C ≤ T_a ≤ 55°C). The selected primer pairs were then aligned with the NR database using BLAST to check for their specificity. Nonspecific candidates were eliminated. The possibility of formation of heterodimers between sequences in the pair, and between the sequences and previously selected primers, was calculated using the software Primer3 [22]. Then the parameters described above were calculated and the pairs were sorted accordingly. The "best" primer pair was selected as a "genus-specific pair."

The parameters described above were then calculated, and the pairs were sorted accordingly. The primer pair with the best fit was selected as a "genus-specific pair."

The sequences of primer pairs for the reference viral genera, designed using the developed algorithm, are presented in Tables 1 and 2.

2.2. Control Samples. The ability of the developed panel to enrich the target cDNA from zoonotic RNA viruses was assessed using high titer solutions of viral RNA (concentration ranging from 10^5 to 10^7 copies per mL) from 24 species of viruses, belonging to 13 viral genera within 12 viral families (Table 1). Viral RNAs were sourced from the collection stored at the Central Research Institute for Epidemiology, Moscow, Russia. All viral RNAs were stored at −70°C till further use for the study. The H_2O sterile (AmpliSens, Russia) was used as a negative control in all experiments.

The control samples cDNA was obtained by reverse transcription reaction performed on 5 μL of the extracted RNA using the Reverta-L RT kit (AmpliSens; total volume of the reaction mixture is 20 μL); after that 5 μL of the reaction mixture containing cDNAs was further used for evaluation of the ability of the primer pair to amplify the targeted region of viruses, both in single and in multiplex PCR format.

2.3. Reaction Mixture and Amplification Mode. The PCR reaction mix (25 μL) was prepared using 5 μL of the cDNA template, 5 μL of H_2O (MilliQ, AmpliSens), 5 μL of PCR mix2 FEP/FRT, 1 μL of 0.2 μM of each primer (in the single-plex format) or 0.08 μM of each primer (total concentration of 3.84 μM in the multiplex format), 2.5 μL of dNTPs (1.76 mM; AmpliSens), and 0.5 μL of TaqF polymerase (AmpliSens). The thermal cycling parameters were initial denaturation at 95°C for 15 min, followed by 45 cycles of 95°C for 15 s, 50°C for 120 s, 72°C for 30 s, and final extension at 72°C for 7 min.

2.4. Specificity of the Developed Panel. PCR products of appropriate lengths were resolved by electrophoresis on 1.5% agarose gel containing ethidium bromide. The amplicons were purified using a QIAquick PCR Purification Kit (Qiagen), following the manufacturer's instructions. The purified PCR products were then sequenced using ABI Prism 3500 sequencer (Applied Biosystems) to confirm the specificity of the reactions in a single-plex format.

2.5. Sample Collection. Bird samples (cloacal swabs and/or feces) were collected from the Enisei Ecological Station, Mirnoe (Russian Federation). The samples were collected from birds captured using mist-net for routine ornithological examination or from droppings left on the ground by geese at their stop-over sites. To prevent contamination, separate

TABLE 1: Viral families and genera covered by the primer panel and control samples of viral RNA used.

Primer set	Family	Genus	Control sample RNA	Acronym
1		*Ebolavirus*	Zaire ebolavirus	ZEBOV
2	Filoviridae	*Marburgvirus*	Marburg virus	MARV
3		*Cuevavirus*	N/A	
4	Arenoviridae	*Mammarenavirus*	Lassa virus	LASV
5	Rhabdoviridae	*Lyssavirus*	Rabies virus	RABV
6		*Ledantevirus*	N/A	
7		*Alphacoronavirus*	N/A	
8	Coronaviridae	*Betacoronavirus*	Middle East respiratory syndrome coronavirus	MERS CoV
9		*Gammacoronavirus*	N/A	
10		*Orbivirus*	Kemerovo virus	KEMV
11	Reoviridae	*Orthoreovirus*	N/A	
12		*Seadornavirus*	N/A	
13	Paramyxoviridae	*Henipavirus*	N/A	
14	Phenuiviridae	*Phlebovirus*	Uukuniemi virus N/A	
15	Hantaviridae	*Hantavirus*	Dobrava virus	DOBV
16	Nairoviridae	*Orthonairovirus*	Crimean-Congo virus hemorrhagic fever virus, Paramushir virus	CCHFV, PRMV
17	Peribunyaviridae	*Orthobunyavirus*	Inkoo virus	INKV
18	Orthomyxoviridae	*Thogotovirus*	N/A	
19	Picornaviridae	*Cardiovirus*	N/A	
20		*Parechovirus*	N/A	
21	Flaviviridae	*Flavivirus*	Tick-borne encephalitis virus, Yellow fever virus, Japanese encephalitis virus	TBEV, YFV, JEV
22	Togaviridae	*Alphavirus*	N/A	

rubber gloves and sterile cotton swabs were used for collection of each sample. The samples were stored at the collection site for up to 30 days at 4–8°C, then for four days at room temperature during transport, and finally at 2–4°C while processing. Samples were stored in the transport medium 0.5 mL tubes for swabs containing storage solution (AmpliSens).

The samples were collected from the following species of birds: Taiga Bean Goose (*Anser fabalis johanseni*), Siberian Thrush (*Geokichla sibirica*), Song Thrush (*Turdus philomelos*), Fieldfare (*Turdus pilaris*), Redwing (*Turdus iliacus*), Black-Throated Thrush (*Turdus atrogularis*), Common Tern (*Sterna hirundo*), Green Sandpiper (*Tringa ochropus*), Common Greenshank (*Tringa nebularia*), Red-Throated Flycatcher (*Ficedula albicilla*), Temminck's Stint (*Calidris temminckii*), and Dusky Warbler (*Phylloscopus fuscatus*). No birds were harmed in this study. A total of 92 bird samples were used for further virome analysis, among which 62 samples belonged to Taiga Bean Goose and 6 to Siberian Thrush.

2.6. RNA Extraction and Reverse Transcription. Total RNA was extracted from 100 μL of the resuspended sample with RNeasy Lipid Tissue Mini Kit (Qiagen) using robotic workstation QIAcube (Qiagen), following the manufacturer's

protocol. The cDNA was obtained by reverse transcription reaction on 10 μL of the extracted RNA using a Reverta-L RT kit (AmpliSens), according to the manufacturer's instructions.

2.7. Testing the Primer Panel with Control Samples. The primer panel was tested with a reference set of samples (Table 1). The results are presented in Figure 1. In all cases, the products of the specified range of lengths were obtained.

The multiplex system was then tested with the same set of viruses and the PCR products were reamplified using the genus-specific primer pairs. In all cases, unspecific amplification was observed as well. However, the reamplification reactions with the genus-specific primers showed the presence of the target products. The multiplex system was first tested with three bat samples infected by several known viruses (sample N1: *Betacoronavirus*, sample N2: *Betacoronavirus*, sample N3: *Orthoreovirus*). The reamplification of the PCR products was carried out with the genus-specific primers (Figure 2). The obtained results clearly demonstrated the presence of the products with target length in all three samples.

TABLE 2: Primers used in the panel along with their structures.

Primer set	Primer name	Sequence 5'-3'
1	ebola_f	GCAATGTTCAAACACTTTGTGARGC
	ebola_r	CTTAACACCATAGCAACGGTTR
2	marburg_f	TGGACGATAGGAAATCGAGCAC
	marburg_r	TGAACTATRTTGCCTGAGTAGTGWG
3	cueva_f	GTGCCAGAACAGTTTGAACTCA
	cueva_r	CCGAATTCTCTGGGTAACACAA
4	mammarena_f	CAATMCTTGAYATGGGWCARGG
	mammarena_r	WGATTTRAACTCTGCAACAAAYCTR
5	lyssa_f	CTKGAYTATGARAARTGGAACA
	lyssa_r	TATGTCGGRCAYARAACCTGRT
6	ledante_f	AAYAATACATGGCCCACWCC
	ledante_r	ARTATTCTCTMARMKCCCARGACAT
7	alphacorona_f	GGYACHACHTCWGGTGATGS
	alphacorona_r	GYTTACGYARRTAACCAWAAWABTC
8	betacorona_f	GTGCWAAGAATAGAGCYCGCAC
	betacorona_r	RTCACAYTTWGGRTAATCCCAACCC
9	gammacorona_f	CCACATCTGCTAATGTTGCR
	gammacorona_r	CAGAAATRTCWGCTACAAGACCYTG
10	orbi_f1	TACCGCARGATMGWATGATGAT
	orbi_f2	TATGTTCCWCARGATCGRATGATG
	orbi_r	TGCGCTCCAWAVCCATTCCA
11	orthoreo_f	GTYTCGGCGCCYCAYACDYT
	orthoreo_r	GCAGTRTGCTCAGTDGARGT
12	seadorna_f	CCRCATGAYGTHATGGCYCC
	seadorna_r	TCACCWGACTTAACWCCWGM
13	henipa_f	GGTCAGARACWYTGGTGGAYGA
	henipa_r	ARTAYGGATCACTRGCCCARTC
14	phlebo_f	GATTYAATCTSTKSARRGCY
	phlebo_r	YTATYWGYTCCAYCCAGTYYTC
15	hanta_f	GCWGATGCAACWAARTGGTC
	hanta_r	YARRTTYCCYTGYARCCART
16	nairo_f	CCTTCTTTTSHGGYATGATGCA
	nairo_r	GAAGTTAACACTGNCGAWGTWGCATG
17	orthobunya_f	CWGAWGARATGATWWSTGARCCWGG
	orthobunya_r	GCACTCCATTTWGACATRTCWG
18	thogoto_f	ATCAARGAYMRRCTGAARAANA
	thogoto_r	TCGATSYGMGGCTTTATDGM
19	cardio_f	MRGGYATGGAYCCMATGGAV
	cardio_r	AAGTTRGARTARTCYACATCRTAGA
20	parecho_f	GGRATYAACCCATAYAARGAYTGGC
	parecho_r	GAYCCTGATGGCATACCRCC
21	flavi_f	CTSCTKTGTGACATMGGDGA
	flavi_r	TACATCTCRTGYGTGGARTTBC
22	alpha_f	ACWCTGTTTGTSAACACWGTVRTYA
	alpha_r	CTYTTYARRGGGTCTGCSACHC

2.8. Preparation and Sequencing of Ion S5 Libraries. The targeted sequences were enriched by multiplex PCR with the designed primer pool described above (Table 2). PCR products were cleaned using carboxyl-coated magnetic particles, commercially available as Sera-Mag Speed Beads (GE Healthcare). The concentrations of the fragments were measured using Qubit dsDNA HS Assay Kit with a Qubit 2.0 fluorimeter (Invitrogen).

The preparation of the amplicon libraries involved phosphorylation of the 5'-end and incorporation of barcoded adapters, followed by amplification of the final library. For this purpose, T4 Polynucleotide Kinase and T4 DNA Ligase (both from New England Biolabs, NEB) were used according to the manufacturer's protocol with slight modification. Amplification was performed using PCR-mix 2 FEP/FRT (AmpliSens).

The two total RNA libraries for Ion S5 high-throughput sequencing were prepared from total RNA of two bird samples (*B23* and *B66*). The first strand of cDNA was synthesized using random primers and Reverta-L RT kit (AmpliSens). The second strand of cDNA was prepared with NEBNext Ultra Second Strand Synthesis Module of Kit #E7530 (NEB). The double stranded DNA was fragmented by Ion Shear Plus Reagent Kit (Thermo Fisher Scientific) and

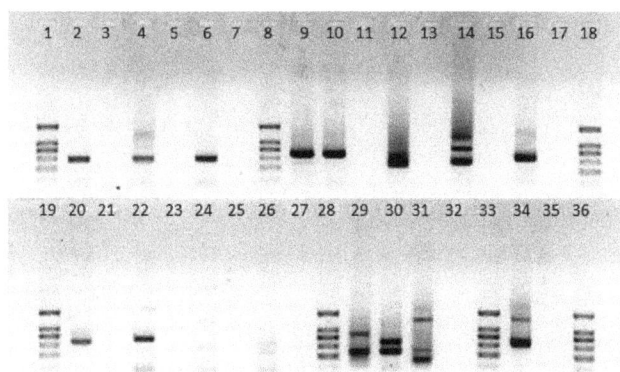

FIGURE 1: Individual primer pairs testing. (**1, 8, 18, 19, 28, 33, 36**) DNA Ladder (100 bp, 200 bp, 300 bp, 400 bp, 500 bp, 800 bp); (**2**) ZEBOV, primers ebola_f/r; (**3**) negative control for primers ebola_f/r; (**4**) MARV, primers marburg_f/r; (**5**) negative control for primers marburg_f/r; (**6**) LASV, primers mammarena_f/r, (**7**) negative control for primers mammarena_f/r; (**9**) CCHFV, primers nairo_f/r; (**10**) PRMV, primers nairo_f/r; (**11**) negative control for primers nairo_f/r; (**12**) INKV, primers orthobunya_f/r; (**13**) negative control for primers orthobunya_f/r; (**14**) DOBV, primers hanta_f/r; (**15**) negative control for primers hanta_f/r; (**16**) KEMV, primers orbi_f1/f2/r; (**17**) negative control for primers orbi_f1/f2/r; (**20**) MERS CoV, primers alphacorona_f/r; (**21**) negative control for primers alphacorona_f/r; (**22**) MERS (*Betacoronavirus*), primers betacorona_1_f/r; (**23**) negative control for primers betacorona_1_f/r; (**24**) MERS (*Betacoronavirus*), primers betacorona_2_f/r; (**25**) negative control for primers betacorona_2_f/r; (**26**) MERS (*Betacoronavirus*), primers gammacorona_f/r; (**27**) negative control for primers gammacorona_f/r; (**29**) TBEV, primers flavi_f/r; (**30**) YFV, primers flavi_f/r; (**31**) JEV, primers flavi_f/r; (**32**) negative control for primers flavi_f/r; (**34**) RABV, primers lyssa_f/r; (**35**) negative control for primers lyssa_f/r.

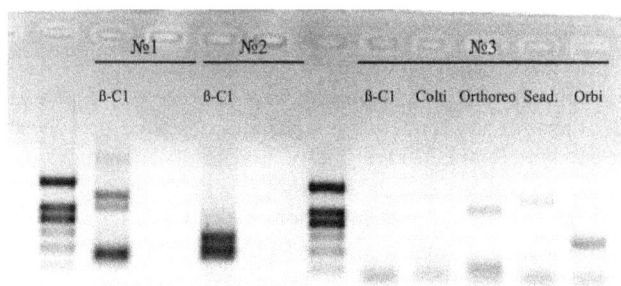

FIGURE 2: Reamplification of the multiplex PCR product; ß-C1: *Betacoronavirus*-specific primers; Colti: coltivirus-specific primers; Orthoreo: *Orthoreovirus*-specific primers; Sead.: Seadornavirus-specific primers; Orbi: orbivirus-specific primers.

libraries preparation was performed using Ion Xpress Plus Fragment Library Kit (Thermo Fisher Scientific) according to the manufacturer's guide.

The quality of final libraries was assessed on the Agilent 2100 Bioanalyzer (Agilent Genomics), employing the Agilent High Sensitivity DNA Kit (Agilent Genomics).

Amplicon libraries were separated by 1.7% agarose gel electrophoresis stained with ethidium bromide, and the fragments of target lengths were cut out and purified using the MinElute Gel Extraction Kit (Qiagen). Size selection of the final total RNA libraries was done using 2% E-Gel™ SizeSelect™ II Agarose Gels (Thermo Fisher Scientific) on the E-Gel electrophoresis system (Thermo Fisher Scientific).

Sequencing was carried out on the Ion S5 platform using Ion 520/530 Kit-Chef reagent sample preparation kit and employing Ion 530 chips on the Ion Chef instrument (Thermo Fisher Scientific).

2.9. Bioinformatics Analysis. Raw sequencing reads obtained from the platform were first filtered using the PRINSEQ-lite tool [23] to eliminate too short (<80 bp) and low-quality (min_mean < 20) fragments. The mean, median, and 10th and 90th percentiles of read lengths distributions for selected unfiltered FASTQ files are shown in the supplementary Table S1. The BWA software [24] was used then to align the filtered reads to the reference birds' genomes database. The ideally aligned reads (full read length and no mismatches) were marked as nonviral reads and were eliminated. The software CD-HIT [21] was used to reduce the redundancy, i.e., the number of reads per sample, by clustering (with a similarity threshold 90%) and selecting the representative sequences for each cluster. Briefly, the CD-HIT algorithm sorts the sequences from long to short and processes them sequentially. The first sequence is automatically classified as the first cluster representative sequence. Then each query sequence from the remaining sequences is compared to the representative sequences identified before it and is classified as redundant or representative based on whether it is similar to one of the existing representative sequences. The described filtering and clustering steps significantly reduced (by ~100 times) the computational time of the further steps. The software BLAST was then employed to first compare the representative sequences (RS) against virus-only nucleotide and protein databases that were collected by selection of virus sequences from GenBank NT and GenBank NR databases, respectively, to identify viral nucleotide candidate RS (nRS) and protein candidate RS (pRS) with E-value cutoffs of 10^{-5} and 10^{-3}, respectively. Since virus-only databases are much smaller than NCBI NT and NR databases, pairwise sequence comparisons are much faster, which maximizes the speed and allows for the more efficient use of computational resources. We subsequently aligned these candidate nRS and pRS to the entire GenBank NT and NR databases, respectively, to eliminate potential false positives (sequences with higher similarity to nonviral reference sequences than to viral ones in the database) among the candidates and to select the true positives. The additional step was applied to select true positives from viral pRS: the pRS aligned to NR database were compared with nRS aligned to NT database to eliminate viral pRS, which correspond to nRS aligning to nonviral nucleotide sequences with a high E-value. To get an idea of the total number of true viral reads belonging to the same virus, the numbers of reads for each RS were eventually summed up.

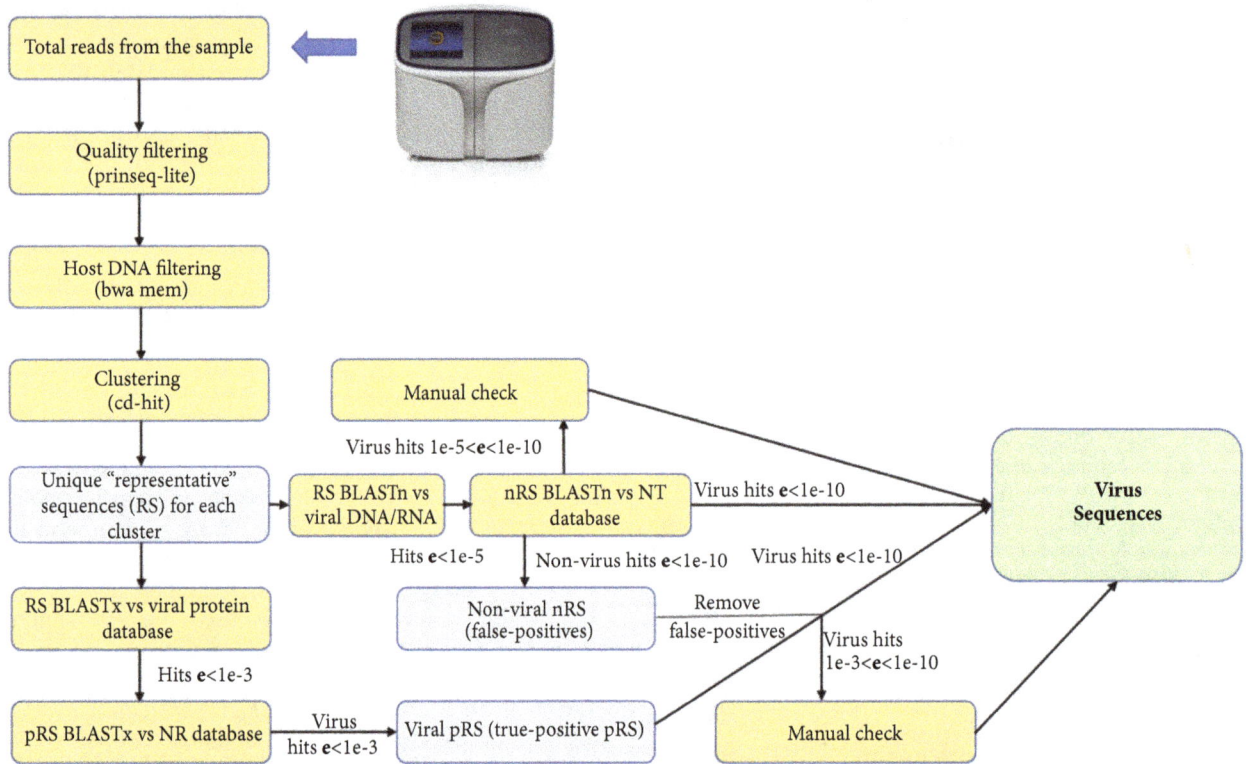

FIGURE 3: A schematic picture of the bioinformatics pipeline developed for the analysis of the NGS data in this study. Specific third-party tools that were employed are shown in parentheses.

A schematic picture of the bioinformatics analysis scheme is presented in Figure 3.

3. Results and Discussion

A panel of 45 primers including 23 forward and 22 reverse primers was designed using the developed algorithm and was synthesized accordingly (Tables 1 and 2). A preliminary analysis using the available control samples (Table 1) demonstrated the ability of the designed primers to perform targeted cDNA enrichment in both single-plex and multiplex formats. This was confirmed by the presence of specific bands of expected lengths in electrophoresis, followed by capillary sequencing (Figures 1 and 2).

Subsequently, we deployed the primer panel to study 70 bird samples (as described in the Methods) and the sequencing results are presented in Table 3 and Figure 4. Only those samples, for which at least 10 viral reads (filtered by quality and length) were identified in the final FASTQ files, are presented in the table. The total number of sequencing reads in such samples is also given to exemplify the percentage of pathogen reads. The alignment of sequencing reads with viral reference sequences was visually inspected to eliminate most of the potential artifacts (such as primer-dimers).

As evident from Table 3, the genera of viruses (samples *B11*, *B23*, and *B24*, highlighted in bold) having a specific primer pair in the panel showed significant amplification, and percentage of the corresponding viral reads ranged

between 4.3% and 43.1%. This confirms that our primer panel can efficiently enrich the target genera. Other sequencing reads belonged to bacteriophages, bacteria, and host species. However, we also observed a significant enrichment in the samples *B27* and *B68*, for which a significant number of reads corresponding to Sanxia water strider virus and Duck adenovirus were, respectively, detected. We scrutinized these results in further detail by carrying out a BLAST analysis of all possible versions of the primers (since they are very degenerated) against the sequencing reads and observed that these findings were very likely due to nonspecific amplification from the primers designed for other genera (*gammacoronal_f* and *flavi_r*), though we have not checked this by a direct experiment with a panel that lacks these primers. Although nonspecific amplification allows an even more exhaustive search, it also introduces potentially undesirable enrichment. This could be a problem, especially when the lengths of obtained amplicons are outside the standard intervals suitable for sequencing on most popular platforms.

We also observed a considerable number of viral reads corresponding to various genera in some samples (*B27*, *B46*, *B49*, *B58*, *B66*, and *B69*), despite the absence of specific primers in the panel for their enrichment. The number of reads varied from 0.00013% (Tunis virus) to 2.2% (Watercress white vein virus). The latter is a plant virus and its presence is expected as the feces of the host birds mainly contained grass. These results are possibly due to a weak, nonspecific PCR amplification.

TABLE 3: Results of the bird samples sequencing with prior enrichment using the primers panel. The number of viral reads and total number of reads per corresponding sample are shown. For three samples (*B11*, *B23*, and *B24*, highlighted in bold) there was a specific primer pair in the panel present for the amplification of the detected genus. Closest viral homologs names and their GenBank IDs are shown.

Bird ID	Viruses (closest homologs) detected	Host specie	GenBank IDs of the detected viruses	Number of viral reads in the sample	Total number of reads obtained for the sample
B11	**Duck-dominant coronavirus|Avian coronavirus|Bird droppings coronavirus**	**Taiga Bean Goose**	**AKQ98474.1, AKQ98475.1, APU51837.1, AIY51827.1, CAH69463.1**	**4,342**	**108,833**
B23	**Duck-dominant coronavirus|Avian coronavirus|Bird droppings coronavirus**	**Taiga Bean Goose**	**AKQ98474.1, AKQ98475.1, APU51837.1, AIY51827.1, CAH69463.1**	**83,730**	**194,156**
B24	**Duck-dominant coronavirus**	**Taiga Bean Goose**	**AKQ98474.1, AKQ98475.1**	**4,554**	**90,430**
B27	Sanxia water strider virus 16	Temminck's Stint	YP_009337377.1	4,062	103,488
B27	Fowl aviadenovirus C|Turkey aviadenovirus B	Temminck's Stint	ACL68145.1, ANB27700.1, ALY06332.1, ALY06333.1	54	103,488
B27	Cimodo virus	Temminck's Stint	YP_009059075.1	160	103,488
B46	Watercress white vein virus | Turnip yellow mosaic virus	Taiga Bean Goose	AFC95826.1, AMH40128.1	636	28,468
B49	Circovirus	Taiga Bean Goose	AEL87792.1	180	149,230
B58	Lake Sarah-associated circular virus-32	Taiga Bean Goose	ALE29729.1	10	42,348
B66	Duck aviadenovirus B	Fieldfare	YP_009047166.1	198	159,604
B68	Duck adenovirus A	Common tern	AGS11269.1, NP_044717.1	95,872	256,549
B69	Tunis virus	Taiga Bean Goose	AMT75434.1	16	126,648

TABLE 4: Comparison of the sequencing results of two samples with and without preenrichment by the primer's panel. In the latter case, the total number of reads was ~4.5 million per sample.

	B23		*B66*	
	With enrichment	Total RNA	With enrichment	Total RNA
Coronaviruses	43.1%	0.2%	-	-
Adenoviruses	-	0.2%	0.1%	0.05%

We then checked whether the obtained viral reads for samples *B11*, *B23*, *B24*, *B27*, and *B68* were due to the amplification with the designed primers in the panel. These five samples were chosen as they indicated the most significant amplification, with 4.0–43.1% of total sequencing reads in the FASTQ files being viral. This was done by repeating a BLAST analysis of all possible versions of the primer sequences against the obtained viral reads for the aforementioned samples and calculating the percentage of those containing at least one primer. We observed that over 99% of the sequences contained the primers validating the effectiveness of the panel.

Finally, in order to confirm the effectiveness of the panel's enrichment, we selected two samples (*B23* and *B66*) for which the presence of viral RNA was shown using amplicon sequencing data (see Table 3). Notably, the *B23* possessed a significant number of reads that correspond to coronaviruses (43.1%) and our panel had specific primers for these genera. As for the *B66* sample, it had a small number of reads that correspond to adenoviruses (0.1%) but we did not design oligonucleotides for them. We then prepared total RNA-seq libraries for these samples, and subsequently sequenced them, yielding ~4.5 million of reads per sample. The percentage of the *coronavirus* reads in the *B23* sample was found to be significantly lower (0.2%) than that in the same sample that was previously enriched by the panel (Table 4). As for the *B66* sample, we identified that 0.05% of reads belong to the *Adenoviridae* family, and most of them were identified as being similar to the Duck and Psittacine adenoviruses. This is similar to the percentage of reads found in the *B66*

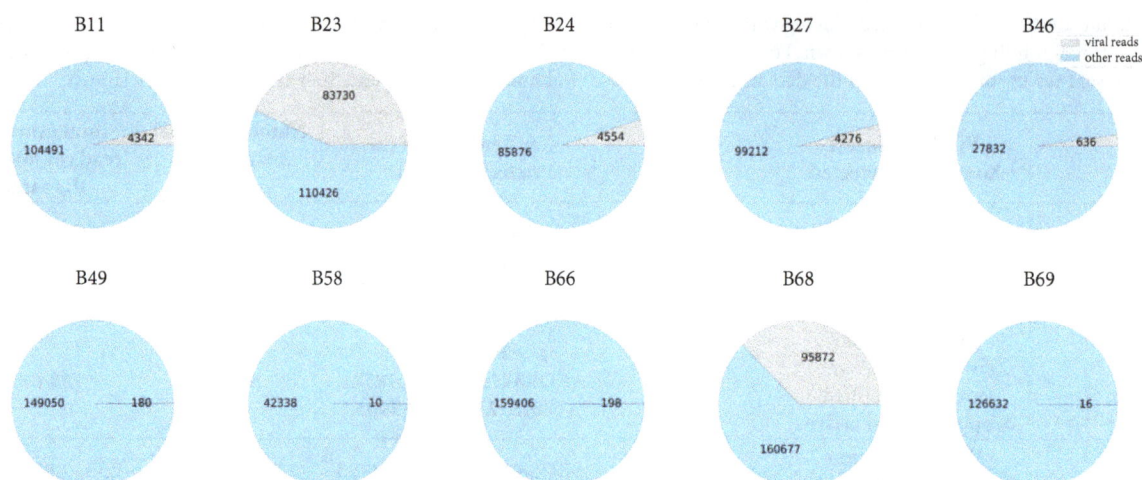

FIGURE 4: A graphical representation of the percentage of the detected viral reads (grey) with respect to the total number of sequencing reads obtained for the samples listed in Table 3.

FASTQ file (0.1%) when the primer panel was applied, i.e., no noticeable enrichment was observed as expected. At the same time, we lost ~0.2% of adenoviruses in the *B23*, but since the amount of data was very different in the two experiments, there was a significant amplification of coronaviruses with almost a half of the reads belonging to these genera; this outcome is not totally surprising. Thus, our approach allows a significant reduction in the cost of sequencing. Besides, for a successful identification of viruses in a preenriched sample, 100,000–200,000 reads per sample are generally enough.

4. Conclusions

In this study, we have presented a method of oligonucleotide design for the enrichment of viral nucleic acids. We used this method to design a primer panel, which showed a high efficiency in the detection and identification of several viruses using NGS sequencing. This is especially important for the detection of viruses known to persist in natural zoonotic reservoirs including birds, bats, and rodents, those with a high genetic diversity, and those which can be potentially dangerous to humans and animals. These factors make the development of rapid test-systems essential for the effective management of potential epidemics.

The described method can be recommended to the researchers investigating diverse viromes across different types of biological samples. We deployed our panel for the screening of a number of bird samples and demonstrated a great efficiency. In future studies, the panel will be expanded to target more diverse viruses and tested with bird samples from other regions.

Disclosure

An earlier version of this work was presented as an abstract at The 43rd FEBS Congress Prague 7-12 July 2018.

Authors' Contributions

Andrey A. Ayginin, Vladimir G. Dedkov, German A. Shipulin, and Kamil Khafizov participated in research design, Ekaterina V. Pimkina, Alina D. Matsvay, Marina V. Safonova, Anna S. Speranskaya, Ekaterina A. Blinova, and Ilya V. Artyushin collected the samples and conducted experiments, Andrey A. Ayginin and Kamil Khafizov developed the algorithm and performed data analysis, Andrey A. Ayginin, Alina D. Matsvay, Marina V. Safonova, Vladimir G. Dedkov, German A. Shipulin, and Kamil Khafizov drafted the manuscript, and Andrey A. Ayginin, Ekaterina V. Pimkina, Alina D. Matsvay, Anna S. Speranskaya, Ekaterina A. Blinova, Marina V. Safonova, Ilya V. Artyushin, Vladimir G. Dedkov, German A. Shipulin, and Kamil Khafizov approved the final manuscript.

Acknowledgments

This work was supported by RSF Grant no. 17-74-20096.

References

[1] B. A. Jones, D. Grace, R. Kock et al., "Zoonosis emergence linked to agricultural intensification and environmental change," *Proceedings of the National Acadamy of Sciences of the United States of America*, vol. 110, no. 21, pp. 8399–8404, 2013.

[2] J. S. Mackenzie and M. Jeggo, "Reservoirs and vectors of emerging viruses," *Current Opinion in Virology*, vol. 3, no. 2, pp. 170–179, 2013.

[3] C. Wang, J. Wang, W. Su et al., "Relationship between domestic and wild birds in live poultry market and a novel human H7N9 virus in China," *The Journal of Infectious Diseases*, vol. 209, no. 1, pp. 34–37, 2014.

[4] V. A. Parvathy, V. P. Swetha, T. E. Sheeja, and B. Sasikumar, "Detection of plant-based adulterants in turmeric powder using DNA barcoding," *Pharmaceutical Biology*, vol. 53, no. 12, pp. 1774–1779, 2015.

[5] T. E. Berry, S. K. Osterrieder, D. C. Murray et al., "DNA metabarcoding for diet analysis and biodiversity: A case study using the endangered Australian sea lion (Neophoca cinerea)," *Ecology and Evolution*, vol. 7, no. 14, pp. 5435–5453, 2017.

[6] S. Jaenicke, C. Ander, T. Bekel et al., "Comparative and joint analysis of two metagenomic datasets from a biogas fermenter obtained by 454-pyrosequencing," *PLoS ONE*, vol. 6, no. 1, Article ID e14519, 2011.

[7] S. Günther and O. Lenz, "Lassa virus," *Critical Reviews in Clinical Laboratory Sciences*, vol. 41, no. 4, pp. 339–390, 2004.

[8] R. Schlaberg, C. Y. Chiu, S. Miller, G. W. Procop, and G. Weinstock, "Validation of metagenomic next-generation sequencing tests for universal pathogen detection," *Archives of Pathology & Laboratory Medicine*, vol. 141, no. 6, pp. 776–786, 2017.

[9] T. Briese, A. Kapoor, N. Mishra et al., "Virome Capture Sequencing Enables Sensitive Viral Diagnosis and Comprehensive Virome Analysis," *mBio*, vol. 6, no. 5, 2015.

[10] D. R. VanDevanter et al., "Detection and analysis of diverse herpes-viral species by consensus primer PCR," *Journal of Clinical Microbiology*, vol. 34, no. 7, pp. 1666–1671, 1996.

[11] S. J. Anthony, J. H. Epstein, K. A. Murray et al., "A strategy to estimate unknown viral diversity in mammals," *MBio*, vol. 4, no. 5, Article ID e00598-13, 2013.

[12] S. Weiss, P. T. Witkowski, B. Auste et al., "Hantavirus in bat, Sierra Leone," *Emerging Infectious Diseases*, vol. 18, no. 1, pp. 159–161, 2012.

[13] C. Drosten et al., "Identification of a novel coronavirus in patients with severe acute respiratory syndrome," *The New England Journal of Medicine*, vol. 348, no. 20, pp. 1967–1976, 1967.

[14] L. Zheng, J. Tang, G. R. G. Clover, M. E. Spackman, A. J. Freeman, and B. C. Rodoni, "Novel genus-specific broad range primers for the detection of furoviruses, hordeiviruses and rymoviruses and their application in field surveys in South-east Australia," *Journal of Virological Methods*, vol. 214, pp. 1–9, 2015.

[15] S. K. Choi, J. K. Choi, W. M. Park, and K. H. Ryu, "RT-PCR detection and identification of three species of cucumoviruses with a genus-specific single pair of primers," *Journal of Virological Methods*, vol. 83, no. 1-2, pp. 67–73, 1999.

[16] M. Pfeffer, B. Proebster, R. M. Kinney, and O.-R. Kaaden, "Genus-specific detection of alphaviruses by a semi-nested reverse transcription-polymerase chain reaction," *The American Journal of Tropical Medicine and Hygiene*, vol. 57, no. 6, pp. 709–718, 1997.

[17] V. G. Dedkov, A. N. Lukashev, A. A. Deviatkin et al., "Retrospective diagnosis of two rabies cases in humans by high throughput sequencing," *Journal of Clinical Virology*, vol. 78, pp. 74–81, 2016.

[18] M. Y. Galperin, X. M. Fernández-Suárez, and D. J. Rigden, "The 24th annual Nucleic Acids Research database issue: a look back and upcoming changes," *Nucleic Acids Research*, vol. 45, no. 9, article 5627, 2017.

[19] B. E. Pickett, E. L. Sadat, Y. Zhang et al., "ViPR: an open bioinformatics database and analysis resource for virology research," *Nucleic Acids Research*, vol. 40, no. 1, pp. D593–D598, 2012.

[20] M. A. Larkin, G. Blackshields, N. P. Brown et al., "Clustal W and clustal X version 2.0," *Bioinformatics*, vol. 23, no. 21, pp. 2947-2948, 2007.

[21] W. Li and A. Godzik, "Cd-hit: a fast program for clustering and comparing large sets of protein or nucleotide sequences," *Bioinformatics*, vol. 22, no. 13, pp. 1658-1659, 2006.

[22] A. Untergasser, I. Cutcutache, T. Koressaar et al., "Primer3-new capabilities and interfaces," *Nucleic Acids Research*, vol. 40, no. 15, p. e115, 2012.

[23] R. Schmieder and R. Edwards, "Quality control and preprocessing of metagenomic datasets," *Bioinformatics*, vol. 27, no. 6, pp. 863-864, 2011.

[24] H. Li and R. Durbin, "Fast and accurate short read alignment with Burrows-Wheeler transform," *Bioinformatics*, vol. 25, no. 14, pp. 1754–1760, 2009.

5

Questioning the Extreme Neurovirulence of Monkey B Virus (*Macacine alphaherpesvirus 1*)

R. Eberle[1] **and L. Jones-Engel**[2]

[1]*Department of Veterinary Pathobiology, Center for Veterinary Health Sciences, Oklahoma State University, Stillwater, OK 74078, USA*
[2]*Department of Anthropology and Center for Studies in Ecology and Demography, University of Washington, Seattle, WA 98195, USA*

Correspondence should be addressed to R. Eberle; r.eberle@okstate.edu

Academic Editor: Anuj Sharma

Monkey B virus (*Macacine alphaherpesvirus* 1; BV) occurs naturally in macaques of the genus *Macaca*, which includes rhesus and long-tailed (cynomolgus) monkeys that are widely used in biomedical research. BV is closely related to the human herpes simplex viruses (HSV), and BV infections in its natural macaque host are quite similar to HSV infections in humans. Zoonotic BV is extremely rare, having been diagnosed in only a handful of North American facilities with the last documented case occurring in 1998. However, BV is notorious for its neurovirulence since zoonotic infections are serious, usually involving the central nervous system, and are frequently fatal. Little is known about factors underlying the extreme neurovirulence of BV in humans. Here we review what is actually known about the molecular biology of BV and viral factors affecting its neurovirulence. Based on what is known about related herpesviruses, areas for future research that may elucidate mechanisms underlying the neurovirulence of this intriguing virus are also reviewed.

1. Introduction

Herpesviruses are ubiquitous viruses, found in a wide variety of species including mammals, birds, and reptiles. Three subfamilies of the Herpesviridae family (Alpha-, Beta- and Gammaherpesvirinae) are found in the order Primates. Of these, alphaherpesviruses typically infect and remain within the peripheral sensory nervous system for the life of their host as part of their natural life cycle. The close and prolonged association of these viruses with their host over its entire lifetime with only rare impairment of nervous system function implies an exquisite degree of host-virus coadaptation. On occasion stability of this commensal symbiotic host-virus relationship can be altered, resulting in severe or even fatal disease often involving the central nervous system (CNS). In cases where an alphaherpesvirus infects a host of another species, the result can be, but is not always, catastrophic. The most notorious example of this is monkey B virus (*Macacine alphaherpesvirus* 1; BV), an alphaherpesvirus enzootic in macaques of the genus *Macaca*. Though exceptionally rare, zoonotic BV infection following exposure to macaques has a mortality rate of ~80%. Here we review what is known about this relatively neglected virus with regard to its infamous neurovirulence.

2. BV in Its Natural Host

Monkey B virus (BV) occurs naturally in all 17 species of macaque monkeys that comprise the genus *Macaca*. Macaques are ecologically adaptable monkeys and are the most numerous and widely distributed nonhuman primate on the planet. The majority of macaque species are distributed throughout Asia and their ubiquity has led to three of these species (*M. mulatta, M. fascicularis,* and *M. nemestrina*) being used as biomedical research models for nearly a century [1–4]. Although known by several names over the years since its initial isolation in 1932 (*Herpesvirus simiae*, monkey B virus, Herpes B, and *Cercopithecine herpesvirus* 1), BV is currently designated as *Macacine alphaherpesvirus* 1 by the International Committee on Taxonomy of Viruses.

From a biological standpoint, in macaques BV is very much like herpes simplex virus (HSV) in humans. Both HSV and BV are normally transmitted horizontally via direct contact and exchange of bodily secretions [3, 5–7]. The prevalence of BV in macaques is related to age, increasing progressively from infant to adult [8–17]. There are very few studies on the prevalence or transmission of BV in free-ranging populations. In captive macaque colonies, very young monkeys (<2 yr of age) usually acquire BV as an oral infection, while in socially and reproductively mature macaques primary BV infections are usually genital. The prevalence of BV in adults of both wild populations and captive breeding colonies typically ranges from 70% to nearly 100%. Only rarely does BV cause lethal infections in healthy macaques, just as HSV rarely causes encephalitis or other serious disease in humans [18].

As with HSV in humans, most primary BV infections occur in mucosal epithelium and do not usually produce overt clinical signs, although lesions are sometimes visible on close inspection [27]. As the virus replicates in epithelial cells, sufficient levels of infectious virus accumulate allowing the virus to invade unmyelinated sensory nerve endings present in the epidermis. Once in sensory neurons, the virus establishes a latent infection in the sensory ganglion, where the viral genome is retained in the nuclei of neurons without entering the lytic viral replicative cycle that occurs in epithelial cells [6, 28–30]. Viral replication in epithelial tissue is eventually controlled and the virus is eliminated by the host adaptive immune response. The only indication that a monkey continues to harbor BV is the presence of circulating antiviral IgG. It has been shown in captive macaques that, in rare instances, usually in infants or the very young, primary infections may not end with the establishment of latency, but rather progress as generalized infections that spread throughout the body and are frequently fatal [31–34].

As is typical of other alphaherpesviruses, BV can periodically reactivate from the latent state in response to various stressful stimuli, resulting in shedding of infectious virus. While lesions may be apparent, most recurrences do not produce clinically apparent lesions; rather, infectious virus is shed asymptomatically. Like HSV in humans, the frequency of BV shedding appears to be fairly low (2-3%) [35–37]. Stress related to social/housing challenges, transportation, immunosuppression, and seasonal breeding have all been linked to reactivation of latent BV [6, 7, 38, 39].

In many ways, BV is the macaque equivalent of human HSV: BV and its macaque hosts have coevolved, resulting in an exquisitely fine-tuned interaction with one another that results in perpetuation of the virus within the host's nervous system with minimal adverse effects on the host but also with occasional shedding of infectious virus that can be transmitted to a naïve host, thereby ensuring perpetuation of the virus. The notorious neurovirulence of BV is therefore not evident in its natural macaque hosts; the neurovirulence of BV only becomes apparent when BV infects other species, particularly humans.

3. Zoonotic BV Infection

In 1932 a young physician, William Brebner, performing poliovirus research with rhesus macaques was bitten on the finger [40–42]. He developed herpetic-like lesions on the finger, and the infection eventually progressed to involve the CNS. The patient died several weeks later from an acute ascending myeloencephalitis. A herpesvirus was isolated from several tissues at autopsy. Although initially identified as HSV, the virus was subsequently shown to be distinct from HSV and was designated as "the B virus" [40, 42].

While the exact number is not available, less than 60 additional cases of pathogenic zoonotic BV infection have occurred sporadically over the last 85 years, all resulting from exposure to laboratory or captive macaques or macaque tissues [2, 4, 5, 43–50]. While zoonotic BV infections are exceedingly rare, the fatality rate is 70–80% and many survivors are left with deteriorative neurologic sequelae. The majority of exposures have been associated with bites or scratches from captive, laboratory-housed macaques. However, additional modes of exposure have been implicated including mucosal membrane contact with macaque urine and/or feces, needlestick injury, and contamination of cuts with material from primary macaque cells in the laboratory [43, 44, 48]. With the sole exception of one spousal person-to-person infection [47], all zoonotic BV infections have involved primate veterinarians, animal care personnel, or laboratory researchers in North America working with macaques or macaque biologics. BV is the single most serious occupational zoonotic concern for persons working with or around macaques.

While the clinical course of zoonotic BV infections can vary, initial symptoms usually develop within 1–3 weeks of an exposure incident [51]. The nature of initial clinical symptoms also varies but usually includes nonspecific flu-like symptoms, vesicular herpetic lesions at the site of exposure, and symptoms indicative of involvement of the peripheral and/or central nervous systems. The infection progressively spreads along sensory nerves into the spinal cord and ascends into the brainstem. Typically, the destruction of nervous tissue as the virus spreads within the CNS results in encephalomyelitis and respiratory failure in terminal stages of the infection. Once the CNS is involved, the final outcome is almost invariably death.

Though most persons known to be infected with BV die, some do survive and some survivors can periodically shed virus after recovery [46, 52–54]. Several cases of zoonotic BV have also occurred in persons who have a history of working with macaques but without any known BV exposure immediately prior to the appearance of clinical signs. Both of these observations suggest that BV latency not only occurs in humans, but that reactivation of latent BV can be associated with clinical disease [47, 54, 55]. Since primary BV and HSV infections in the natural host species are usually asymptomatic, the potential exists for asymptomatic zoonotic BV infections to occur as well. However, there has only been one study that tested persons working with captive macaques for serological evidence of BV infection [56]. None were detected, suggesting that asymptomatic infections are likely uncommon, if they do occur.

A puzzling aspect of zoonotic BV infections is the notable lack of any fatal or even clinically evident BV infections in Asia where BV-positive macaques and humans have copious close interactions, and exposure to macaque bodily fluids through bites, scratches, and mucosal splashes is common [11, 19, 57–59]. The human-macaque interface is diverse and deep in Asia, in part because of cultural and religious beliefs that provide a context for tolerance and a measure of protection for these ubiquitous monkeys. Macaques, particularly the abundant rhesus, long-tailed and pigtail monkeys, are found at the thousands of temples and shrines located throughout a broad geographic swath extending east from Afghanistan to Japan and south through the Indonesian archipelago. Millions of people who live and work at these sites, as well as those who worship, have frequent contact with macaques. Additionally, many of these sacred sites are also international tourist destinations, drawing hundreds of thousands of visitors each year who come to appreciate the culture and to feed and interact with the monkeys. Human exposures are routine, with macaques aggressively pursuing food handouts while climbing on visitors. Bites and scratches commonly occur, especially to international tourists who lack experience with monkeys, when humans either fail to relinquish food or behave in a manner the monkeys deem threatening. In a retrospective study of French tourists seeking medical treatment for an animal bite received in Southeast Asia, most reported that the injuring animal was a monkey [60]. Studies have shown that between 6 and 40% of visitors to a monkey temple will be bitten, and thus it is not surprising that zoonotic transmission of a primate retrovirus (simian foamy virus) has been documented following exposure to macaques in Asia [20, 61–63].

In addition to the hundreds of monkey temples across Asia, tens of thousands of macaques are free-ranging in urban areas such as Singapore, Hong Kong, Delhi, and the famous wild monkey parks of Japan. Macaques are also commonly found as pets, and a centuries-old tradition of keeping and training performing monkeys continues in China and Japan. Finally, it should be noted that Indonesia, Thailand, Malaysia, Singapore, Vietnam, Cambodia, Laos, Philippines, China, and Japan all have active biomedical research programs and/or primate breeding research centers which collectively employ thousands of workers and involve tens of thousands of macaques each year. Many of these breeding facilities operate under conditions of extreme animal overcrowding with husbandry and handling protocols that are substandard (Jones-Engel, pers. observ.). Despite frequent contact between humans and free-ranging, temple, pet, or urban macaques in Asia, fatal cases of BV have only occurred in the US and Canada following contact with captive macaques. This geographic restriction of zoonotic BV infections has long been and remains a puzzle.

One immediate question is whether or not BV is even zoonotically transmitted in Asia. There is no question that individuals in communities living near macaques or who work in SE Asian monkey forests have a history of extensive macaque contact and injury [19]. If such persons had experienced BV infection over their years in close contact with wild macaques, their antiviral serum antibodies should differ in their virus-specificity from that of persons never exposed to BV. When an HSV infected person is infected with an antigenically related virus, an anamnestic response will occur to antigens shared by the two viruses, while a *de novo* response will occur to antigens specific to the second virus. Thus, detection of BV-specific antibodies is a difficult problem, as the BV-specific antibody response develops more slowly and may be overshadowed by the immediate and strong response to cross-reactive antigens. Consequently, persons infected with HSV who had experienced an asymptomatic BV infection would be expected to have higher levels of antibodies directed against antigens shared by all primate alphaherpesviruses than would be present in sera of persons only infected with HSV.

Limited testing compared the relative reactivity of sera from persons working in monkey forests with that of persons having no known contact with monkeys (negative controls) and patients that died of zoonotic BV infection (positive controls) (Figure 1). When sera were tested by ELISA against HSV and multiple simian virus antigens, it was evident that a few monkey forest workers had higher levels of reactivity with simian virus antigens than was evident in most other monkey forest workers or negative control sera (Figure 1(a)). Such elevated antibody levels directed against cross-reactive alphaherpesvirus antigens suggests that these individuals have experienced an infection with a virus antigenically related to but different from HSV. Further analysis by sensitive competition ELISA [23, 24] confirmed that the reactivity of these sera was consistent with that of having been infected with BV (Figure 1(b)). Given the absence of any history consistent with typical BV infection (i.e., infections with neurological involvement), it is possible that these persons experienced asymptomatic BV infections. However, if asymptomatic BV infections do occur in Asia, then the lack of apparent asymptomatic BV infections in the US presents a different enigma.

When assessing the neurovirulence of BV, it is important to recognize that, within Asia where hundreds of thousands of macaques come into daily contact with millions of people, there is no conclusive evidence of zoonotic infections, neurological or otherwise. Genetic differences in human subjects (Asian versus non-Asian background) would seem an unlikely explanation for the lack of fatal BV infections in Asia since many non-Asian tourists visiting monkey forests in Asia and non-Asian military troops serving in Asia have experienced bites and scratches from macaques without any resulting zoonotic BV infections [11, 19, 61, 64]. Similarly, inaccurate diagnosis of zoonotic BV infections in rural areas with limited healthcare seems unlikely explanation as tens of thousands of macaques are free-ranging in large metropolitan areas in Asia where access to healthcare, diagnostics, and case follow-up are readily available (e.g., Singapore, Hong Kong, and Kyoto). It is even less likely that clinicians in a tourist's home country would fail to diagnose BV when presented with a history of a macaque bite and neurological symptoms.

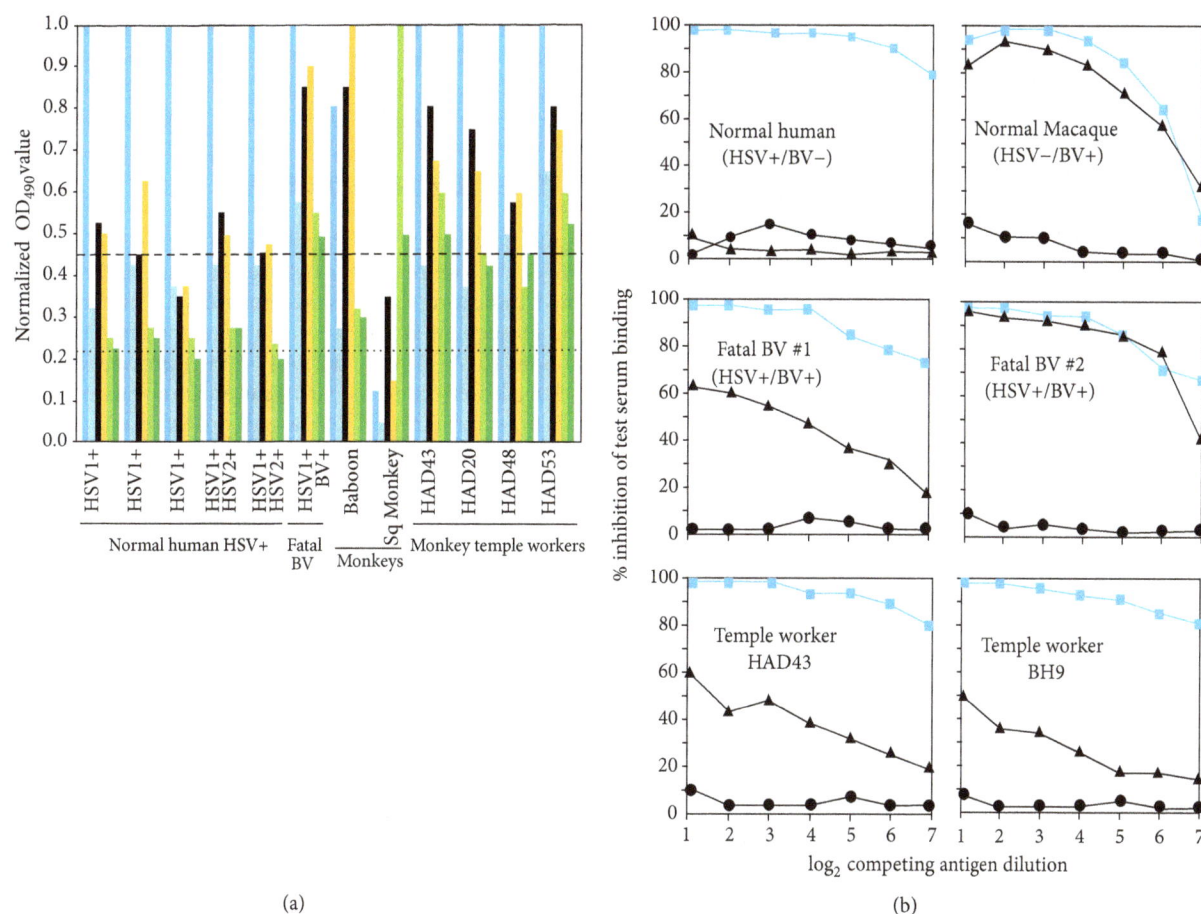

(a)

(b)

FIGURE 1: Evidence of possible asymptomatic BV infections in Asia. (a) Sera from individuals working at monkey forests in SE Asia [19, 20] were tested by ELISA as described [21, 22] against HSV1 (dark blue), HSV2 (light blue), BV (red), HVP2 (orange), squirrel monkey herpesvirus (light green), and spider monkey herpesvirus (dark green) antigens. HSV1 OD values were normalized to 1.0 to assess relative levels of reactivity with cross-reactive antigens. Average levels of cross-reactivity with BV and HVP2 in normal HSV-positive control sera (individuals with no known contact with monkeys) are indicated by the dashed line, and average levels of cross-reactivity with the two S. American monkey viruses are indicated by the dotted line. The four sera from monkey forest workers and serum from a fatal case of zoonotic BV infection have higher levels of cross-reactivity with all simian virus antigens than do control sera. (b) Competition ELISAs were performed as described [23, 24] to determine if sera from monkey forest workers with high levels of cross-reactivity were consistent with having been infected with BV. Soluble antigens (extracts of cells infected with HSV1 (blue), BV (red), or uninfected cells (black)) were used to compete the binding of serum to HSV1 antigen coated onto the ELISA plates. Binding of control HSV1-positive serum was inhibited only by soluble HSV1 antigen, not by BV or control antigens. Binding of BV-positive macaque serum (HSV-negative) to the solid phase HSV1 antigen was equally competed by soluble HSV1 and BV antigens. Binding of sera from two patients that died of zoonotic BV infection (both HSV1-positive) were competed by both HSV1 and BV soluble antigens, although competition by BV antigen was less than by HSV1 antigen. Binding competition for sera from two monkey forest workers (both HSV1-positive) was similar to that of zoonotic BV patient sera.

Despite being exposed to populations of macaques known to be BV positive, no cases of zoonotic BV have been reported among international tourists [65].

Perhaps a more likely explanation lies in the monkeys, that is, captive versus free-ranging. Do captive macaques shed BV more frequently as a result of some husbandry practices? When they are shedding do they shed more virus? Do free-ranging monkeys preferentially shed virus (or more virus) genitally rather than orally, while captive monkeys shed more orally? All these are questions that have been examined only superficially or not at all. It is particularly intriguing that amongst the dozens of primate breeding facilities that

have operated in Asia for decades, some of which contain up to 10,000 macaques, there have been no reported cases of zoonotic BV. The macaques housed in these facilities are exported and are a source of animals used in biomedical research in North America. Other possibilities such as recombinant BV in captive monkeys that arose through past practices of cohousing of different species during capture and shipping have also been raised. The lack of BV isolates from free-ranging macaques for comparison to BV isolates from captive macaques and isolates recovered from zoonotic cases will be necessary to address these and many other aspects of BV neurovirulence.

4. Model Systems for Zoonotic BV Infection

Rabbits have historically been used as an animal model for
BV infections. Until recently, all testing of antivirals for anti-
BV activity was conducted using rabbits [66–70]. Rabbits
are however not an ideal model system given their size, the
relative paucity of immunological reagents, and the difficulty
of housing and handling infected animals under stringent
biohazard conditions. Infant mice were found to be susceptible to BV and using this model, the spread of BV in an axonal-
transsynaptic manner was demonstrated [71, 72]. However,
this model has a number of inherent drawbacks (immature
immune system, size, and dependable numbers/availability)
and has not been used further. Infection of young adult
mice by intramuscular (i.m.) injection (similar to a bite
wound) found substantial variation in the neurovirulence of
various strains of BV isolated from rhesus monkeys, but this
model system was not highly reproducible [73]. However,
inoculation of young adult Balb/c mice by skin scarification
of the flank was found to produce disease very similar to
that seen in humans and to be very reproducible [74]. This
mouse model has recently been used for testing efficacy of
antiviral drugs and molecular studies on BV [75–77]. Lesions
in the brainstem of BV infected mice are characterized by
perivascular cuffing with mononuclear cells, discrete foci of
neuronal necrosis, gliosis, and discrete areas of destruction
of white matter within reticular tracts, accompanied by large
foamy macrophages (gitter cells) similar to those present
in spinal cord lesions. Viral antigen is also present within
neurons and glial cells, and the severity of inflammation
is related to the amount of viral antigen present [73]. The
inflammatory response to infection has been linked to the
lethality of HSV encephalitis in mice [78, 79], and an
aggressive inflammatory response in neural tissue may well
contribute to the lethality of BV infections in both mice and
humans.

In this mouse model, all BV isolates from rhesus
macaques and an isolate from a long-tailed macaque (*M.
fascicularis*) were found to have similar LD$_{50}$ values of
approximately 10^4 PFU [77]. In contrast, isolates from pigtail
(*M. nemestrina*) and lion-tailed macaques (*M. silenus*) were
not lethal (at 10^6 PFU) despite producing clinical signs of neurological involvement. This is interesting when one considers
that most if not all cases of zoonotic BV have been associated
with exposure to rhesus or long-tailed macaques rather than
pigtail macaques (lion-tailed macaques are endangered and
not used in biomedical research).

As mentioned above, the neurovirulence of BV actually
relates to its neurovirulence in nonnatural host species. In
this regard, it is interesting that no zoonotic infections due to
the two viruses most closely related to BV, HVP2 of baboons
(*Papio* spp.) and SA8 of vervets (*Cercopithecus aethiops*),
have been reported (with one probable exception [50]). Both
baboons and vervets have long been used in biomedical
research and exposure incidents have certainly occurred. It
thus appears that when SA8 or HVP2 are transmitted to
humans they both undergo abortive infections. It is thus
interesting that most HVP2 isolates have been shown to be
just as neurovirulent as BV in mice [74, 80] and to be the cause

of a lethal neurological infection in a black-and-white colobus
monkey (*Colobus guereza*) [81]. Given the lower biosafety
rating of HVP2 (BSL2 versus BSL4 for BV), HVP2 is an
attractive model for BV cross-species infections [74, 76].

5. Molecular Aspects of BV

From the time of its original isolation in 1932, extensive
antigenic cross-reactivity between BV and HSV has been
noted, indicating that these viruses are closely related [42, 82–
85]. Subsequent studies revealed that alphaherpesviruses of
baboons (HVP2), vervets (SA8), and chimpanzees (ChHV)
and to a lesser extent the viruses of squirrel monkeys (HVS1)
and spider monkeys (HVA1) are all closely related [23, 83, 85–
90]. Phylogenetic analyses of the alphaherpesviruses based on
gene sequences have defined three major clades of primate
alphaherpesviruses consisting of the hominid viruses (HSV1,
HSV2, and ChHV), cercopithecine (African and Asian)
monkey viruses (BV, HVP2, and SA8), and the platyrrhine (S.
American) monkey viruses (HVS1 and HVA1) [91–93]. Based
on the close relatedness of BV and HSV, the relative lack of
research on the simian viruses, and the biohazard concerns in
working with infectious BV, comparatively little experimental
molecular work with BV has been published. Thus, most
of what is "known" about BV structure, protein functions,
and viral replication is actually extrapolated from what is
known for HSV. However, as more work is done with BV and
related simian viruses, significant differences between these
viruses and HSV become more apparent.

BV has the typical virion structure of alphaherpesviruses,
the genome being enclosed within an icosahedral capsid
that is embedded in an amorphous protein tegument and
surrounded by a lipid membrane envelope [51, 94]. Like HSV,
the lytic replication cycle of BV is rapid with extracellular
progeny virus appearing ~6–8 hrs after infection (PI) [95].
And as for HSV, synthesis of BV proteins appears to follow
the immediate early/early/late gene expression paradigm.

In 1971, an isolate of BV from a rhesus macaque was
adapted to replicate in primary rabbit cells, and this strain
(E2490) now serves as the "standard" or "laboratory" BV
strain [69, 96]. The genome sequence of this strain has
been determined [97–99]. Recently, genome sequences of
a number of additional BV strains from various macaque
species have also been determined [77, 100]. BV genomes
range in size from 154,958 to 157,447 bp, the differences being
largely due to variation in the number of iterations of repeated
sequence units in specific areas of the genome. The BV
genome has a very high G + C content (~75%) and its genetic
arrangement is orthologous to that of HSV (Figure 2). Based
on PCR/sequencing of a small region of the BV genome,
different "genotypes" of BV were identified that correlated
with the macaque species the virus was isolated from [24,
101, 102]. Comparison of complete genome sequences of
BV isolates from different macaque species confirmed the
division of BV into host species-based genotypes [77]. While
sequence identity among BV isolates from rhesus macaques
or between isolates from pigtail macaques is >99%, sequence
identity among different BV genotypes is only ~89–95%.
Comparing the genome sequences of all BV isolates, most

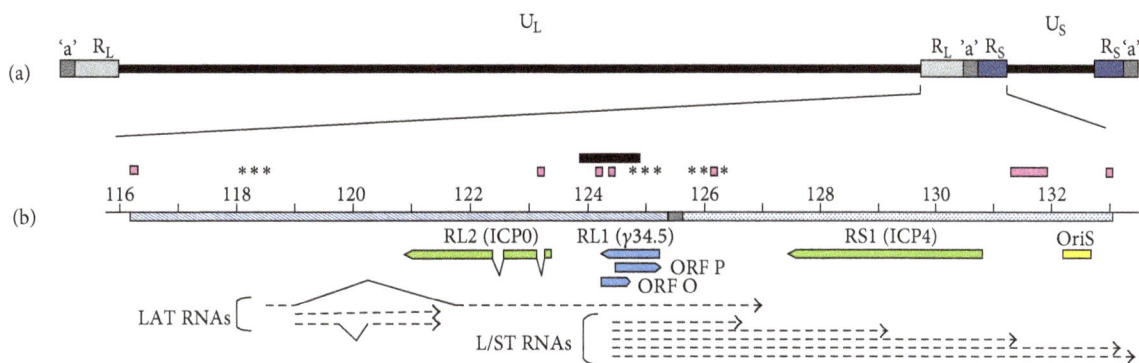

FIGURE 2: Genomic organization of BV. The BV genome is comprised of two unique regions (U_L and U_S) in which open reading frames homologous to the UL1–UL56 and US1–US12 genes of HSV are located, respectively (a). The U_L and U_S regions are each flanked by repeat regions (R_L an R_S, resp.) with the 'a' repeat present at the ends of the genome and between the internal copies of R_L and R_S. The R_L and R_S regions are enlarged in (b) to indicate the position of the following features discussed in the text: predicted ORFs (green), HSV ORFs not found in BV (blue), the origin of DNA replication in R_S (yellow), miRNAs (asterisks), islands of reiterated sequences (magenta), and the region deleted in the E90ΔRL1 mutant (red).

coding sequences, miRNAs, and small RNAs are highly conserved [77, 100, 103, 104]. The most prominent differences are located in areas of the long and short repeat regions (R_L and R_S, resp.) of the genome that do not encode proteins, miRNAs, or small RNAs. Within these areas, there are islands of reiterated sequences. While the primary sequence of these reiterated repeat units and the number of iterations are not conserved among all BV isolates, the positions of these repeat islands are conserved suggesting they likely serve some unknown function.

The genome of BV (as well as HVP2 and SA8) is very similar to that of HSV2 and ChHV in its genetic organization, with homologs of almost every HSV gene being present in the same order and orientation in BV [77, 92, 99, 105, 106]. There are some minor differences like the grouping of some genes into different cotranscriptional units [107]. However, there is one major difference, that being the lack of a detectable homolog of the RL1 (γ34.5) and ORF P genes in the simian viruses [92, 99, 105, 106]. This was somewhat unexpected as both of these genes have been shown to be involved in neurovirulence of HSV (see below). It should be noted however that none of the alphaherpesviruses of nonprimate animals have homologs of the RL1 or ORF P genes either.

Based on DNA sequence data, variation in predicted amino acid (AA) sequence identity of homologous BV and HSV2 proteins averages 62.5% [99]. In contrast, average AA sequence identity values are approximately 95% among BV strains, 87% between BV and HVP2, and 83% between BV and SA8 [100, 105, 106]. This level of AA sequence homology is consistent both with previous studies that detected antigenic cross-reactivity of almost all BV proteins with homologous proteins of HSV [83, 87, 108–111] and with the extensive antigenic cross-reactivity observed between BV and HSV in ELISA, western blot, and neutralization assays [84–86, 112–115].

The highly conserved nature of most HSV, ChHV, and simian virus proteins argues for the homologous proteins of each virus having similar functions. Certainly this is true for

structural capsid proteins (which as a functional group are the most conserved proteins) and viral enzymes. However, a number of BV proteins have regions of dissimilarity relative to other simian viruses and even among different genotypes of BV. Given the interaction of viral immediate early (IE) proteins with host cell proteins to facilitate expression of the viral DNA and initiate the lytic replication cycle, it might be expected that the IE proteins would be highly conserved. However, these regulatory IE proteins are actually some of the least conserved, both among BV genotypes and between BV and other primate viruses. By virtue of their expression on the surface of virions and infected cells, glycoproteins and other membrane associated proteins are another group of proteins that likely interact with elements of host cells. While some are strongly conserved (>90% AA sequence identity), others are very poorly conserved (<62% AA identity). Consistent with this, a number of glycoproteins have some degree of virus-specific antigenicity. The gB (UL27) and gD (US6) glycoproteins are major immunogens of BV, and while both are structurally conserved and have many cross-reactive epitopes, each also has some degree of antigenic BV-specificity [70, 87, 108, 109, 116, 117]. Both the gG (US4) and gC (UL44) glycoproteins are much less conserved and are largely BV-specific antigens with respect to HSV, but still exhibit some antigenic cross-reactivity with the homologous glycoproteins of HVP2 and SA8 [25, 109, 110, 116, 118–120]. Regardless of the degree of conservation/divergence of BV proteins from those of other related viruses, with one exception there are no studies where the involvement of specific BV proteins in neurovirulence has been examined. The one exception is the UL41 gene which encodes the virion host shutoff (VHS) protein. Deletion of this ORF does not cause a significant reduction in the LD_{50} of BV in mice [75].

While BV encodes homologs of all the various HSV proteins mentioned above, little is known about these BV proteins regarding functional equivalency to their HSV counterparts. BV glycoproteins gC (UL44) and gD (US6) as well as VHS (UL41) have been shown to have similar structural and functional properties to their HSV homologs [75, 117, 120–122]. While AA homology suggests that BV proteins function much as their HSV homologs do, the functional equivalency of all other BV proteins has not been directly examined. As one example, the BV ICP0 (RL2) homolog has the characteristic RING finger domain and many other structural motifs of the HSV ICP0 (phosphorylation sites, USP7/ND10 localization region, nuclear localization signal, and multiple SIM-like sequences [123]). While this certainly indicates that the BV ICP0 protein is structurally very similar to the HSV ICP0 protein, the actual functional equivalency of BV ICP0 has yet to be demonstrated. Furthermore, while these various structural motifs are evident, even minor differences in their primary AA sequence could have an effect on their differential function in epithelial versus neuronal cells or macaque versus human-macaque cells.

Although not examined in BV, the UL39 gene is interesting with regard to host-specific neurovirulence. Despite the lack of any clinical differences in its natural baboon host, phylogenetic analyses and testing in mice place HVP2 isolates into two distinct subtypes [26, 80, 124]. One subtype (HVP2ap) produces no clinical signs of infection in mice following infection with as much as 10^6 PFU but does induce an adaptive immune response. In contrast, isolates of the second subtype (HVP2nv) are extremely neurovirulent in mice, having an LD_{50} of ~10^4 PFU (like BV). This dichotomous mouse-specific neurovirulence phenotype of HVP2 isolates allowed mapping of the neurovirulence locus. Recombinant HVP2ap/nv viruses were constructed and tested for neurovirulence in mice. Correlation of the neurovirulence phenotype with genome sequence analyses (defining which parts of the genome were derived from HVP2ap versus HVP2nv) identified a limited region of 3-4 genes that was associated with the neurovirulence phenotype. Based on this, the UL39 gene was the most likely candidate for the "neurovirulence gene," and this was ultimately confirmed by construction and testing of UL39 ORF-specific recombinant viruses [125]. Thus, replacing the UL39ap coding sequence with the UL39nv coding sequence makes an HVP2ap virus neurovirulent, and vice versa.

The UL39 gene encodes the large subunit of the ribonucleotide reductase protein (R1). UL39 has been associated with neurovirulence in HSV (the ability to replicate in nondividing nerve cells) and is one of several genes deleted from prototype HSV gene delivery vectors [126]. While the C-terminal ~75% of the R1 protein is highly conserved and has homology to mammalian ribonucleotide reductase proteins, the N-terminal regions of the HSV, HVP2, and BV R1 proteins are unrelated to other known proteins and (in HSV) are not essential for ribonucleotide reductase enzymatic activity [127, 128]. It is this N-terminal region that is distinct in the two HVP2 subtypes, implying that the N-terminal region of the UL39 protein in some way determines the neurovirulence of HVP2 in mice. Interestingly, this region of BV UL39 exhibits similarly extensive sequence variation between BV isolates from rhesus/long-tailed macaques (that are neurovirulent in mice) and pigtail/lion-tailed macaque isolates (that are

not lethal in mice). It remains to be seen if UL39 underlies neurovirulence of BV in mice as it does in HVP2.

The HSV R1 protein is involved in evasion of cell death by preventing necroptosis in human but not mouse cells [129–131]. In mouse cells, the HSV R1 protein interacts with receptor interacting kinase 1 (RIP1) and RIP3 via their RIP homotypic interaction motifs (RHIMs) which is also present in the N-terminal region of HSV R1, and this interaction ultimately leads to formation of necrosomes and death of the infected cell. In human cells, R1 disrupts the interaction between RIP1 and RIP3, also in a RHIM-dependent manner, thereby preventing necroptosis. Both the BV and HVP2 R1 proteins contain this RHIM motif, and the sequence in this small area is highly conserved. There is however one subtype-specific AA substitution in the RHIM of HVP2ap/nv R1, but the AA residue present in nonneurovirulent HVP2ap isolates is the same as that present in all BV isolates that are lethal in mice, suggesting that this AA may not be responsible for the HVP2 neurovirulence phenotype.

6. Does BV Have a Functional Homolog of the HSV RL1 (γ34.5) Neurovirulence Gene?

In HSV both the RL1 (γ34.5) gene encoding the ICP34.5 (RL1) protein and the ORF P gene (on the opposite strand and overlapping the RL1 gene) have been shown to be primary determinants of neurovirulence in mice [132–137]. Given the neurovirulent reputation of BV, the finding that BV lacks homologs of both the RL1 and ORF P genes was not expected. The HSV RL1 coding sequence starts approximately 200 bp from the internal copy of the 'a' repeat (Figure 2). However, no ATG initiation codon is apparent within 500 bp of the 'a' repeat in any BV strain (or in HVP2 or SA8). Similarly, no potential termination codon is present in any of the simian viruses near the initiation point of the L/ST RNAs where the HSV RL1 termination codon is located. Furthermore, no predicted AA sequence homology exists in the "RL1 region" in any of the simian viruses. Thus, multiple investigators have been unable to identify a simian virus homolog of the RL1 or ORF P genes [77, 99, 100, 105, 106]. Despite the lack of a discernable simian homolog of the HSV RL1 gene (or an overlapping ORF P gene on the opposite strand), the RL1 region between the RL2 start codon and the 'a' repeat of the simian virus genomes (1844–2146 bp) is about the same size as in HSV and ChHV (2048–2154 bp). This suggests that despite the lack of discernable homologs of the RL1 and ORF P genes, this region of the simian virus genomes serves some function. While there are no apparent ORFs in this region of BV, there are two islands of reiterated sequences, and RNA structural analysis of this region (which includes the $5'$ part of the L/ST RNAs) indicates a plethora of potential stem-loop secondary structures. The sequence in this region is highly conserved among 15 strains of BV from rhesus macaques but not between BV isolates from different macaque species. Whether or not this region encodes functions similar to those of HSV is not known.

Comparing the RL1 region sequences of simian virus genomes, there are some conserved features. As in HSV2 and ChHV, the three simian viruses all have three miRNAs, a

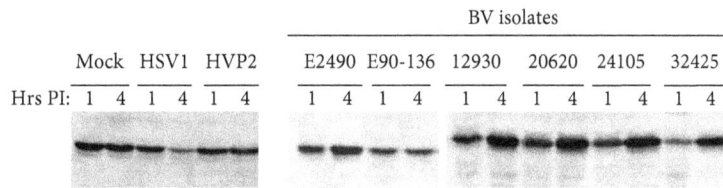

FIGURE 3: Lack of eIF2α dephosphorylation by BV. Cells were harvested at 1 or 4 hrs PI and western blots were performed with antibody directed against phosphorylated eIF2α (Cell Signaling Technologies; Danvers, MA) as described [25]. No change in the level of phosphorylated eIF2α was evident in mock infected cells and the amount of phosphorylated eIF2α decreased from 1 to 4 hrs PI in HSV1 infected cells. In contrast, phosphorylated eIF2α levels increased in BV infected cells.

potential TATA sequence, and both ICP4 and SP1 binding site motifs that are likely control elements for transcription of L/ST RNAs [138]. There is also a potential ORF P start codon located approximately 760–815 bp 5′ of these putative L/ST transcriptional control elements in all three simian viruses (in HSV the ORF P start codon is 3′ of the L/ST control elements). The translated sequence from this start codon in BV is conserved only for the initial four codons (M-A-A-R/E), after which no discernable sequence homology exists. Whether this possibly represents an actual start codon to a spliced gene or is simply the result of sequence similarity due to the extremely high G + C content of this region (producing a strong bias towards high-GC codons) is unknown. It may also be that this potentially conserved AA sequence is completely irrelevant, conserved DNA sequence instead representing part of the conserved transcriptional start site of the L/ST RNAs.

HSV mutants lacking the RL1 or ORF P genes are attenuated in a number of mouse model systems, and they fail to spread within the nervous system even when inoculated directly into the brain [132–134, 137]. The ICP34.5 protein plays a crucial role in allowing HSV to evade the host innate immune response by blocking MHC II expression on the surface of infected cells. When infected, cells initiate an antiviral interferon response that primarily affects neighboring uninfected cells making them more resistant to infection, and ICP34.5 deletion mutants are very sensitive to this host antiviral IFN-α/β response [139–141]. Another host cell response to infection is activation of double-stranded RNA-dependent protein kinase (PKR). PKR acts to phosphorylate translation initiation factor eIF-2α resulting in cessation of protein synthesis in the cell. The HSV ICP34.5 protein dephosphorylates eIF-2α, thus counteracting eIF-2α phosphorylation-induced autophagy [142–146]. The C-terminal region of ICP34.5 has homology with GADD34 protein which facilitates its interaction with the MyD116 and PCNA cell proteins to form a DNA-binding complex [139, 146, 147]. ICP34.5 thus appears to be of central importance to the HSV replicative cycle in many ways. Given the importance of ICP34.5 functions in HSV, the close relatedness of BV and HSV, and the similar size of the RL1 region of the genomes, it is reasonable to hypothesize that this region of the genome may serve some similar function(s) in all these viruses. However, unlike HSV none of the simian viruses display the ICP34.5 function of eIF-2α dephosphorylation

following infection (Figure 3). Quite the opposite, accumulation of phosphorylated eIF-2α is readily evident in BV infected cells. How BV continues to replicate while eIF-2α is phosphorylated is not known.

Using the deletion/replacement approach described for other genes [75, 125], a BV mutant (E90ΔRL1) lacking 1162 bp in the RL1 region but retaining 5′ transcriptional control elements of the RL2 (ICP0) gene and 2 of 3 miRNAs located adjacent to the 'a' repeat was constructed. This mutant grows as well as the parental wild-type virus in Vero cells, indicating that this region of the genome is not essential for BV replication in vitro. When proteins synthesized at various times PI were examined (1-2, 4–6, 10–12, and 4–24 hrs PI), no differences were detectable between the parental wild-type virus and the E90ΔRL1 mutant. In primary mouse skin fibroblasts infected at a low multiplicity of infection (MOI; 0.3 PFU/cell), wild-type BV forms small plaques by 24 hrs PI and subsequently spreads to adjacent cells involving the entire cell monolayer by 48 hrs PI (Figure 4). In contrast, while the E90ΔRL1 mutant also forms small plaques by 24 hrs PI, these fail to spread with time. Quantitation of infectious virus produced after low MOI infection reflected this, in that while the E90ΔRL1 mutant does replicate, the amount of infectious progeny produced at 24 hrs PI is significantly less than that produced by wild-type BV. Since Vero cells do not produce IFN-β while primary mouse cells do, this suggests that deletion of the RL1 region from the BV genome renders the virus susceptible to the host IFN-β response. The E90ΔRL1 mutant does however effectively suppress the host IFN-β response when cells are infected with a high MOI, suggesting that low MOI infection with the E90ΔRL1 mutant allows adjacent uninfected cells to initiate an effective IFN-β response that the mutant is unable to overcome, preventing further spread of the virus. In this respect, the BV RL1 region deletion mutant appears similar to ICP34.5 mutants of HSV.

The E90ΔRL1 mutant was also tested in mice using the skin scarification model to assess what effect this region has on neurovirulence. As mentioned above, HSV mutants lacking the RL1 gene are not neurovirulent in mice and fail to spread within the nervous system. In contrast, the neurovirulence of the E90ΔRL1 mutant was actually slightly increased relative to that of the parental wild-type virus, the mutant having an LD$_{50}$ of $10^{3.7}$ PFU compared to $10^{4.4}$ PFU for the parental virus. Even so, the time to death/euthanasia of infected mice was the same for both viruses (5.5–6 days

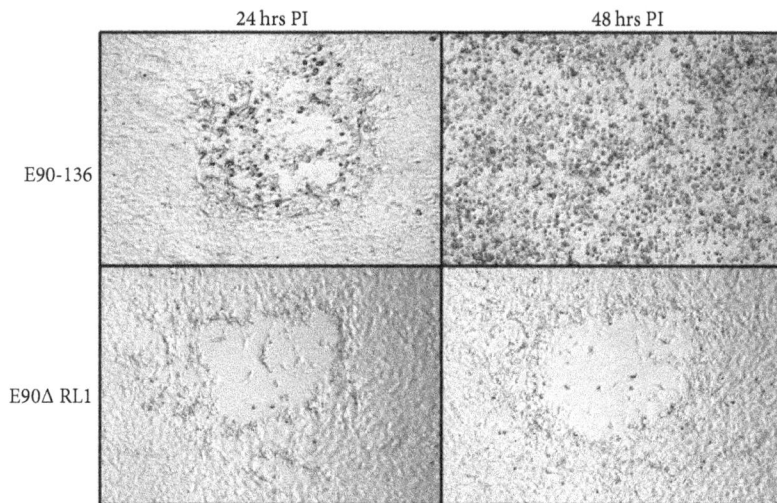

24 hrs PI   48 hrs PI

E90-136

E90Δ RL1

FIGURE 4: Deletion of the RL1 region affects BV spread in primary mouse cells. Primary murine skin fibroblast cells were prepared, cultured, and infected as described [26]. At low MOI (0.3 PFU/cell) wild-type BV (E90-136) forms plaques by 24 hr PI and rapidly spreads over the next 24 hrs, while the E90ΔRL1 deletion mutant fails to spread after 24 hrs PI.

PI). Thus, the RL1 region of BV does not appear to encode all the same functions ascribed to the γ34.5 protein of HSV and is not a major determinant of BV neurovirulence.

7. What Else Could Underlie the Extreme Neurovirulence of BV in Non-Macaque Hosts?

One possibility that has been raised to explain the restriction of zoonotic BV cases to North America is that some BV isolates circulating in these captive macaques are potentially recombinant viruses, the recombinant viruses having arisen due to past practices of cocaging monkeys of different species during importation. Sequencing of multiple BV isolates from different US rhesus breeding colonies failed to detect any such recombinants [77]. However, none of the isolates examined were from zoonotic BV cases. Comparative genome sequencing of BV isolates from zoonotic cases and from monkeys could determine if there are specific characteristics (including recombinants) that are associated with zoonotic isolates but not present in all monkey isolates. In addition, sequencing of BV isolated from free-ranging (noncaptive) monkeys would serve to identify the presence of recombinant viruses in North American captive macaques.

In assessing the host-specific nature of BV neurovirulence, differences that occur in how the virus behaves in the natural versus nonnatural host obviously need to be examined. There are really two critical points where differences in host-virus interactions in humans and macaques would most probably affect neurovirulence/clinical disease. The first is the ability of BV to invade the nervous system. In the normal course of pathogenesis, viral replication in epithelial tissue at the site of inoculation is needed to produce sufficient levels of infectious progeny virus to allow invasion of sensory neurons innervating the site (this is not necessary if sufficiently high levels of infectious virus are transmitted to

allow direct infection of sensory neurons) [148–151]. Second, once within a sensory neuron, the linked processes of viral replication, establishment of latency, and reactivation from latency could affect the spread of BV within the nervous system.

Replication at the Site of Infection. The occurrence of herpetic lesions at injury sites in zoonotic BV patients suggests that BV can replicate effectively in human epithelial tissue. However, the rarity of zoonotic BV infections relative to the number of annual exposure incidents that occur and the apparent lack or rarity of asymptomatic zoonotic infections could indicate that zoonotic transmission of BV does not always lead to an active or clinically apparent infection in many or even most cases. This could be due to any number of things including (1) monkeys not shedding virus at the time of contact; (2) too low levels of virus transmitted to overcome preexisting (cross-reactive) immunity to HSV; or (3) innate host resistance resulting in inefficient or abortive replication of BV in human epithelial cells relative to its ability to replicate in macaque cells. While it has been shown that HSV replication in rhesus cells can be very inefficient or abortive [152–154], such has not been shown for BV replication in human cells. A failure of BV to replicate well in humans at the original site of infection resulting in insufficient levels of virus to invade sensory neurons could result in the majority of exposure incidents not leading to active zoonotic BV infections, such cases only resulting when high enough levels of infectious virus are transmitted to allow infection of sensory neurons without need for further amplification of virus by local replication.

Recent studies have begun to investigate the comparative replication of BV in macaque versus human cells. It has been shown that while the HSV gD glycoprotein binds host cell proteins HVEM, nectin 1 and nectin 2 to facilitate viral entry, the BV gD glycoprotein only binds nectin 1 and nectin 2 in both human and macaque cells [121, 122, 155]. While a single amino acid mutation was identified in the external domain of gD that affected the stability of binding to nectin 1, comparison of gD sequences from 19 clinical BV strains isolated from humans and macaques found that this mutation did not correlate with zoonosis [117], indicating that differing stability of gD binding to nectin 1 is not related to the ability of BV to infect human versus macaque cells. Consistent with this, the gD glycoprotein has been shown to be altogether dispensable for BV entry into both macaque and human cells [155].

The HSV IE protein ICP47 (US12) mediates downregulation of MHC expression on the surface of infected cells, thus likely evading activation of host antiviral T cells and altering susceptibility of infected cells to killing by natural killer (NK) cells [156]. The BV ICP47 protein lacks the TAP-binding domain of the HSV ICP47 and thus BV fails to downregulate MHC expression in both human and macaque cells, suggesting that the differences in BV and HSV evasion of activation of antiviral T cells and susceptibility to NK cells are not responsible for any differential pathogenicity of BV in humans versus macaques [157]. Similarly, PI3K-dependent Akt phosphorylation (which promotes survival of the infected cell and inhibits apoptosis) is not markedly different in macaque and human fibroblasts [158]. Thus, there is no evidence to date to suggest that BV replicates much differently in human versus macaque epithelial cells.

Replication, Latency, and Reactivation in Neurons. Virtually nothing is known regarding details of the establishment of BV latency or reactivation from latency. However, based on what is known about HSV, some predictions can be made about what might occur differently in these aspects of BV in its natural versus nonnatural host. When HSV infects a neuron, the viral envelope fuses with the cell plasma membrane, releasing the nucleocapsid and tegument proteins into the cytoplasm. The nucleocapsid (or at least the viral DNA) is transported to the nucleus where the viral DNA is immediately coated with histones and cellular repressor proteins to prevent viral IE gene expression and entry into the lytic replication cycle, resulting in latency [159, 160]. To counteract this, the viral tegument protein VP16 (UL48) recruits several host cell proteins to form complexes at IE gene promotors that facilitate expression of the viral IE genes and progression into the lytic replication cycle [159]. At the same time, the ICP0 (RL2) IE protein, which is also present in the tegument, degrades host cell proteins involved in repressing viral gene expression via its E3 ubiquitin ligase activity. ICP0 also competitively binds to certain components of repressor complexes, thus destabilizing the repressor complexes and tilting the balance against entry into the lytic replication cycle and favoring latency [123, 161]. This fine balance between lytic replication in neurons and establishment of latency represents an exquisite degree of coadaptation between HSV and its human host, allowing both to coexist. It is likely that BV follows this same paradigm in macaques, becoming latent in sensory neurons with the host adaptive immune response clearing the initial infection in epithelial tissue. Anything that alters this fine balance between lytic replication and

repression of the BV genome in human neurons could well result in a very different outcome of infection compared to that seen in macaques.

As mentioned previously, there is evidence supporting the ability of BV to establish latent infections in humans and to reactivate at later times just as occurs in macaques. Even so, slight alterations in the most basic molecular aspects of these processes could have a radical effect on the ultimate outcome of BV infections in humans. It may be that in human neurons BV usually overcomes the innate preemptive response of the neuron to effectively repress viral IE gene expression and establish latency. This would result in lytic replication of BV in human neurons with production of progeny virus and subsequent spread of the virus to other neurons and/or accessory cells. Given the apparently central role played by the multifunctional ICP0 protein in the establishment of latency [123, 161], variant interaction of the BV ICP0 protein with macaque versus human cell factors could well be a critical factor.

When reactivated from latency, progeny virions (or virion components) are transported anterograde down the axon where the virus exits the neuron and undergoes lytic replication in epithelial tissue [148, 162]. While details of how reactivation from latency occurs are not known, reactivation undoubtedly once again involves altered interactions between the latent viral genome and host cell factors affecting IE gene transcription. Since HSV latency associated transcripts (LAT) and both small RNAs and miRNAs appear to be primarily involved in maintaining latency [138, 160], differential expression and/or function of homologous BV RNAs in macaque versus human neurons could alter the stability of the latent state in the two species. While some miRNAs and small RNAs have been identified and mapped in BV [103, 104], nothing is known about BV LATs or functions of these RNAs.

Since reactivation from latency must involve replication of the virus in the neuron, it has been hypothesized that replication and production of progeny virus in neurons is much less efficient than in epithelial cells, thereby sparing widespread destruction of host neurons [163]. This could well be the case in macaques, but not when BV reactivates in human neurons. Instead, BV may replicate much more efficiently in human neurons compared to macaque neurons, resulting in production of more virus within the nervous system and more efficient spread of BV within the human nervous system as seen in fatal zoonotic infections.

A similar possibility is that while BV may become latent in humans, it is reactivated much more readily in humans than in macaques (days as opposed to months or years). This would be consistent with the variable time (days to several weeks) between exposure incidents and the first appearance of clinical symptoms in zoonotic BV patients [5, 46, 51]. In the natural host, it is likely that only small amounts of infectious virus are produced in neurons following reactivation from latency and progeny virions are transported anterograde in the axon down to the original epithelial site of infection where further replication occurs until cleared by an adaptive immune response. If reactivation of BV from latency is much more efficient in human neurons, it is conceivable that BV could eventually overload the host/virus balance with successive waves of newly replicated virus infecting many more neurons than occurs in the natural macaque host.

Another possibility is that in humans BV is more readily transported down dendrites than in macaques, resulting in more efficient spread of the virus within the human nervous system. Interestingly, in pseudorabies virus (PRV; a porcine alphaherpesvirus), there does appear to be some virus-specificity in attachment of virions to dynein motor proteins (for axonal transport) versus kinesin motor proteins (for axonal and/or dendritic transport) [164]. Binding to kinesin motors involves the gE (US8), gI (US7), and US9 proteins of PRV, while tegument proteins UL36, UL37, and US3 impart affinity for dynein motors. Thus, even slightly altered specificity of any of the homologous BV proteins for macaque versus human dynein or kinesin motor proteins could affect the neurovirulence of BV in humans by altering the spread of infection from that which occurs in the natural macaque host. The failure to establish latency in human neurons, altered stability of latency, and altered spread of the virus within the nervous system are all consistent with the very serious CNS infection versus no infection picture of zoonotic BV infection that seems to occur in humans.

8. Conclusions

BV is ubiquitous in populations of captive and free-ranging macaques and despite many exposure incidents every year; zoonotic infections are extremely rare and have only been documented in North America. Notwithstanding, BV is notorious for its extreme neurovirulence in the handful of humans who have been infected. Biological aspects of BV infection in its natural macaque host are very similar to that of HSV in humans, including primary replication in epithelial tissue, invasion of sensory neurons, establishment of latency in sensory ganglia, and periodic reactivation from latency in response to stress allowing transmission of the virus to a new host. Phylogenetic analysis of the primate alphaherpesviruses suggests that these viruses have likely coevolved with their hosts, not surprising given the exquisite details that must be involved in virus-host interactions to maintain the virus within the nervous system for the lifespan of its host without serious adverse consequences while still allowing transmission and perpetuation of the virus within the host species. Given that nonhuman primates are our closest phylogenetic relatives, it is not surprising that BV should be very much like HSV with regard to the virus-host interactions and mechanisms involved in maintaining the virus-host relationship in a balanced state. The orthologous nature of the BV and HSV genomes and similarity of encoded proteins support this. Based on comparative sequence analyses, it also appears that BV encodes LATs, miRNAs, and small RNAs that would be involved in the intricate regulation of viral latency in neurons as in HSV.

Due to the hazardous and restrictive nature of performing research with infectious BV, very little experimental or molecular research has been done on this intriguing virus. To date the only genetic characteristic that differs dramatically between BV and HSV is the lack of homologs of the RL1 (γ34.5) and ORF P genes in BV. Despite lacking these genes, this region of the simian virus genome remains nearly the same size as in HSV. Although both the RL1 and ORF P genes are important determinants of HSV neurovirulence in mice, deletion of this region of the BV genome has little effect on its neurovirulence in mice.

BV has attained its reputation as having extreme neurovirulence due to the high mortality associated with the approximately 60 zoonotic cases that have occurred since its identification 85 years ago. However, for comparison HSV causes ~500 cases of encephalitis each year in the US, and without treatment is ~70% fatal with only ~5% of patients fully recovering [18], characteristics that are very similar to that of zoonotic BV. The neurovirulence of BV is only apparent when it infects non-macaques. While there are some differences between HSV and BV, to date no differences in the replication of BV *in vitro* in human versus macaque cells have been identified that might account for the divergent neurovirulence of BV in these two species. Given the delicate balance that exists in neurons between repression of gene expression to establish latency and lytic replication, even slight differences in any of the multitude of host-virus interactions affecting this balance could ultimately alter the pathogenesis of BV in a nonnatural host species, resulting in very different outcomes of infection in macaques versus humans. Considerably more research into molecular aspects of host-virus interactions in macaque versus human cells, both epithelial and neural, needs to be pursued to better understand the extreme neurovirulence exhibited by BV in humans.

Acknowledgments

The authors wish to thank Drs. C. Jones, K. Ohsawa, and J. d'Offay for helpful discussions and critical review of this manuscript and DA Leib for eIF2 western blots. This work was supported by PHS Grant R24 OD022013.

References

[1] D. Elmore and R. Eberle, "Monkey B virus (Cercopithecine herpesvirus 1)," *Comparative Medicine*, vol. 58, no. 1, pp. 11–21, 2008.

[2] J. L. Huff and P. A. Barry, "B-virus (Cercopithecine herpesvirus 1) infection in humans and macaques: Potential for zoonotic disease," *Emerging Infectious Diseases*, vol. 9, no. 2, pp. 246–250, 2003.

[3] S. A. Keeble, G. J. Christofinis, and W. Wood, "Natural Virus-B infection in rhesus monkeys," *The Journal of Pathology*, vol. 76, no. 1, pp. 189–199, 1958.

[4] A. E. Palmer, "Herpesvirus simiae: historical perspective," *Journal of Medical Primatology*, pp. 16–99, 1987.

[5] B. J. Weigler, "Biology of B Virus in Macaque and Human Hosts: A Review," *Clinical Infectious Diseases*, vol. 14, no. 2, pp. 555–567, 1992.

[6] H. T. Zwartouw and E. A. Boulter, "Excretion of B virus in monkeys and evidence of genital infection," *Laboratory Animals*, vol. 18, no. 1, pp. 65–70, 1984.

[7] H. T. Zwartouw, J. A. Macarthur, E. A. Boulter, J. H. Seamer, J. H. Marston, and A. S. Chamove, "Transmission of B virus infection between monkeys especially in relation to breeding colonies," *Laboratory Animals*, vol. 18, no. 2, pp. 125–130, 1984.

[8] M. R. Andrade, J. Yee, P. Barry et al., "Prevalence of antibodies to selected viruses in a long-term closed breeding colony of rhesus macaques (Macaca mulatta) in Brazil," *American Journal of Primatology*, vol. 59, no. 3, pp. 123–128, 2003.

[9] R. F. Di Giacomo and K. V. Shah, "Virtual absence of infection with Herpesvirus simiae in colony-reared rhesus monkeys (Macaca mulatta), with a literature review on antibody prevalence in natural and laboratory rhesus populations.," *Laboratory Animals*, vol. 22, no. 1, pp. 61–67, 1972.

[10] K. Jensen, F. Alvarado-Ramy, J. González-Martínez, E. Kraiselburd, and J. Rullán, "B-Virus and Free-Ranging Macaques, Puerto Rico," *Emerging Infectious Diseases*, vol. 10, no. 3, pp. 494–496, 2004.

[11] L. Jones-Engel, G. A. Engel, J. Heidrich et al., "Temple monkeys and health implications of commensalism, Kathmandu, Nepal," *Emerging Infectious Diseases*, vol. 12, no. 6, pp. 900–906, 2006.

[12] M. J. Kessler and J. K. Hilliard, "Seroprevalence of B Virus (Herpesvirus simiae) antibodies in a naturally formed group of rhesus macaques," *Journal of Medical Primatology*, vol. 19, no. 2, pp. 155–160, 1990.

[13] F. Lee, Y.-J. Lin, M.-C. Deng, T.-Y. Lee, and C.-C. Huang, "Prevalence of antibody reaction with cercopithecine herpesvirus 1 antigen in Macaca cyclopis, Macaca fascicularis, and Papio anubis in Taiwan," *Journal of Medical Primatology*, vol. 36, no. 6, pp. 343–347, 2007.

[14] M.-H. Lee, M. K. Rostal, T. Hughes et al., "Macacine herpesvirus 1 in long-tailed macaques, Malaysia, 2009-2011," *Emerging Infectious Diseases*, vol. 21, no. 7, pp. 1107–1113, 2015.

[15] Q. Lin, G.-L. Yuan, L. Ai, J. Li, and H.-L. Li, "Seroprevalence of BV (Macacine herpesvirus 1) in bred cynomolgus monkeys in Cambodia," *Journal of Veterinary Medical Science*, vol. 74, no. 3, pp. 355-356, 2012.

[16] R. P. Orcutt, G. J. Pucak, H. L. Foster, J. T. Kilcourse, and T. Ferrell, "Multiple testing for the detection of B virus antibody in specially handled rhesus monkeys after capture from virgin trapping grounds," *Laboratory Animals*, vol. 26, no. 1, pp. 70–74, 1976.

[17] B. J. Weigler, J. A. Roberts, D. W. Hird, N. W. Lerche, and J. K. Hilliard, "A cross sectional survey for B virus antibody in a colony of group housed rhesus macaques," *Laboratory Animals*, vol. 40, no. 3, pp. 257–261, 1990.

[18] R. J. Whitley and J. W. Gnann, "Viral encephalitis: familiar infections and emerging pathogens," *The Lancet*, vol. 359, no. 9305, pp. 507–513, 2002.

[19] G. A. Engel, L. Jones-Engel, M. A. Schillaci et al., "Human exposure to herpesvirus B-seropositive Macaques, Bali, Indonesia," *Emerging Infectious Diseases*, vol. 8, no. 8, pp. 789–795, 2002.

[20] L. Jones-Engel, G. A. Engel, M. A. Schillaci et al., "Primate-to-human retroviral transmission in Asia," *Emerging Infectious Diseases*, vol. 11, no. 7, pp. 1028–1035, 2005.

[21] R. Eberle and J. K. Hilliard, "Serological evidence for variation in the incidence of herpesvirus infections in different species of apes," *Journal of Clinical Microbiology*, vol. 27, no. 6, pp. 1357–1366, 1989.

[22] R. Eberle, "Evidence for an alpha-herpesvirus indigenous to mountain gorillas.," *Journal of Medical Primatology*, vol. 21, no. 5, pp. 246–251, 1992.

[23] E. Luebcke, E. Dubovi, D. Black, K. Ohsawa, and R. Eberle, "Isolation and characterization of a chimpanzee alphaherpesvirus," *Journal of General Virology*, vol. 87, no. 1, pp. 11–19, 2006.

[24] S. A. Thompson, J. K. Hilliard, D. Kittel et al., "Retrospective analysis of an outbreak of B virus infection in a colony of DeBrazza's monkeys (Cercopithecus neglectus)," *Comparative Medicine*, vol. 50, no. 6, pp. 649–657, 2000.

[25] E. L. Blewett, D. Black, and R. Eberle, "Characterization of virus-specific and cross-reactive monoclonal antibodies to Herpesvirus simiae (B virus)," *Journal of General Virology*, vol. 77, no. 11, pp. 2787–2793, 1996.

[26] K. M. Rogers, D. H. Black, and R. Eberle, "Primary mouse dermal fibroblast cell cultures as an in vitro model system for the differential pathogenicity of cross-species herpesvirus papio 2 infections," *Archives of Virology*, vol. 152, no. 3, pp. 543–552, 2007.

[27] S. A. Keeble, "B virus infection in monkeys," *Annals of the New York Academy of Sciences*, vol. 85, no. 3, pp. 960–969, 1960.

[28] E. A. Boulter, "The isolation of Monkey B virus (Herpesvirus simiae) from the trigeminal ganglia of a healthy seropositive rhesus monkey," *Journal of Biological Standardization*, vol. 3, no. 3, pp. 279-280, 1975.

[29] J. L. Melnick and D. D. Banker, "Isolation of B virus (herpes group) from the central nervous system of a rhesus monkey," *The Journal of Experimental Medicine*, vol. 100, no. 2, pp. 181–194, 1954.

[30] A. D. Vizoso, "Recovery of herpes simiae (B virus) from both primary and latent infections in rhesus monkeys," *Journal of Experimental Pathology*, vol. 56, no. 6, pp. 485–488, 1975.

[31] D. C. Anderson, R. B. Swenson, J. L. Orkin, S. S. Kalter, and H. M. McClure, "Primary Herpesvirus simiae (B-virus) infection in infant macaques," *Laboratory Animals*, vol. 44, no. 5, pp. 526–530, 1994.

[32] C. S. Carlson, M. G. O'Sullivan, M. J. Jayo et al., "Fatal Disseminated Cercopithecine Herpesvirus 1 (Herpes B) Infection in Cynomolgus Monkeys (Macaca fascicularis)," *Veterinary Pathology*, vol. 34, no. 5, pp. 405–414, 1997.

[33] M. D. Daniel, F. G. Garcia, L. V. Melendez, R. D. Hunt, J. O'Connor, and D. Silva, "Multiple Herpesvirus simiae isolation from a rhesus monkey which died of cerebral infarction," *Laboratory Animals*, vol. 25, no. 3, pp. 303–308, 1975.

[34] M. A. Simon, M. D. Daniel, D. Lee-Parritz, N. W. King, and D. J. Ringler, "Disseminated B virus infection in a cynomolgus monkey," *Laboratory Animals*, vol. 43, no. 6, pp. 545–550, 1993.

[35] J. L. Huff, R. Eberle, J. Capitanio, S. S. Zhou, and P. A. Barry, "Differential detection of B virus and rhesus cytomegalovirus in rhesus macaques," *Journal of General Virology*, vol. 84, no. 1, pp. 83–92, 2003.

[36] B. J. Weigler, D. W. Hird, J. K. Hilliard et al., "Epidemiology of Cercopithecine Herpesvirus 1 (B Virus) Infection and Shedding in a Large Breeding Cohort of Rhesus Macaques," *The Journal of Infectious Diseases*, vol. 167, no. 2, pp. 257–263, 1993.

[37] E. C. Weir, P. N. Bhatt, R. O. Jacoby, J. K. Hilliard, and S. Morgenstern, "Infrequent shedding and transmission of Herpesvirus simiae from seropositive macaques," *Laboratory Animals*, vol. 43, no. 6, pp. 541–544, 1993.

[38] G. J. Chellman, V. S. Lukas, E. M. Eugui, K. P. Altera, S. J. Almquist, and J. K. Hilliard, "Activation of B virus (Herpesvirus simiae) in chronically immunosuppressed cynomolgus monkeys," *Laboratory Animals*, vol. 42, no. 2, pp. 146–151, 1992.

[39] F. Mitsunaga, S. Nakamura, T. Hayashi, and R. Eberle, "Changes in the titer of anti-B virus antibody in captive macaques (Macaca fuscata, M. mulatta, M. fascicularis)," *Comparative Medicine*, vol. 57, no. 1, pp. 120–124, 2007.

[40] F. P. Gay and M. Holden, "The herpes encephalitis problem, ii," *The Journal of Infectious Diseases*, vol. 53, no. 3, pp. 287–303, 1933.

[41] J. D. Pimentel, "Herpes B virus – "B" is for Brebner: Dr. William Bartlet Brebner (1903-1932)," *Canadian Medical Association Journal*, vol. 178, no. 6, pp. 734–734, 2008.

[42] A. B. Sabin, "Acute ascending myelitis following a monkey bite, with the isolation of a virus capable of reproducing the disease," *The Journal of Experimental Medicine*, vol. 59, no. 2, pp. 115–136, 1934.

[43] Fatal Cercopithecine herpesvirus 1 (B virus) infection following a mucocutaneous exposure and interim recommendations for worker protection, MMWR 47:1073-1076, 1083, 1998.

[44] A. W. Artenstein, C. B. Hicks, B. S. Goodwin Jr., and J. K. Hilliard, "Human infection with B virus following a needlestick injury," *Reviews of Infectious Diseases*, vol. 13, no. 2, pp. 288–291, 1991.

[45] D. S. Davenport, D. R. Johnson, G. P. Holmes, D. A. Jewett, S. C. Ross, and J. K. Hilliard, "Diagnosis and management of human b virus (herpesvims simiae) infections in michigan," *Clinical Infectious Diseases*, vol. 19, no. 1, pp. 33–41, 1994.

[46] W. L. Davidson and K. Hummeler, "B Virus Infection in Man," *Annals of the New York Academy of Sciences*, vol. 85, no. 3, pp. 970–979, 1960.

[47] G. P. Holmes, J. K. Hilliard, K. C. Klontz et al., "B virus (Herpesvirus simiae) infection in humans: Epidemiologic investigation of a cluster," *Annals of Internal Medicine*, vol. 112, no. 11, pp. 833–839, 1990.

[48] K. Hummeler, W. L. Davidson, W. Henle, A. C. Laboccetta, and H. G. Ruch, "Encephalomyelitis due to infection with Herpesvirus simiae (herpes B virus); a report of two fatal, laboratory-acquired cases," *The New England Journal of Medicine*, vol. 261, no. 2, pp. 64–68, 1959.

[49] F. P. Nagler and M. Klotz, "A fatal B virus infection in a person subject to recurrent herpes labialis," *Canadian Medical Association Journal*, pp. 79–743, 1958.

[50] J. M. M. Nsabimana, M. Moutschen, E. Thiry, and F. Meurens, *Cahiers/Santé*, Infection humaine par le virus B du singe en Afrique. Cahiers Sante 1, 3-8, 2008.

[51] R. J. Whitely, J. K. Hilliard, Cercopithecine herpesvirus (B virus), In: D. M. Knipe, P. M. Howley (eds) Fields Virology, Lippincott Williams and Wilkins, Philadelphia, PA, USA, pp 2835-2848, 2001.

[52] G. E. Breen, S. G. Lamb, and A. T. Otaki, "Monkey-bite encephalomyelitis report of a case—with recovery," *British Medical Journal*, vol. 2, no. 5087, pp. 22-23, 1958.

[53] B. L. Bryan, C. D. Espana, R. W. Emmons, N. Vijayan, and P. D. Hoeprich, "Recovery from encephalomyelitis caused by herpesvirus simiae: report of a case," *JAMA Internal Medicine*, vol. 135, no. 6, pp. 868–870, 1975.

[54] J. Fierer, P. Bazeley, and A. I. Braude, "Herpes B virus encephalomyelitis presenting as ophthalmic zoster: A possible latent infection reactivated," *Annals of Internal Medicine*, vol. 79, no. 2, pp. 225–228, 1973.

[55] C. Calvo, S. Friedlander, J. K. Hilliard et al., "Case Report: Reactivation of latent B virus (Macacine herpesvirus 1) presenting as bilateral uveitis, retinal vasculitis and necrotizing herpetic retinitis," *Investigative Ophthalmology & Visual Science*, pp. 52–2975, 2011.

[56] A. G. Freifeld, J. Hilliard, J. Southers et al., "A controlled seroprevalence survey of primate handlers for evidence of asymptomatic herpes b virus infection," *The Journal of Infectious Diseases*, vol. 171, no. 4, pp. 1031–1034, 1995.

[57] K. L. Craig, M. K. Hasan, D. L. Jackson et al., "A seminomadic population in Bangladesh with extensive exposure to macaques does not exhibit high levels of zoonotic simian foamy virus infection," *Journal of Virology*, vol. 89, no. 14, pp. 7414–7416, 2015.

[58] W. F. Johnston, J. Yeh, R. Nierenberg, and G. Procopio, "Exposure to Macaque Monkey Bite," *The Journal of Emergency Medicine*, vol. 49, no. 5, pp. 634–637, 2015.

[59] M. A. Schillaci, L. Jones-Engel, G. A. Engel et al., "Prevalence of enzootic simian viruses among urban performance monkeys in Indonesia," *Tropical Medicine & International Health*, vol. 10, no. 12, pp. 1305–1314, 2005.

[60] P. Gautret, B. Jesse, L. Dacheux et al., "Correction to: Rabies in Nonhuman Primates and Potential for Transmission to Humans: A Literature Review and Examination of Selected French National Data (PLoS Negl Trop Dis, 9, 5)," *PLOS Neglected Tropical Diseases*, vol. 9, no. 5, Article ID e0003799, 2015.

[61] G. A. Engel, C. T. Small, K. Soliven et al., "Zoonotic simian foamy virus in Bangladesh reflects diverse patterns of transmission and co-infection," *Emerging Microbes & Infections*, vol. 2, no. 9, pp. e58–e58, 2013.

[62] A. Fuentes and S. Gamerl, "Disproportionate participation by age/sex classes in aggressive interactions between long-tailed macaques (Macaca fascicularis) and human tourists at Padangtegal monkey forest, Bali, Indonesia," *American Journal of Primatology*, vol. 66, no. 2, pp. 197–204, 2005.

[63] B. P. Wheatley, The Sacred Monkeys of Bali, Waveland Press, Prospect Heights, IL, USA, 1999.

[64] L. E. Mease and K. A. Baker, "Monkey bites among US military members, Afghanistan, 2011," *Emerging Infectious Diseases*, vol. 18, no. 10, pp. 1647–1649, 2012.

[65] N. J. Riesland and H. Wilde, "Expert Review of Evidence Bases for Managing Monkey Bites in Travelers," *Journal of Travel Medicine*, vol. 22, no. 4, pp. 259–262, 2015.

[66] A. M. Bennett, M. J. Slomka, D. W. G. Brown, G. Lloyd, and M. Mackett, "Protection against herpes B virus infection in rabbits with a recombinant vaccinia virus expressing glycoprotein D," *Journal of Medical Virology*, vol. 57, no. 1, pp. 47–56, 1999.

[67] E. A. Boulter and D. P. Grant, "Latent infection of monkeys with B virus and prophylactic studies in a rabbit model of this disease," *Journal of Antimicrobial Chemotherapy*, vol. 3, pp. 107–113, 1977.

[68] E. A. Boulter, H. T. Zwartouw, and B. Thornton, "Postexposure immunoprophylaxis against B virus (herpesvirus simiae) infection," *British Medical Journal (Clinical Research ed.)*, vol. 283, no. 6305, p. 1495, 1981.

[69] R. N. Hull and J. C. Nash, "Immunization against b virus infection: Preparation of an experimental vaccine," *American Journal of Epidemiology*, vol. 71, no. 1, pp. 15–28, 1960.

[70] L. Perelygina, I. Patrusheva, H. Zurkuhlen, and J. K. Hilliard, "Characterization of B virus glycoprotein antibodies induced by DNA immunization," *Archives of Virology*, vol. 147, no. 11, pp. 2057–2073, 2002.

[71] G. Gosztonyi, D. Falke, and H. Ludwig, "Axonal and transsynaptic (transneuronal) spread of Herpesvirus simiae (B virus) in experimentally infected mice," *Histology and Histopathology*, vol. 7, no. 1, pp. 63–74, 1992.

[72] G. Gosztonyi, D. Falke, and H. Ludwig, "Axonal-transsynaptic spread as the basic pathogenetic mechanism in B virus infection of the nervous system.," *Journal of Medical Primatology*, vol. 21, no. 1, pp. 42-43, 1992.

[73] J. W. Ritchey, M. E. Payton, and R. Eberle, "Clinicopathological characterization of monkey B virus (cercopithecine herpesvirus 1) infection in mice," *Journal of Comparative Pathology*, vol. 132, no. 2-3, pp. 202–217, 2005.

[74] K. M. Rogers, J. W. Ritchey, M. Payton, D. H. Black, and R. Eberle, "Neuropathogenesis of herpesvirus papio 2 in mice parallels infection with Cercopithecine herpesvirus 1 (B virus) in humans," *Journal of General Virology*, vol. 87, no. 2, pp. 267–276, 2006.

[75] D. Black, J. Ritchey, M. Payton, and R. Eberle, "Role of the virion host shutoff protein in neurovirulence of monkey B virus (Macacine herpesvirus 1)," *Virologica Sinica*, vol. 29, no. 5, pp. 274–283, 2014.

[76] L. A. Brush, D. H. Black, K. A. McCormack et al., "Papiine herpesvirus 2 as a predictive model for drug sensitivity of Macacine herpesvirus 1 (monkey B virus)," *Comparative Medicine*, vol. 64, no. 5, pp. 386–393, 2014.

[77] R. Eberle, L. K. Maxwell, S. Nicholson, D. Black, and L. Jones-Engel, "Genome sequence variation among isolates of monkey B virus (Macacine alphaherpesvirus 1) from captive macaques," *Virology*, vol. 508, pp. 26–35, 2017.

[78] E. A. Kurt-Jones, M. Chan, S. Zhou et al., "Herpes simplex virus 1 interaction with Toll-like receptor 2 contributes to lethal encephalitis," *Proceedings of the National Acadamy of Sciences of the United States of America*, vol. 101, no. 5, pp. 1315–1320, 2004.

[79] P. Lundberg, C. Ramakrishna, J. Brown et al., "The immune response to herpes simplex virus type 1 infection in susceptible mice is a major cause of central nervous system pathology resulting in fatal encephalitis," *Journal of Virology*, vol. 82, no. 14, pp. 7078–7088, 2008.

[80] K. M. Rogers, K. A. Ealey, J. W. Ritchey, D. H. Black, and R. Eberle, "Pathogenicity of different baboon Herpesvirus papio 2 isolates is characterized by either extreme neurovirulence or complete apathogenicity," *Journal of Virology*, vol. 77, no. 20, pp. 10731–10739, 2003.

[81] B. V. Troan, L. Perelygina, I. Patrusheva et al., "Naturally transmitted herpesvirus papio-2 infection in a black and white colobus monkey," *Journal of the American Veterinary Medical Association*, vol. 231, no. 12, pp. 1878–1883, 2007.

[82] R. Eberle and J. Hilliard, "The simian herpesviruses," *Infectious Agents and Disease*, vol. 4, no. 2, pp. 55–70, 1995.

[83] J. K. Hilliard, D. Black, and R. Eberle, "Simian alphaherpesviruses and their relation to the human herpes simplex viruses," *Archives of Virology*, vol. 109, no. 1-2, pp. 83–102, 1989.

[84] D. Katz, J. K. Hilliard, R. Eberle, and S. L. Lipper, "ELISA for detection of group-common and virus-specific antibodies in human and simian sera induced by herpes simplex and related simian viruses," *Journal of Virological Methods*, vol. 14, no. 2, pp. 99–109, 1986.

[85] Y. Ueda, I. Tagaya, and K. Shiroki, "Immunological relationship between herpes simplex virus and B virus," *Archiv für die Gesamte Virusforschung*, vol. 24, no. 3, pp. 231–244, 1968.

[86] E. A. Boulter, S. S. Kalter, R. L. Heberling, J. E. Guajardo, and T. L. Lester, "A comparison of neutralization tests for the detection of antibodies to Herpesvirus simiae (monkey B virus)," *Laboratory Animals*, vol. 32, no. 2, pp. 150–152, 1982.

[87] R. Eberle, D. Black, and J. K. Hilliard, "Relatedness of glycoproteins expressed on the surface of simian herpesvirus virions and infected cells to specific HSV glycoproteins," *Archives of Virology*, vol. 109, no. 3-4, pp. 233–252, 1989.

[88] R. D. Henkel, H. M. McClure, P. Krug, D. Katz, and J. K. Hilliard, "Serological evidence of alpha herpesvirus infection in sooty mangabeys," *Journal of Medical Primatology*, vol. 31, no. 3, pp. 120–128, 2002.

[89] B. Roizman, "The Herpesviruses. Albert S. Kaplan, Ed. Academic Press, New York, 1973. xvi, 740 pp., illus. %1," *Science*, vol. 184, no. 4143, pp. 1277-1278, 1974.

[90] S.-W. Mou, J. K. Hilliard, C.-H. Song, and R. Eberle, "Comparison of the primate alphaherpesviruses - I. Characterization of two Herpesviruses from spider monkeys and squirrel monkeys and viral polypeptides synthesized in infected cells," *Archives of Virology*, vol. 91, no. 1-2, pp. 117–133, 1986.

[91] D. J. McGeoch, F. J. Rixon, and A. J. Davison, "Topics in herpesvirus genomics and evolution," *Virus Research*, vol. 117, no. 1, pp. 90–104, 2006.

[92] A. Severini, S. D. Tyler, G. A. Peters, D. Black, and R. Eberle, "Genome sequence of a chimpanzee herpesvirus and its relation to other primate alphaherpesviruses," *Archives of Virology*, vol. 158, no. 8, pp. 1825–1828, 2013.

[93] J. O. Wertheim, M. D. Smith, D. M. Smith, K. Scheffler, and S. L. Kosakovsky Pond, "Evolutionary origins of human herpes simplex viruses 1 and 2," *Molecular Biology and Evolution*, vol. 31, no. 9, pp. 2356–2364, 2014.

[94] A. Arvin, G. Campadelli-Fiume, E. Mocarski et al., "Human herpesviruses: Biology, therapy, and immunoprophylaxis," *Human Herpesviruses: Biology, Therapy, and Immunoprophylaxis*, pp. 1–1410, 2007.

[95] J. K. Hilliard, R. Eberle, S. L. Lipper, R. M. Munoz, and S. A. Weiss, "Herpesvirus simiae (B virus): Replication of the virus and identification of viral polypeptides in infected cells," *Archives of Virology*, vol. 93, no. 3-4, pp. 185–198, 1987.

[96] R. N. Hull, "B virus vaccine," *Laboratory Animal Science*, vol. 21, pp. 1068–1071, 1971.

[97] K. Ohsawa, D. H. Black, H. Sato, and R. Eberle, "Sequence and genetic arrangement of the Us region of the monkey B virus (Cercopithecine Herpesvirus 1) genome and comparison with the Us regions of other primate herpesviruses," *Journal of Virology*, vol. 76, no. 3, pp. 1516–1520, 2002.

[98] K. Ohsawa, D. H. Black, H. Sato, K. Rogers, and R. Eberle, "Sequence and genetic arrangement of the UL region of the monkey B virus (Cercopithecine herpesvirus 1) genome and comparison with the UL region of other primate herpesviruses," *Archives of Virology*, vol. 148, no. 5, pp. 989–997, 2003.

[99] L. Perelygina, L. Zhu, H. Zurkuhlen, R. Mills, M. Borodovsky, and J. K. Hilliard, "Complete sequence and comparative analysis of the genome of herpes B virus (Cercopithecine herpesvirus 1) from a rhesus monkey," *Journal of Virology*, vol. 77, no. 11, pp. 6167–6177, 2003.

[100] K. Ohsawa, D. Black, M. Ohsawa, and R. Eberle, "Genome sequence of a pathogenic isolate of monkey B virus (species Macacine herpesvirus 1)," *Archives of Virology*, vol. 159, no. 10, pp. 2819–2821, 2014.

[101] K. Ohsawa, D. H. Black, R. Torii, H. Sato, and R. Eberle, "Detection of a unique genotype of monkey B virus (Cercopithecine herpesvirus 1) indigenous to native Japanese macaques (Macaca fuscata)," *Comparative Medicine*, vol. 52, no. 6, pp. 555–559, 2002.

[102] A. L. Smith, D. H. Black, and R. Eberle, "Molecular evidence for distinct genotypes of monkey B virus (herpesvirus simiae) which are related to the macaque host species," *Journal of Virology*, vol. 72, no. 11, pp. 9224–9232, 1998.

[103] M. A. Amen and A. Griffiths, "Identification and expression analysis of herpes B virus-encoded small RNAs," *Journal of Virology*, vol. 85, no. 14, pp. 7296–7311, 2011.

[104] M. I. Besecker, M. E. Harden, G. Li, X.-J. Wang, and A. Griffiths, "Discovery of herpes B virus-encoded MicroRNAs," *Journal of Virology*, vol. 83, no. 7, pp. 3413–3416, 2009.

[105] S. D. Tyler, G. A. Peters, and A. Severini, "Complete genome sequence of cercopithecine herpesvirus 2 (SA8) and comparison with other simplex viruses," *Virology*, vol. 331, no. 2, pp. 429–440, 2005.

[106] S. D. Tyler and A. Severini, "The complete genome sequence of herpesvirus papio 2 (Cercopithecine herpesvirus 16) shows evidence of recombination events among various progenitor herpesviruses," *Journal of Virology*, vol. 80, no. 3, pp. 1214–1221, 2006.

[107] R. Eberle and D. H. Black, Molecular aspects of monkey B virus and implications for diagnostic test development, Recent Res Devel Virol, vol. 1, pp. 85-94, 1999.

[108] L. Perelygina, H. Zurkuhlen, I. Patrusheva, and J. K. Hilliard, "Identification of a herpes B virus-specific glycoprotein D immunodominant epitope recognized by natural and foreign hosts," *The Journal of Infectious Diseases*, vol. 186, no. 4, pp. 453–461, 2002.

[109] L. Perelygina, I. Patrusheva, S. Hombaiah et al., "Production of herpes B virus recombinant glycoproteins and evaluation of their diagnostic potential," *Journal of Clinical Microbiology*, vol. 43, no. 2, pp. 620–628, 2005.

[110] M. J. Slomka, L. Harrington, C. Arnold, J. P. N. Norcott, and D. W. G. Brown, "Complete nucleotide sequence of the herpesvirus simiae glycoprotein G gene and its expression as an immunogenic fusion protein in bacteria," *Journal of General Virology*, vol. 76, no. 9, pp. 2161–2168, 1995.

[111] K. Tanabayashi, R. Mukai, and A. Yamada, "Detection of B virus antibody in monkey sera using glycoprotein D expressed in mammalian cells," *Journal of Clinical Microbiology*, vol. 39, no. 9, pp. 3025–3030, 2001.

[112] R. L. Heberling and S. S. Kalter, "A dot-immunobinding assay on nitrocellulose with psoralen inactivated Herpesvirus simiae (B virus).," *Laboratory animal science Chicago*, vol. 37, no. 3, pp. 304–308, 1987.

[113] D. Katz, W. Shi, P. W. Krug, R. Henkel, H. McClure, and J. K. Hilliard, "Antibody cross-reactivity of alphaherpesviruses as mirrored in naturally infected primates," *Archives of Virology*, vol. 147, no. 5, pp. 929–941, 2002.

[114] D. Katz, W. Shi, P. W. Krug, and J. K. Hilliard, "Alphaherpesvirus antigen quantitation to optimize the diagnosis of herpes B virus infection," *Journal of Virological Methods*, vol. 103, no. 1, pp. 15–25, 2002.

[115] G. L. Van Hoosier Jr. and J. L. Melnick, "Neutralizing antibodies in human sera to Herpesvirus simiae (B virus)," *Texas Reports on Biology and Medicine*, vol. 19, pp. 376–380, 1961.

[116] D. Katz, W. Shi, M. S. Gowda et al., "Identification of unique B virus (Macacine Herpesvirus 1) epitopes of zoonotic and macaque isolates using monoclonal antibodies," *PLoS ONE*, vol. 12, no. 8, Article ID e0182355, 2017.

[117] I. Patrusheva, L. Perelygina, I. Torshin, J. LeCher, and J. Hilliard, "B virus (Macacine herpesvirus 1) divergence: Variations in glycoprotein D from clinical and laboratory isolates diversify virus entry strategies," *Journal of Virology*, vol. 90, no. 20, pp. 9420–9432, 2016.

[118] E. Linwood Blewett, J. T. Saliki, and R. Eberle, "Development of a competitive ELISA for detection of primates infected with monkey B virus (Herpesvirus simiae)," *Journal of Virological Methods*, vol. 77, no. 1, pp. 59–67, 1999.

[119] L. M. Cropper, D. N. Lees, R. Patt, I. R. Sharp, and D. Brown, "Monoclonal antibodies for the identification of herpesvirus simiae (B virus)," *Archives of Virology*, vol. 123, no. 3-4, pp. 267–277, 1992.

[120] H. P. Huemer, C. Wechselberger, A. M. Bennett, D. Falke, and L. Harrington, "Cloning and expression of the complement receptor glycoprotein C from Herpesvirus simiae (herpes B virus): Protection from complement-mediated cell lysis," *Journal of General Virology*, vol. 84, no. 5, pp. 1091–1100, 2003.

[121] Q. Fan, M. Amen, M. Harden, A. Severini, A. Griffiths, and R. Longnecker, "Herpes B virus utilizes human nectin-1 but not HVEM or PILRα for cell-cell fusion and virus entry," *Journal of Virology*, vol. 86, no. 8, pp. 4468–4476, 2012.

[122] L. Li, Z. Qiu, Y. Li et al., "Herpes B virus gD interaction with its human receptor - An in silico analysis approach," *Theoretical Biology and Medical Modelling*, vol. 11, no. 1, article no. 27, 2014.

[123] C. Boutell and R. D. Everett, "Regulation of alphaherpesvirus infections by the ICP0 family of proteins," *Journal of General Virology*, vol. 94, no. 3, pp. 465–481, 2013.

[124] K. M. Rogers, R. F. Wolf, G. L. White, and R. Eberle, "Experimental infection of baboons (Papio cynocephalus anubis) with apathogenic and neurovirulent subtypes of Herpesvirus papio 2," *Comparative Medicine*, vol. 55, no. 5, pp. 425–430, 2005.

[125] D. Black, K. Ohsawa, S. Tyler, L. Maxwell, and R. Eberle, "A single viral gene determines lethal cross-species neurovirulence of baboon herpesvirus HVP2," *Virology*, vol. 452-453, pp. 86–94, 2014.

[126] T. Todo, "Active immunotherapy oncolytic virus therapy using HSV-1," *Advances in Experimental Medicine and Biology*, vol. 746, pp. 178–186, 2012.

[127] J. Conner, J. Macfarlane, H. Lankinen, and H. Marsden, "The unique N terminus of the herpes simplex virus type 1 large subunit is not required for ribonucleotide reductase activity," *Journal of General Virology*, vol. 73, no. 1, pp. 103–112, 1992.

[128] D. Lembo and W. Brune, "Tinkering with a viral ribonucleotide reductase," *Trends in Biochemical Sciences*, vol. 34, no. 1, pp. 25–32, 2009.

[129] H. Guo, S. Omoto, P. A. Harris et al., "Herpes simplex virus suppresses necroptosis in human cells," *Cell Host & Microbe*, vol. 17, no. 2, pp. 243–251, 2015.

[130] Z. Huang, S.-Q. Wu, Y. Liang et al., "RIP1/RIP3 binding to HSV-1 ICP6 initiates necroptosis to restrict virus propagation in mice," *Cell Host & Microbe*, vol. 17, no. 2, pp. 229–242, 2015.

[131] X. Wang, Y. Li, S. Liu et al., "Direct activation of RIP3/MLKL-dependent necrosis by herpes simplex virus 1 (HSV-1) protein

ICP6 triggers host antiviral defense," *Proceedings of the National Acadamy of Sciences of the United States of America*, vol. 111, no. 43, pp. 15438–15443, 2014.

[132] C. A. Bolovan, N. M. Sawtell, and R. L. Thompson, "ICP34.5 mutants of herpes simplex virus type 1 strain 17syn+ are attenuated for neurovirulence in mice and for replication in confluent primary mouse embryo cell cultures," *Journal of Virology*, vol. 68, no. 1, pp. 48–55, 1994.

[133] J. Chou, E. R. Kern, R. J. Whitley, and B. Roizman, "Mapping of herpes simplex virus-1 neurovirulence to γ134.5, a gene nonessential for growth in culture," *Science*, vol. 250, no. 4985, pp. 1262–1266, 1990.

[134] L. Y. Lee and P. A. Schaffer, "A virus with a mutation in the ICP4-binding site in the L/ST promoter of herpes simplex virus type 1, but not a virus with a mutation in open reading frame P, exhibits cell-type-specific expression of γ134.5 transcripts and latency-associated transcripts," *Journal of Virology*, vol. 72, no. 5, pp. 4250–4264, 1998.

[135] N. S. Markovitz, D. Baunoch, and B. Roizman, "The range and distribution of murine central nervous system cells infected with the γ134.5- Mutant of herpes simplex virus 1," *Journal of Virology*, vol. 71, no. 7, pp. 5560–5569, 1997.

[136] B. Roizman and N. Markovitz, "Herpes simplex virus virulence: the functions of the gamma (1)34.5 gene," *Journal of NeuroVirology*, vol. 3 Suppl, p. S1, 1997.

[137] R. J. Whitley, E. R. Kern, S. Chatterjee, J. Chou, and B. Roizman, "Replication, establishment of latency, and induced reactivation of herpes simplex virus γ1 34.5 deletion mutants in rodent models," *The Journal of Clinical Investigation*, vol. 91, no. 6, pp. 2837–2843, 1993.

[138] D. Phelan, E. R. Barrozo, and D. C. Bloom, "HSV1 latent transcription and non-coding RNA: A critical retrospective," *Journal of Neuroimmunology*, vol. 308, pp. 65–101, 2017.

[139] G. Cheng, M.-E. Brett, and B. He, "Val193 and Phe195 of the γ134.5 protein of herpes simplex virus 1 are required for viral resistance to interferon-α/β," *Virology*, vol. 290, no. 1, pp. 115–120, 2001.

[140] X. Jing, M. Cerveny, K. Yang, and B. He, "Replication of herpes simplex virus 1 depends on the γ134. 5 functions that facilitate virus response to interferon and egress in the different stages of productive infection," *Journal of Virology*, vol. 78, no. 14, pp. 7653–7666, 2004.

[141] J. Trgovcich, D. Johnson, and B. Roizman, "Cell surface major histocompatibility complex class II proteins are regulated by the products of the γ34.5 and UL41 genes of herpes simplex virus 1," *Journal of Virology*, vol. 76, no. 14, pp. 6974–6986, 2002.

[142] J. Chou and B. Roizman, "The γ134.5 gene of herpes simplex virus 1 precludes neuroblastoma cells from triggering total shutoff of protein synthesis characteristic of programed cell death in neuronal cells," *Proceedings of the National Acadamy of Sciences of the United States of America*, vol. 89, no. 8, pp. 3266–3270, 1992.

[143] J. Chou and B. Roizman, "Herpes simplex virus 1 γ134.5 gene function, which blocks the host response to infection, maps in the homologous domain of the genes expressed during growth arrest and DNA damage," *Proceedings of the National Acadamy of Sciences of the United States of America*, vol. 91, no. 12, pp. 5247–5251, 1994.

[144] J. Chou, J.-J. Chen, M. Gross, and B. Roizman, "Association of a Mr 90,000 phosphoprotein with protein kinase PKR in cells exhibiting enhanced phosphorylation of translation initiation factor eIF-2α and premature shutoff of protein synthesis after

infection with γ134.5- mutants of herpes simplex virus," *Proceedings of the National Acadamy of Sciences of the United States of America*, vol. 92, no. 23, pp. 10516–10520, 1995.

[145] P. A. M. Gobeil and D. A. Leib, "Herpes simplex virus gamma34.5 interferes with autophagosome maturation and antigen presentation in dendritic cells," *mBio*, vol. 3, no. 5, pp. e00267–e00212, 2012.

[146] B. He, M. Gross, and B. Roizman, "The γ134.5 protein of herpes simplex virus 1 complexes with protein phosphatase 1α to dephosphorylate the α subunit of the eukaryotic translation initiation factor 2 and preclude the shutoff of protein synthesis by double-stranded RNA-activated protein kinase," *Proceedings of the National Acadamy of Sciences of the United States of America*, vol. 94, no. 3, pp. 843–848, 1997.

[147] B. He, M. Gross, and B. Roizman, "The γ134.5 Protein of herpes simplex virus I has the structural and functional attributes of a protein phosphatase I regulatory subunit and is present in a high molecular weight complex with the enzyme in infected cells," *The Journal of Biological Chemistry*, vol. 273, no. 33, pp. 20737–20743, 1998.

[148] A. Simmons and A. A. Nash, "Zosteriform spread of herpes simplex virus as a model of recrudescence and its use to investigate the role of immune cells in prevention of recurrent disease," *Journal of Virology*, vol. 52, no. 3, pp. 816–821, 1984.

[149] Y. Tsalenchuck, T. Tzur, I. Steiner, and A. Panet, "Different modes of herpes simplex virus type 1 spread in brain and skin tissues," *Journal of NeuroVirology*, vol. 20, no. 1, pp. 18–27, 2014.

[150] L. M. Wakim, C. M. Jones, T. Gebhardt, C. M. Preston, and F. R. Carbone, "CD8+ T-cell attenuation of cutaneous herpes simplex virus infection reduces the average viral copy number of the ensuing latent infection," *Immunology & Cell Biology*, vol. 86, no. 8, pp. 666–675, 2008.

[151] M. Yamada, Y. Arao, F. Uno, and S. Nii, "Mechanism of Differences in Pathogenicity between Two Variants of a Laboratory Strain of Herpes Simplex Virus Type 1," *Microbiology and Immunology*, vol. 30, no. 12, pp. 1259–1270, 1986.

[152] Y. Minamishima and Y. Eizuru, "Susceptibility of Primate Diploid Cells to Human Herpesviruses," *Microbiology and Immunology*, vol. 21, no. 11, pp. 667–671, 1977.

[153] S. Nii, "Abortive infection of LLC-MK2 cells by Herpes simplex virus.," *Biken Journal, Journal of the Research Institute for Microbial Diseases*, vol. 15, no. 1, pp. 43–47, 1972.

[154] M. Yamada, "Replication of herpes simplex virus in two cell systems derived from rhesus monkeys," *Biken Journal, Journal of the Research Institute for Microbial Diseases*, vol. 26, no. 1, pp. 35–47, 1983.

[155] L. Perelygina, I. Patrusheva, M. Vasireddi, N. Brock, and J. Hilliard, "Virus (Macacine herpesvirus 1) glycoprotein D is functional but dispensable for virus entry into macaque and human skin cells," *Journal of Virology*, vol. 89, no. 10, pp. 5515–5524, 2015.

[156] M. L. van de Weijer, R. D. Luteijn, and E. J. H. J. Wiertz, "Viral immune evasion: Lessons in MHC class I antigen presentation," *Seminars in Immunology*, vol. 27, no. 2, pp. 125–137, 2015.

[157] M. Vasireddi and J. Hilliard, "Herpes B virus, macacine herpesvirus 1, breaks simplex virus tradition via major histocompatibility complex class I expression in cells from human and macaque hosts," *Journal of Virology*, vol. 86, no. 23, pp. 12503–12511, 2012.

[158] M. Vasireddi and J. K. Hilliard, "Regulation of PI3K/Akt dependent apoptotic markers during b virus infection of human

and macaque fibroblasts," *PLoS ONE*, vol. 12, no. 5, Article ID e0178314, 2017.

[159] B. Roizman, G. Zhou, and T. Du, "Checkpoints in productive and latent infections with herpes simplex virus 1: conceptualization of the issues.," *Journal of NeuroVirology*, vol. 17, no. 6, pp. 512–517, 2011.

[160] B. Roizman and R. J. Whitley, "An inquiry into the molecular basis of HSV latency and reactivation," *Annual Review of Microbiology*, vol. 67, pp. 355–374, 2013.

[161] S. Efstathiou and C. M. Preston, "Towards an understanding of the molecular basis of herpes simplex virus latency," *Virus Research*, vol. 111, no. 2, pp. 108–119, 2005.

[162] W. A. Blyth, D. A. Harbour, and T. J. Hill, "Pathogenesis of zosteriform spread of herpes simplex virus in the mouse," *Journal of General Virology*, vol. 65, no. 9, pp. 1477–1486, 1984.

[163] B. Roizman and G. Zhou, "The 3 facets of regulation of herpes simplex virus gene expression: A critical inquiry," *Virology*, vol. 479-480, pp. 562–567, 2015.

[164] T. Kramer and L. W. Enquist, "Directional spread of alphaherpesviruses in the nervous system," *Viruses*, vol. 5, no. 2, pp. 678–707, 2013.

6

Molecular Characterization of Chicken Anemia Virus Circulating in Chicken Flocks in Egypt

Mohammed AboElkhair,[1,2] Alaa G. Abd El-Razak,[3] and Abd Elnaby Y. Metwally[4]

[1] Department of Virology, Faculty of Veterinary Medicine, University of Sadat City, Sadat City 32897, Minoufiya, Egypt
[2] Research Center for Animal Hygiene and Food Safety, Obihiro University of Agriculture and Veterinary Medicine, Inada 2-11, Hokkaido, Obihiro 080-8555, Japan
[3] Department of Bird and Rabbits Medicine, Faculty of Veterinary Medicine, University of Sadat City, Sadat City 32897, Minoufiya, Egypt
[4] Animal Health Research Institute, Kafr El Sheikh Provincial Laboratory, Kafr El Sheikh, Egypt

Correspondence should be addressed to Mohammed AboElkhair; maboelkhair2004@yahoo.com

Academic Editor: Finn S. Pedersen

Introduction. Although many previous studies reported detection of chicken anemia virus (CAV) in Egypt since 1990, genomic characterization of this circulating CAV has not been published. In the present study, four nucleotide sequences of detected CAV were genetically characterized. *Methods.* These nucleotide sequences were obtained from commercial chicken flocks in two different locations of Egypt during 2010. The target region for sequencing was 675 bp nucleotide of partial coding region of VP1 protein. The nucleotide and deduced amino acid sequences of the detected CAV were aligned and compared to worldwide CAV isolates including commonly used vaccine strains. Phylogenetic analysis of these sequences was also carried out. *Results.* Our results showed that all the Egyptian CAV sequences were grouped in one group with viruses from diverse geographic regions. This group is characterized by amino acids profile ^{75}I, ^{97}L, ^{139}Q, and ^{144}Q in VP1. The phylogenetic and amino acid analyses of deduced amino acid indicated that the detected CAV sequences differ from CAV vaccine strains. *Conclusion.* This is the first report that describes molecular characterization of circulating CAV in Egypt. The study showed that the detected CAV, in Egypt are field viruses and unrelated to vaccine strains.

1. Introduction

Chicken anemia virus (CAV) is an economically important pathogen with a worldwide distribution. CAV is a small DNA virus with a closed circular, negative, single stranded DNA genome. It belongs to genus *Gyrovirus* of family Circoviridae [1]. The genome consists of three partially overlapping open reading frames encoding three viral proteins: VP1 (51.6 kDa), the major viral capsid protein, VP2 (24 kDa), a novel dual specificity protein phosphatase [2] that also probably acts as scaffolding protein during virion assembly [3], and VP3 (13.6 kDa), also called apoptin, which has been shown to have apoptotic activity in transformed cell lines [4]. VP1 shows the highest nucleotide variability; therefore, it is usually used for genetic characterization and molecular studies of CAV [5, 6].

Infection with CAV constitutes a serious economic threat, especially to the broiler industry and the producers of specific pathogen free (SPF) eggs. The clinical signs are mainly noticed in young chicks of 10–14 days of age, which acquire the infection vertically. Chickens older than 2-3 weeks of age are also susceptible to infection but only develop a subclinical disease evidenced by poor vaccine response [7]. The disease is characterized by aplastic anemia and generalized lymphoid atrophy with concomitant immunosuppression and frequent association with secondary viral, bacterial, parasitic, or fungal infections [7]. Mortalities and morbidities due to CAV infection may reach 55% and 80%, respectively [8].

In Egypt, many previous publications have reported detection of CAV in chicken population (cited in [9–11]); however, genomic characterization from these isolates has not been published. The aim of this study was to identify CAV obtained from farms with problems associated with immunosuppression and to determine their relationship with vaccine and other reference strains.

TABLE 1: Samples collected for the current study.

Province	Numbers of the flocks	Type of samples	Age of the flock
Sharkia	Three	Tissue homogenates	12–35 days
Kafr El Sheikh	One	Tissue homogenate	25 days
Minoufiya	One	Liver	30 days

2. Materials and Methods

2.1. Samples Collection. Tissue homogenates were collected from Sharkia and Kafr El Sheikh provinces. The homogenates contained thymus loops, bone marrow, bursa of Fabricius, liver, spleen, and intestines samples. Tissue homogenates of Sharkia province were collected from three commercial broiler flocks. The flocks ranged in age from 12 to 35 days representing different breeds and localities in the province. Tissue homogenate of Kafr El Sheikh Province was only collected from one commercial broiler flock aged 25 days. Five liver samples were also collected from a commercial broiler chicken flock aged 30 days from Minoufiya province. All flocks of collected samples were showing clinical signs and lesions indicative of CAV infection [10]. The places, numbers of flocks, and age of flocks of selected samples are listed in Table 1. All samples were stored frozen at −70°C for subsequent DNA extraction.

2.2. Sample Preparation. Tissues were homogenized in a mortar with sterile sand and phosphate-buffered saline. Cell debris and sand were eliminated by centrifugation, and the supernatants were collected and stored at −70°C.

2.3. DNA Extraction and PCR Amplification. DNA was extracted from the supernatant of liver and tissue homogenates by QIAamp DNA mini kit (Qiagen Inc., Valencia, CA) according to the manufacturer instructions. The oligonucleotide primers 5′-GAC TGT AAG ATG GCA AGA CGA GCT C-3′ and 5′-GGC TGA AGG ATC CCT CAT TC-3′ were used to amplify a 675 bp DNA fragment of Vp1 [12]; from nucleotides 823 to 1498, numbering is corresponding to the Del-Ros strain (GenBank AF313470). The PCR assay was performed in a final volume of 50 μL Reddy-Mix, 18 μL PCR grade water, 1 μL of each primer, and 5 μL template. The amplification was performed under the following conditions: one cycle of initial denaturation step at 95°C for 15 min followed by 30 cycles of 95°C for 1 min, 56°C for 1 min, and 72°C for 1 min representing denaturation, annealing, and extension steps, respectively, and finally one cycle of final extension step at 72°C for 5 min. The amplified products were analyzed using electrophoresis unit. They were loaded to 1% agarose stained by ethidium bromide, visualized under 304 nm ultraviolet (UV Transilluminator, Major Science), and photographed by a gel documentation system using Canon power-shot camera.

2.4. Nucleotide Sequence Analysis. Sequencing was performed in both directions with virus specific primers. Sequences were analyzed using BioEdit program [13]. This program was also used to read the sequencing electropherograms to exclude nucleotide ambiguity. The phylogenetic analysis was based on the deduced amino acids of 579 nucleotides encompassing hypervariable region of vp1. The detected sequences were compared with others deposited in GenBank by multiple alignment with the Clustal W included in Bioedit software. Phylogenetic relationships were evaluated by the Neighbor Joining method present in the MEGA version 6 software [14] with 1,000 bootstrap replications. Sequence data were submitted to GenBank with accession numbers KJ955377 to KJ955380 for the Egy-1 CAV to the Egy-4 CAV, respectively.

2.5. Attempted Isolation of the Virus. Isolation of CAV from the tissue homogenate of the PCR-positive samples was attempted in embryonated SPF eggs through yolk sac inoculation [7]. Tissue samples were prepared according to [15]. Briefly, the homogenate was mixed with an equal volume of chloroform for 15 min in a shaker. Three times of repeated freezing and thawing were applied and then the homogenate was centrifuged for 20 min at 3000 rpm. The supernatants were used for SPF egg inoculation. Each homogenate was injected in 5 SPF eggs (100 μL/egg). After 14 days, all embryos tissues were homogenized. DNA extraction and PCR amplification were carried out from the supernatant of these tissue homogenates in the same condition as described above. The whole isolation attempt was repeated once.

3. Results

3.1. Samples and Clinical Signs. All affected birds were at age of 12 to 35 days. All affected flocks showed signs of anemia, generalized weakness, depression, pale comb and wattles, growth retardation, and high mortality rates. The postmortem examination revealed pale and enlarged liver and spleen, mild to severe thymus atrophy, and atrophied bursa of Fabricius.

3.2. PCR Amplification. Analysis of PCR amplification of the extracted DNA from tissue samples by agarose gel electrophoresis indicated DNA bands of corrected size as expected with a length of 675 bp. The authenticity of PCR amplification was confirmed by the nucleotide sequencing. All of the liver samples from the flock in Minoufiya province showed negative results. Also, all SPF embryo homogenates were PCR negative.

3.3. Nucleotide Sequence Analysis. The four nucleotide sequences of detected CAV displayed a limited diversity. Total nucleotide variation among the sequences ranged from

TABLE 2: Nucleotide and deduced amino acid difference and identity matrices among Egyptian CAV sequences.

(a) Nucleotide sequence difference count matrix

	Egy-1 CAV	Egy-2 CAV	Egy-3 CAV	Egy-4 CAV
Egy-1 CAV	ID			
Egy-2 CAV	19	ID		
Egy-3 CAV	29	22	ID	
Egy-4 CAV	1	18	28	ID

(b) Amino acid sequence identity matrix

	Egy-1 CAV	Egy-2 CAV	Egy-3 CAV	Egy-4 CAV
Egy-1 CAV	ID			
Egy-2 CAV	99.4%	ID		
Egy-3 CAV	98.9%	99.4%	ID	
Egy-4 CAV	99.4%	100%	99.4%	ID

1 to 29 nucleotides (Table 2(a)). They showed 94.9–99.8% similarity between them. Egy-3 CAV sequence showed the lowest similarity 94.9–96.2% with the other CAV sequences. Egy-1 CAV and Egy-4 CAV showed the highest similarity 99.8%. Compared to isolates from other geographical places around the world, two Egyptian CAV sequences (Egy-1 CAV and Egy-4 CAV) were found to have maximum homology with an Argentinean isolate, Arg0021-3, by 99% and 100%, respectively, whereas the Egy-2 CAV showed 98% homology with a Cameroon strain, CMR09-731, and the Egy-3 CAV was 99% similar to a Cameroon strain, CMR09-485.

3.4. Amino Acids Sequence Analysis. The four detected CAV sequences showed 98.9% to 100% identity with each other at the level of amino acid sequence (Table 2 (b)). The maximum difference was between Egy-3 CAV and Egy-1 CAV. These two sequences (Egy-3 CAV and Egy-1 CAV) varied only in two amino acids. The deduced amino acid sequences of the Egyptian CAV sequences and some vaccine strains were aligned. The analysis was carried out to outline the shared amino acid residues between detected viruses and some vaccine strains (Cux-1, Del-Ros, and 26PA) (Table 3). Also, other strains from all over the world were included. The Egyptian CAV sequences showed consensus amino acid sequence at positions 75, 97, 139, and 144 of VP1. At position 22, however, Egy-1 CAV, Egy-2 CAV, and Egy-4 CAV had histidine (H), but Egy-3 CAV had asparagine (N) instead of H. As shown in Table 3, all Egyptian CAV sequences showed sequence difference with regard to vaccine strains. At position 75, the Egyptian CAV had isoleucine (I) instead of valine (V), at position 97, they had leucine (L) instead of methionine (M), at position 139, they had glutamine (Q) instead of lysine (K), and, at position 144, they also had Q instead of glutamic acid (E), N, or aspartic acid (D).

3.5. Phylogenetic Analysis. The deduced amino acid sequences of the partial vp1 sequence of Egyptian CAV were compared with those of other sequences deposited in the GenBank. All detected CAVs in Egypt were grouped together

in one group (Figure 1). The topology of the phylogenetic tree revealed the presence of three groups that were defined in this study as I, II, and III. The tree topology also showed that the Egyptian sequences were related to different sequences such as NIE/19.04/118/Nigeria, CMR09-731 and CMR09-485/Cameroon, CL37/Chile, CAV-B/India, AN-China 23/China, C1A-1/USA, Arg0021-3/Argentina, and BD-3/Bangladesh which were classified as group II according to [16]. However, different commonly used vaccine strains, for example, Nobilis P4, Del-Ros, 26PA, and Cux-1, grouped with other sequences in groups I and III (Figure 1).

4. Discussion

It was reported that CAV spread among chicken in Egypt since the early 1980s when several outbreaks occurred in many breeds [9]. The presence of CAV was confirmed by detection of both CAV antibodies and genome in both meat and egg type chicken flocks [9–11]. However, the molecular characterization from these viruses has not been published. Currently, it is so important to characterize circulating CAVs circulating in Egypt to improve methods of virus control and to determine the relationship of circulating CAV with vaccine strains and other CAV strains. Particularly, a large number of isolates have been fully or partially sequenced. These isolates were obtained in many countries, for example, Bangladesh, Brazil, China, Malaysia, Slovenia, the United States [1], and Argentina [6]. Also, a number of CAV sequences have been reported in African continent, for example, Nigeria [5], Central African Republic, and Cameroon [17], and more recently from South Africa [18]. Comparison of all sequence data indicates that these isolates can be divided into 3 or 4 distinct groups [1]. Vp1 gene sequence is commonly used to determine the relationship of different CAV isolates due to the fact that most of the amino acid substitutions between isolates lie in vp1 gene and more specifically in the N-terminal half of vp1 gene [6, 19]. Moreover, a hypervariable region spanning from amino acid positions 139 to 151 in Vp1 was identified [20]. Islam et al. [16] found that five of 16 commonly variable amino acid positions of the whole vp1 fall within this small region. Therefore, in the present study, we used partial sequencing of vp1 including hypervariable region as a tool to study the molecular characterization of Egyptian CAV sequences. Although the Egyptian detected CAVs showed up to 5.1% difference at the nucleotide sequence level (Table 2(b)), they are almost identical at the amino acid level. This indicated that they differed only by silent mutations.

According to a previous study [16], CAV isolates can be grouped into three different groups based on the amino acid residues at positions of 75, 97, 139, and 144 of amino acid sequence of VP1 protein. In the current study, all detected CAV sequences showed the same amino acid profiles [75]I, [97]L, [139]Q, and [144]Q. Furthermore, the phylogenetic analysis indicated that all detected Egyptian CAV sequences belong to group II based on Islam et al. classification [16]. The members of this group are from very diverse geographic origins. Also,

TABLE 3: Amino substitution in VP1 sequence of CAV isolates.

Isolate	Amino acid positions									
	22	48	**75**	83	**97**	125	**139**	141	**144**	157
Consensus	H	A	V	I	M	I	K	Q	Q	V
Egy-1 CAV/Egypt	·	·	I	·	L	·	Q	·	·	·
Egy-2 CAV/Egypt	·	·	I	·	L	·	Q	·	·	·
Egy-3 CAV/Egypt	N	·	I	·	L	·	Q	·	·	·
Egy-4 CAV/Egypt	·	·	I	·	L	·	Q	·	·	·
Cux-1 M Germany	·	·	·	·	·	·	·	·	D	·
Cux-1 N Germany	·	·	·	·	·	·	·	·	D	·
Del-Ros/USA	·	·	·	·	·	·	·	·	N	·
ConnB/USA	·	·	·	·	·	·	·	·	E	·
26PA/USA	·	·	·	·	·	·	·	·	E	M
SMSC-1/Malaysia	·	·	I	·	L	·	·	·	·	·
CIA-1/USA	N	·	I	·	L	·	Q	·	·	·
A2/Japan	·	·	·	·	·	·	·	E	E	M
AF448446/China	·	·	·	·	·	·	·	·	E	·
BD-3/Bangladesh	·	·	I	·	L	·	Q	·	·	·
NIE/19.04/118/Nigeria	·	·	I	·	L	·	Q	·	·	·
Isolate704/Australia	·	·	I	·	L	·	Q	·	·	·
ArgA0021-3/Argentina	·	·	I	·	L	·	Q	·	·	·
AN-China 23/China	N	·	I	·	L	·	Q	·	·	·
CMR09-731/Cameroon	·	·	I	·	L	·	Q	·	·	·
CL37/Chile	·	·	I	·	L	·	Q	·	·	·

most of strains isolated from African continent are included in this group.

Interestingly, Egy-3 CAV has a unique amino acid substitution at position 22 which is similar to CIA-1 and AN-China 23 isolates. It had N instead of H at this position. van Santen et al. [21] considered this residue to be important for distinguishing of CAV strains.

It was suggested that the genetic grouping of CAV strains might be related to different biological properties of these strains. Renshaw et al. [20] suggested that ^{139}Q and ^{144}Q could affect the rate of replication or spread of infection in cultured cells. They have proved that presence of these two amino acids is associated with decreased rate of spread in cell culture. Based on this finding, all detected Egyptian CAVs could have a reduced ability to spread in cell culture.

Also, all detected Egyptian CAVs had threonine in position 89 instead of alanine. It was suggested that this substitution is associated with attenuation [5]. Others [22], however, suggested that the previous mutation should be combined with ^{75}I, ^{125}L, ^{141}L, and ^{144}E to produce attenuation. No one of Egyptian detected CAV sequences displayed this combination.

Although the evidence of use of live attenuated CAV vaccines occurring in the Egyptian poultry industry is not readily available, the topology of the phylogenetic tree showed that the CAV Egyptian sequences are in a distant relationship with different vaccine strains commonly used, for example, Nobilis P4, Del-Ros, and Cux-1. All Egyptian CAV sequences are

included in group II, whereas vaccine strains are located in groups I and III.

Failure of isolation of CAV in SPF eggs may be due to the low virus concentration in the inoculum or due to the presence of CAV antibodies in the inoculated SPF eggs. It was reported that SPF eggs might contain CAV antibodies [1]. Also, the failure of detection of CAV DNA in livers of Minoufiya chicken flock could be due to inability of the used primers to amplify the proposed CAV because of mutations within the primer location, as we used in this study only one pair of primer set. It was proposed that mutation in location of the primer could lead to loss of detection of some CAV strains [5].

There are some CAV sequences from Egypt (unpublished report) available in the GenBank with accession numbers HM460879.1 to HM460883.1. However, these sequences shared only around 124 nucleotides of VP1 with our sequence. So, the alignment with our sequences was difficult.

5. Conclusion

This is the first report that describes the molecular characterization of circulating CAV in Egyptian poultry farms. Although the number of samples was limited, our phylogenetic analysis revealed that CAV strains detected in Egypt were in one group that showed similarity to several strains all over the world, particularly to those circulating in African and South American continents. The results presented in this

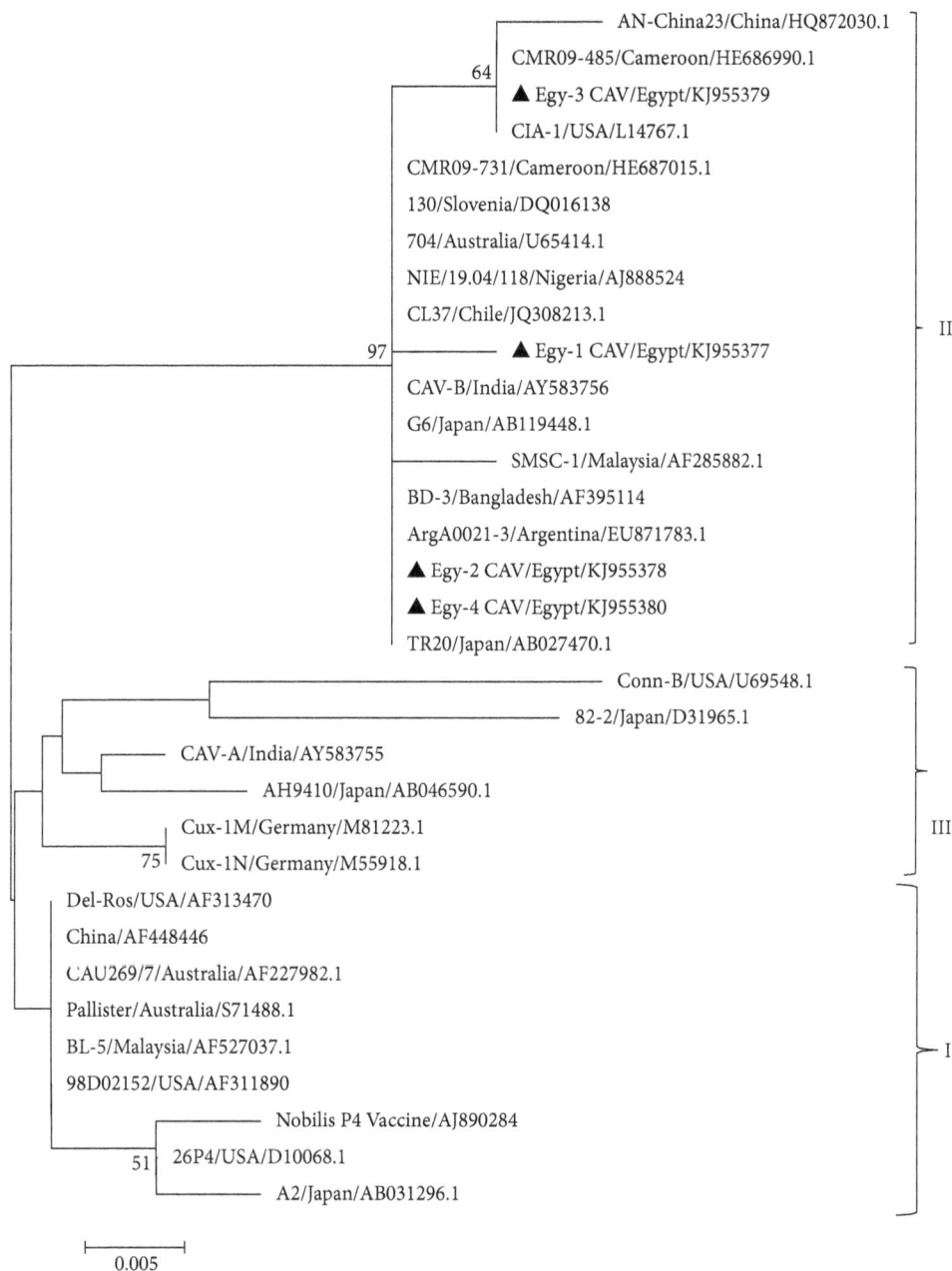

FIGURE 1: Phylogenetic relationship among 33 different CAV isolates based on partial amino acid sequences of VP1. The tree was constructed by the Neighbor Joining algorithm. Relevant nodes with significant bootstrap values (>50%) over 1000 replicates are indicated. Egyptian detected CAVs are marked in black triangles. The horizontal lines indicate the relative nucleotide distance between samples.

study clearly showed that the detected CAV sequences belong to field viruses and are not vaccine strains.

Acknowledgments

The authors would like to thank Dr. Nazim A.A for his assistance in sample collection. Also, they thank Trinuh QD, Obihiro University of Agricultural and Veterinary Medicine, Japan, for his assistance, and El-Naggar RF for her technical assistance.

References

[1] K. A. Schat, "Chicken anemia virus," *Current Topics in Microbiology and Immunology*, vol. 331, pp. 151–183, 2009.

[2] M. A. Peters, D. C. Jackson, B. S. Crabb, and G. F. Browning, "Chicken anemia virus VP2 is a novel dual specificity protein phosphatase," *Journal of Biological Chemistry*, vol. 277, no. 42, pp. 39566–39573, 2002.

[3] M. H. M. Noteborn, C. A. J. Verschueren, G. Koch, and A. J. Van Der Eb, "Simultaneous expression of recombinant baculovirus-encoded chicken anaemia virus (CAV) proteins VP1 and VP2 is required for formation of the CAV-specific neutralizing

epitope," *Journal of General Virology*, vol. 79, no. 12, pp. 3073–3077, 1998.

[4] M. H. M. Noteborn, G. F. de Boer, D. J. van Roozelaar et al., "Characterization of cloned chicken anemia virus DNA that contains all elements for the infectious replication cycle," *Journal of Virology*, vol. 65, no. 6, pp. 3131–3139, 1991.

[5] M. F. Ducatez, A. A. Owoade, J. O. Abiola, and C. P. Muller, "Molecular epidemiology of chicken anemia virus in Nigeria," *Archives of Virology*, vol. 151, no. 1, pp. 97–111, 2006.

[6] M. I. Craig, A. Rimondi, M. Delamer et al., "Molecular characterization of chicken infectious anemia virus circulating in Argentina during 2007," *Avian Diseases*, vol. 53, no. 3, pp. 331–335, 2009.

[7] K. A. Schat, "Chicken infectious anemia," in *Diseases of Poultry*, Y. M. Saif, H. J. Barnes, J. R. Glisson, A. M. Fadly, L. R. McDougald, and E. Swayne, Eds., pp. 182–202, Iowa State University Press, Ames, Iowa, USA, 11th edition, 2003.

[8] G. H. Lai, M. K. Lin, Y. Y. Lien et al., "Expression and characterization of highly antigenic domains of chicken anemia virus viral VP2 and VP3 subunit proteins in a recombinant E. coli for sero-diagnostic applications," *BMC veterinary research*, vol. 9, p. 161, 2013.

[9] H. A. Hussein, M. Z. Sabry, E. A. El-Ibiary, M. El-Safty, and A. I. Abd El-Hady, "Chicken infectious anaemia virus in Egypt: molecular diagnosis by PCR and isolation of the virus from infected flocks," *Arab Journal of Biotechnology*, vol. 5, no. 2, pp. 263–274, 2002.

[10] M. Hegazy, F. M. Abdallah, L. K. Abd-El Samie, and A. A. Nazim, "Chicken infectious anemia virus (CIAV) in broilers and laying hens in Sharkia Province, Egypt," *Journal of American Science*, vol. 6, pp. 752–758, 2010.

[11] M. A. Mohamed, "Chicken infectious anemia status in commercial broiler chickens flocks in assiut-upper Egypt: occurrence, molecular analysis using PCR-RFLP and apoptosis effect on affected tissues," *International Journal of Poultry Science*, vol. 9, no. 6, pp. 591–598, 2010.

[12] D. Todd, K. A. Mawhinney, and M. S. McNulty, "Detection and differentiation of chicken anemia virus isolates by using the polymerase chain reaction," *Journal of Clinical Microbiology*, vol. 30, no. 7, pp. 1661–1666, 1992.

[13] T. A. Hall, "BioEdit: a user-friendly biological sequence alignment editor and analysis for Windows 95/98/NT," *Nucleic Acids Symposium Series*, vol. 41, pp. 95–98, 1999.

[14] K. Tamura, G. Stecher, D. Peterson, A. Filipski, and S. Kumar, "MEGA6: molecular evolutionary genetics analysis version 6.0," *Molecular Biology and Evolution*, vol. 30, no. 12, pp. 2725–2729, 2013.

[15] W. Zhou, B. Shen, B. Yang et al., "Isolation and identification of chicken infectious anemia virus in China," *Avian Diseases*, vol. 41, no. 2, pp. 361–364, 1997.

[16] M. R. Islam, R. Johne, R. Raue, D. Todd, and H. Müller, "Sequence analysis of the full-length cloned DNA of a chicken anaemia virus (CAV) strain from Bangladesh: evidence for genetic grouping of CAV strains based on the deduced VP1 amino acid sequences," *Journal of Veterinary Medicine B*, vol. 49, no. 7, pp. 332–337, 2002.

[17] C. J. Snoeck, G. F. Komoyo, B. P. Mbee et al., "Epidemiology of chicken anemia virus in Central African Republic and Cameroon," *Virology Journal*, vol. 9, pp. 189–197, 2012.

[18] H. E. M. Smuts, "Novel gyroviruses, including chicken anaemia virus, in clinical and chicken samples from South Africa," *Advances in Virology*, vol. 2014, Article ID 321284, 7 pages, 2014.

[19] Z. Hailemariam, A. R. Omar, M. Hair-Bejo, and T. C. Giap, "Detection and characterization of chicken anemia virus from commercial broiler breeder chickens," *Virology Journal*, vol. 5, article 128, 2008.

[20] R. W. Renshaw, C. Soiné, T. Weinkle et al., "A hypervariable region in VP1 of chicken infectious anemia virus mediates rate of spread and cell tropism in tissue culture," *Journal of Virology*, vol. 70, no. 12, pp. 8872–8878, 1996.

[21] V. L. van Santen, L. Li, F. J. Hoerr, and L. H. Lauerman, "Genetic characterization of chicken anemia virus from commercial broiler chickens in Alabama," *Avian Diseases*, vol. 45, no. 2, pp. 373–388, 2001.

[22] D. Todd, A. N. J. Scott, N. W. Ball, B. J. Borghmans, and B. M. Adair, "Molecular basis of the attenuation exhibited by molecularly cloned highly passaged chicken anemia virus isolates," *Journal of Virology*, vol. 76, no. 16, pp. 8472–8474, 2002.

7

Global Status of *Porcine circovirus* Type 2 and its Associated Diseases in Sub-Saharan Africa

Kayode O. Afolabi,[1,2] **Benson C. Iweriebor,**[1,2] **Anthony I. Okoh,**[1,2] **and Larry C. Obi**[1,2,3]

[1]*SAMRC Microbial Water Quality Monitoring Centre, University of Fort Hare, Private Bag X1314,*
  Alice 5700, Eastern Cape, South Africa
[2]*Applied and Environmental Microbiology Research Group (AEMREG), Department of Biochemistry and Microbiology,*
  University of Fort Hare, Private Bag X1314, Alice 5700, Eastern Cape, South Africa
[3]*Academic and Research Division, University of Fort Hare, Private Bag X1314, Alice, Eastern Cape, South Africa*

Correspondence should be addressed to Kayode O. Afolabi; kayodeolayinkaafolabi@gmail.com

Academic Editor: Trudy Morrison

Globally, *Porcine circovirus* type 2 (PCV2) is a recognized viral pathogen of great economic value in pig farming. It is the major cause of ravaging postweaning multisystemic wasting syndrome (PMWS) and many other disease syndromes generally regarded as *Porcine circovirus* associated diseases (PCVAD) in Europe. PCV2 infections, specifically PMWS, had impacted huge economic loss on swine production at different regions of the world. It has been studied and reported at different parts of the globe including: North and South America, Europe, Asia, Oceania, Middle East, and the Caribbean. However, till date, this virus and its associated diseases have been grossly understudied in sub-Sahara African region and the entire continent at large. Two out of forty-nine, representing just about 4% of countries that make up sub-Sahara Africa presently, have limited records on reported cases and occurrence of the viral pathogen despite the ubiquitous nature of the virus. This review presents an overview of the discovery of *Porcine circovirus* and its associated diseases in global pig herds and emphasizes the latest trends in PCV2 vaccines and antiviral drugs development and the information gaps that exist on the occurrence of this important viral pathogen in swine herds of sub-Saharan Africa countries. This will serve as wake-up call for immediate and relevant actions by stakeholders in the region.

1. Introduction

Pig rearing is one of the fastest growing livestock sector worldwide [1] as it is a valuable source of animal protein globally and the industry contributes largely to the economy of many countries [2]. Despite the huge economic potentials of piggery business, many farms are faced with myriads of problems orchestrated by diseases that have the capacity to decimate herds. In as much as many opportunities abound in pig rearing especially for small scale farmers, their efforts to improve on their production capacity are hampered by great loss of animals to diseases [3]. Furthermore, the problem becomes more complicated by limited information on the relative frequency of occurrence of the different diseases and their detrimental effects on pig production, most especially in developing countries of Africa [4]. Swine diseases of economic importance range between bacterial, viral, fungal, and protozoan origins. According to Vidigal et al. [5], swine infectious pathogens have greatly caught the attention of researchers from early 1990s when a lot of pig-producing countries experienced very huge economic losses as a result of emerging viral disease-causing agents such as *Porcine circovirus* type 2 (PCV2).

PCV2 has been known as a universal viral pathogen because of its presence in most, if not all the swine herds [6]. Its global prevalence and status have brought about its seropositivity rate of 20–80% in pigs coupled with very high incidence rate of 60% that is accompanied by general mortality rate of 3–10% and culling rate of 40% in seriously affected pig farms [7]. PCV2 is the main etiologic entity implicated in postweaning multisystemic wasting syndrome (PMWS) with other remaining *Porcine circovirus* associated diseases (PCVADs) [8]. It has also been established to be a necessary agent in the pathogenesis of PCVADs, but not a sufficient cause of the diseases that are known to be of great economic importance in pigs production worldwide [9, 10].

2. Historical Background, Classification, and Genomic Organization of *Porcine circovirus*

2.1. Overview of Initial Discovery and Subsequent Retrospective Studies of Porcine circovirus in Global Swine Herds. The initial discovery of *Porcine circovirus* (PCV) in Germany occurred in a continuous pig kidney cell line (PK-15 ATCC-CCL31) as a picornavirus-like contaminant and without any cytopathic effect, with initial assumption of having an RNA genome [11]. However, subsequent observations led to its description as a minute, nonenveloped, and icosahedral shaped virus possessing a genome with circular single-stranded DNA [12]. Experimentally, the PCV obtained from the PK-15 cell line did not produce any ailment in pigs [13, 14]. Subsequently in 1991 at Saskatchewan, Canada, another PCV emerged in a sporadic disease called PMWS which was characterized by weight loss, breathing discomfort, jaundice, and peculiar microscopic lesions in lymphoid tissues of infected pigs [15, 16].

Ellis [17] expressed the initial bias view of some investigators with "hope" of discovering a novel porcine lentivirus from the diseased pigs since they presented an AIDS-like syndrome. They hypothesized that a lentivirus caused the immunosuppression and allowed an observable, disease-causing proliferation of an endemically infectious agent proposed to be "new" circovirus [18]. However, the disease condition was further investigated by its first discoverers: Dr. John Harding, a swine consultant veterinarian in a private practice, and Dr. Edward Clark, a veterinary pathologist at University of Saskatchewan, Canada. Subsequently, a new DNA-virus with similar morphology to the PK-15 originated PCV was discovered from PMWS-affected pigs not only in North America but also in European countries [19–21] and has virtually been described in all continents of the world. Further examination of PMWS-associated PCV showed notable variations when compared with initially defined PCV [22, 23], and in a bid to differentiate the nonpathogenic PCV from pathogenic PMWS-associated PCV, the nonpathogenic strain was called *Porcine circovirus* type 1 (PCV1), while the latter was named *Porcine circovirus* type 2 (PCV2) [24].

Through PCV2 serological studies, it was observed that PCV2 infection is present globally, whereas the prevalence of its associated diseases is much lower; hence, the commonest form of PCV2 manifestation is the subclinical infection [25, 26]. However through various retrospective studies, the pathogenic PCV2 was observed to be in existence in swine herds from different regions of the world earlier before the PMWS outbreak in 1998 [27]. Jacobsen et al. [28] attempted to unravel the origin, spread, and pathogenesis of PCV2 and its diseases in northern Germany confirmed that the existence of PCV2 in pigs dated back to 1962 based on archived samples taken for necropsy within the period of 1961 and 1998 with

TABLE 1: Retrospective studies on earlier occurrence of PCV2 in pigs from some countries of the world.

Country	Sampling period	Reference
Northern Germany	1961–1998	[28]
Belgium	1969	[35]
UK	1970–1997	[36]
Northern Ireland	1970-1971	[37]
Northern Ireland	1973–1999	[38]
Canada	1985	[39]
Spain	1985–1997	[40]

the use of in situ hybridization techniques and polymerase chain reaction (PCR). Furthermore, it was discovered that the relative incidence of detectable viral nucleic acid and existence of PCV2-related lesions was significantly different by the subsequent years.

Total incidence of PCV2 infection was actually minimal within the period of 1961 to 1984, ranging from 0 to 11.7% but increased between 1985 and 1998 within the range of 14.3–53.3%. Also, PCV2-associated diseases were first seen in 1985 archived samples, while sequence analyses of some selected PCV2 DNA segments also showed high homology with currently existing PCV2 strains [28]. This retrospective study by Jacobsen et al. [28] is the foremost report on the detection of PCV2 in pigs worldwide. Many other retrospective studies had also confirmed the existence of the virus in swine from different countries prior to its official detection in 1998 (Table 1). However, associated diseases like PMWS and porcine dermatitis and nephritis syndrome (PDNS) were not diagnosed in the archived samples prior to 1985, implying that PCV2 infection solely is insufficient to bring about the onset of PCV2-associated diseases.

The overall epidemiological data so far thus shows PCV2 to have probably been in existence in the swine population across the universe for more than five decades [27–29].

2.2. Classification of Circoviruses. Historically, family Circoviridae comprises two genera, namely, *Gyrovirus* and *Circovirus* based on their morphology and genomic organization [30, 31], as established in the last published (ninth) report of International Committee on Taxonomy of Viruses (ICTV) of the year 2009 [32] with 11 species in the genus *Circovirus* which include *Canary circovirus, Pigeon circovirus, Duck circovirus, Finch circovirus, Goose circovirus, Beak and feather disease virus, Gull circovirus, Starling circovirus, Swan circovirus, Porcine circovirus type 1,* and *Porcine circovirus type 2*. Genus *Gyrovirus* consists of only *Chicken anaemia virus*, with different genome organizations compared to that of *Circovirus*. Due to the genomic organization and replication strategy of viruses listed in the genus *Circovirus*, they are known to have close relationship to the plant viruses called nanoviruses and geminiviruses, with characteristic stem loop structure situated at their origin of replication and the similarity of their replication proteins [33]. It had been asserted that circoviruses are the possible genetic intermediates between nanoviruses and geminiviruses [34].

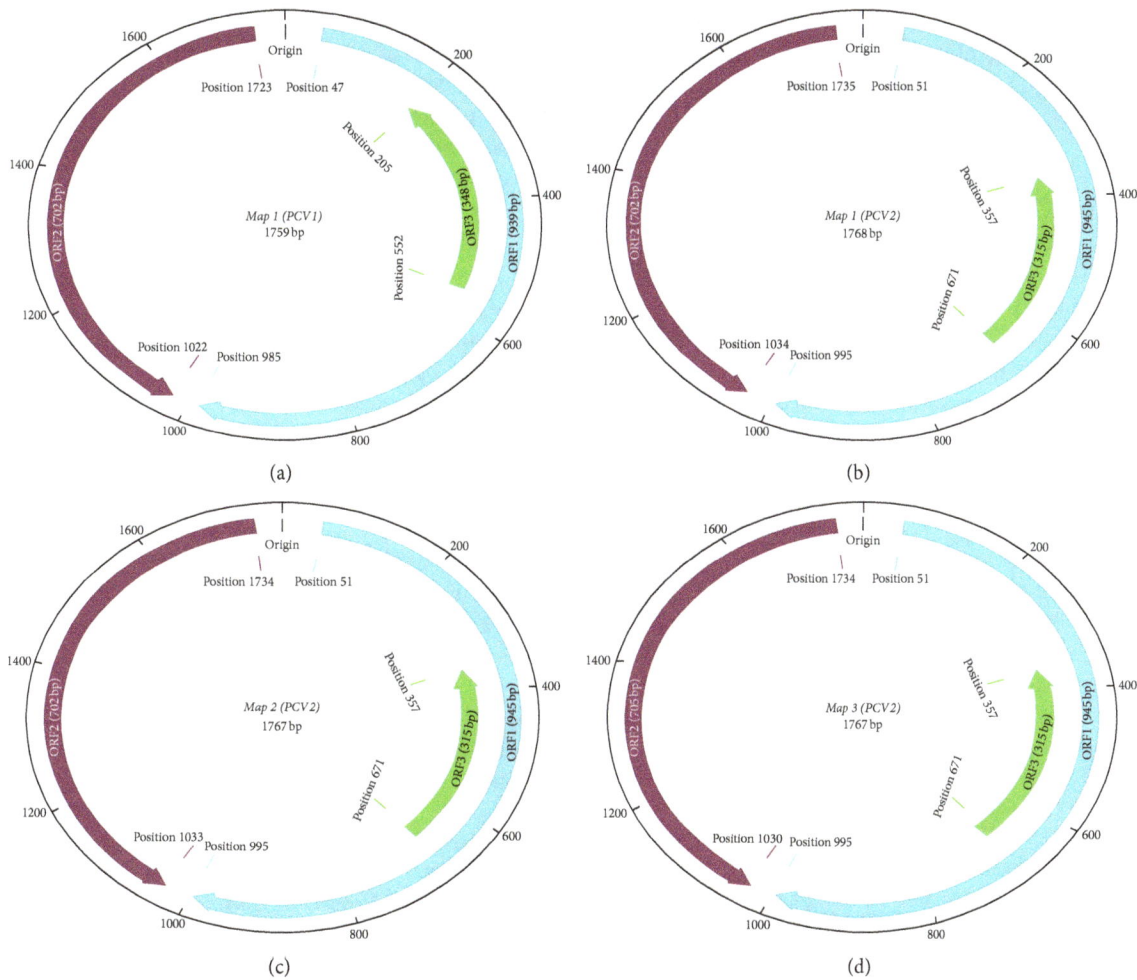

FIGURE 1: Genome organization of *Porcine circovirus* (NB: map (a) is for PCV1, while maps (b), (c), and (d) are for PCV2a and 2e; PCV2b and PCV2c and 2d, resp.), adapted from Zhai et al. [46].

However in a latest development, the taxonomy of Circoviridae has been revisited due to the discovery of new viruses and reevaluation of genomic features that characterize members of the family. In a current ratification by ICTV (2016), genus *Gyrovirus* has been reassigned to the family Anelloviridae while genus *Circovirus* and a new genus, *Cyclovirus,* were grouped together in family Circoviridae, consisting of twenty-seven (27) and forty-three (43) species, respectively [41]. Cycloviruses were discovered in 2010 as a group of viruses with very high relatedness to circoviruses, having genomic features that are closely related to them, and were tentatively named cycloviruses to differentiate them from the circoviruses [42, 43]. The establishment of the two groups in family Circoviridae becomes justifiable due to phylogenetic and genomic differences that exist between them vis-à-vis the host range differences [41].

2.3. Genomic Organization of Porcine circovirus. Presently, PCVs are the smallest viruses found in animals. The diameter of their virions ranges from 17 to 21 nanometres in size [12]. Their genomes consist of single-stranded DNA that is circular

in nature with about 1759 (PCV1) and 1767-1768 (PCV2) nucleotides sequence [12, 44]. PCV1 has only one genome map (Figure 1), which consists of two main open reading frames (ORFs) coding for replication initiating proteins and the structural capsid protein. The locations of the promoters of the genes (*Prep* and *Pcap)* have been determined. The capsid gene promoter is situated within the *rep* open reading frame (ORF1) precisely nucleotide position 1328 to 1252, while the replicase gene promoter is located at the intergenic area towards upstream of the replicase gene at nucleotide position 640 to 796 and forms a kind of overlapping at the origin of replication of PCV1 [45].

PCV2 genome organization is of three types: Maps 1 to 3 (Figure 1), corresponding to PCV2a and PCV2e; PCV2b; and PCV2c and PCV2d genotypes, respectively [46]. It also possesses three main ORFs: ORF1 (945 nucleotides at positions 51 to 995) which codes for replication proteins that controls replication process of the virus [47]; ORF-2 (702 or 705 nucleotides at positions 1734/1735 to 1030/1033/1034) which codes for the immunogenic structural protein (Cap) that determines the virus antigenicity [48]; and ORF3 (315 nucleotides at positions 671 to 357) which was reported to encode PCV2 protein that causes apoptosis in vitro and also involved in the pathogenicity of the virus in mice during an in vivo study [49, 50]. Furthermore, through a latest study by [51], a novel insight that gives deeper understanding of the biological function of PCV2 ORF3 was obtained when a nuclear export sequence (NES) was localized at the N-terminus of ORF3 that codes for protein which plays critical role in nuclear export activity. In another relatively recent study, a newly discovered viral protein from ORF4 (with 180 nucleotides on positions 386 to 565) was reported. The open reading frame is not really essential for PCV2 replication; however, according to He et al. [52], it has a function of bringing down caspase activity and also helps in CD4 (+) and CD8 (+) T-lymphocytes' regulation at the time of PCV2 infection.

3. *Porcine circovirus* Type 2 (PCV2)

3.1. Genotypic Classification of Porcine circovirus Type 2.
According to Ojok et al. [53], no virulence specific DNA polymorphism has been recognized in PCV2; however, characterization of the virus is important for epidemiological purposes. Based on phylogenetic studies and polymerase chain reaction-restriction fragment length polymorphism (PCR-RFLP), a prototype for classifying PCV2 was given that earlier divided the strains of the virus into five genogroups, namely, PCV2a to 2e [54]. However, through phylogenetic analysis that was based on cap gene and complete genome of PCV2 (Figure 2), the virus has been classified into four different genotypes which are PCV2a with five clusters, PCV2b with three clusters, PCV2c, and PCV2d [55–57]. PCV2a and 2b are known to have worldwide distribution, with PCV2b being the predominant genotype detected since 2003. The third type, PCV2c, was first reported in Denmark from an archived material [58] and, recently, it was discovered from live feral pigs in Brazil [59] and also from various field samples obtained from sick pigs in China [60]. The fourth genotype, PCV2d, was reported from China [56]; more recently it has been found dominating in most cases of PCV2 infections in the United State [61], South Korean pig population [62], and globally [63].

Based on latest argument of Chae [64], the classification of PCV2d is not in agreement with the standardized nomenclature rules for new PCV2 genogroups as stipulated by the European Union consortium on PCV-AD [57]. Classification of novel PCV2 genotypes is expected to fulfill two main requirements which are (a) having cut-off value on pairwise sequence comparisons (PASC) analysis of ≥0.0351 and (b) p-distance cut-off value of ≥0.035 [57, 65]. The p-distance that was obtained between PCV2b and PCV2d was 0.057 while the PASC value was just 0.020; hence, PCV2d according to Chae [64] does not meet up with the criteria by which it should be classified as a different genotype. As a result of this, it was proposed that PCV2d should be renamed as mutant *Porcine circovirus* type 2b (mPCV2b) on the account of the naming system laid down by the European Union consortium which serves to prevent any possible scientific confusion as regarding the PCV2 genotype names [64]. However, based

on the p-distance value of 0.055 ± 0.008 between PCV2d and PCV2b that is greater than the earlier stated PCV2 genotype definition cut-off of 0.035, Xiao et al. [63] in a similar investigation, supported classification of PCV2d as an independent genotype without putting PASC cut-off value into consideration.

3.2. PCV2 Genotypes and Their Pathogenicity.
It has been confirmed that both PCV2a and PCV2b are causing swine diseases with different levels of severity [66, 67], whereas PCV2c was discovered in Denmark from healthy pigs [58]. Earlier on before 2003, both PCV2a and 2b were usually prevalent in Europe and China, while in Canada and the United States, only PCV2a was common [68]. However, an observable spontaneous shift in the prevalence of PCV2a compared to PCV2b in commercial swine populations has occurred globally since 2003 with simultaneous increment in the severity of clinical PCVAD according to many available research findings [69–72]. Irrespective of the notable shift, however, there has not been any remarkable difference in pathogenicity observed between PCV2a and 2b experimentally [73] as their study using conventional specific-pathogen-free (SPF) pig model observed no appreciable difference in the virulence of the two viruses in pigs that were experimentally infected with them.

Also in a similar study conducted by Lager et al. [74] using germ-free experimental pigs that were infected with PCV2a or PCV2b infectious clone, it was reported that the pathological manifestations and viral antigen load observed in the two treatments were not really different, even though the pigs that were infected with PCV2b had quicker onset of diseases and higher overall morbidity/mortality of 100% than those infected with PCV2a which was just 25%. Similarly, in a meta-analysis experiment which focused on determining the contributory factors that culminate in development of PMWS experimentally, it was observed that inoculating the pigs with PCV2b among four other factors favoured more successful reproduction of PMWS in the pigs [75]. However, the fact remains that the disease had been successfully induced in healthy pigs using either PCV2a or 2b, though, there is possibility for the observable difference in virulence between the two main genogroups, to be a function of one among several other potential factors that influence the development of the PCVADs [70].

Notwithstanding several arguments and counterarguments on virulence potentials between the two major genotypes, series of findings have shown that there is no similarity in the antigenic composition of the two genotypes [76, 77]. Sequences disparities that exist between them are usually seen at the viral structural capsid gene as well as a specific signature sequence motif that differentiates the two were observed in the genomes of the two major genotypes of the virus [78, 79]. Furthermore, reported isolation of more virulent recombinant PCV2b strains (mPCV2b) from cases of vaccine failure from countries like China [56, 80] and United States of America [81, 82] and recently from Republic of South Korea [83], Brazil [84], Uruguay [85], and Germany [86] has become a serious cause for concern due to the corresponding

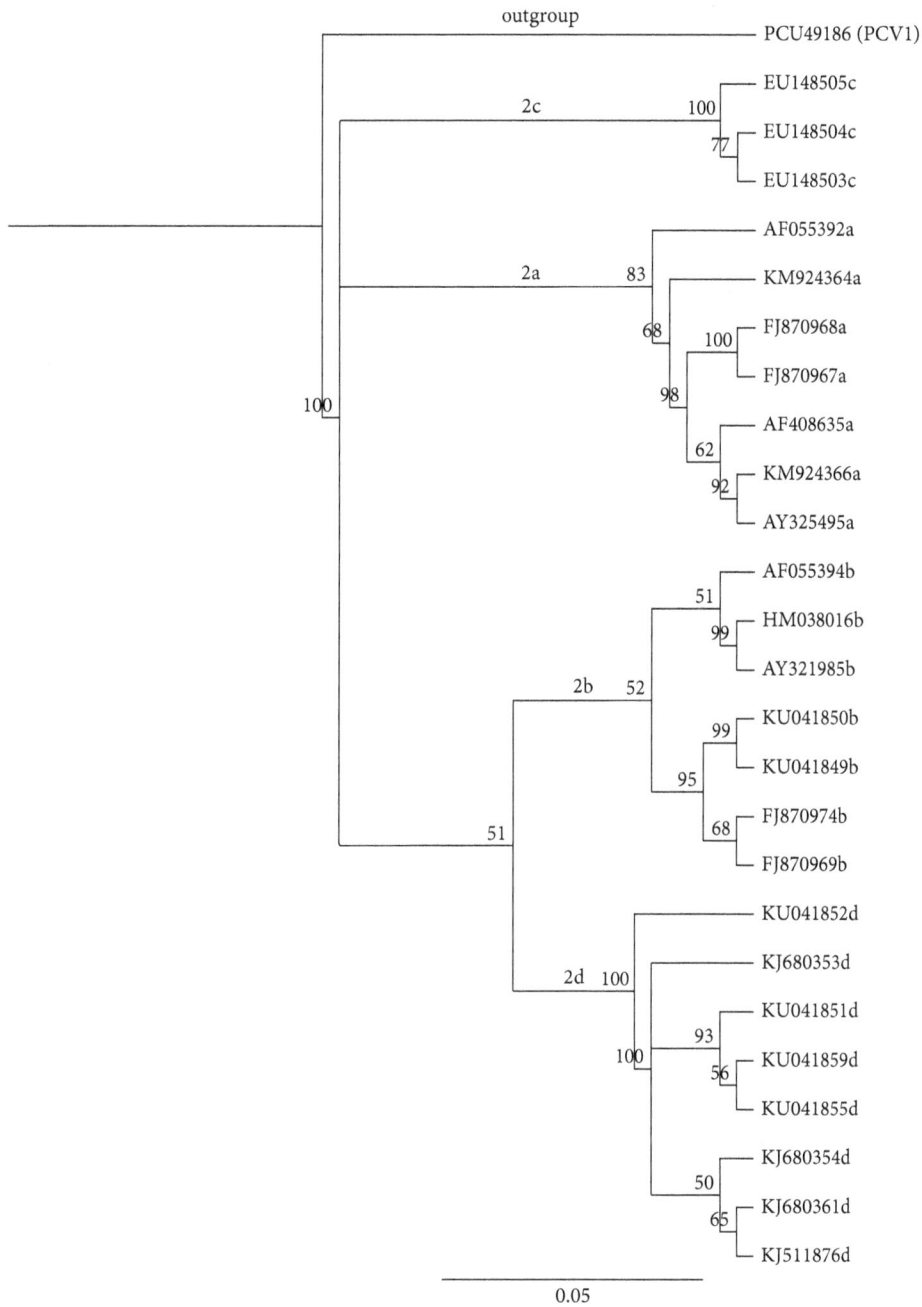

FIGURE 2: Four main genotypes of PCV2 as shown by phylogenetic tree that was constructed based on neighbor-joining method for complete genomes of some PCV2 sequences obtained from NCBI Genbank; genotypes of the virus were written on the main branches of the tree and PCV1 was used as outgroup (NB: the tree was constructed using Geneious 9.1.5, Biomatters Ltd. Boostrap values obtained from 1000 replicates are shown at the major nodes).

increase in virulence and very fast spread. Series of latest findings on the escalation of genetic differences in PCV2 according to Constans et al. [69] and subsequently confirmed by Reiner et al. [87] suggests that current vaccines that are based on PCV2a may be the driving force behind the viral selection and evolution with resultant emergence of more virulent PCV2b strains as reported in cases from fields.

3.3. Pathology, Concurrent Infections with Other Pathogens, and Transmission Modes of PCV2 and Its Associated Diseases

3.3.1. Clinical Pathology of PCV2 and Its Associated Diseases. PCV2 and its associated diseases primarily affect pigs in their late nursery stage and growers, ranging between 7 and 16 weeks old due to presumed protective influence of maternal antibody in younger piglets [88]. Clinicopathological manifestations of PCV2 infection are wasting (i.e., loss of weight), unthriftiness, skin paleness, jaundice, enlarged lymph nodes, and diarrhoea [25, 89, 90]. PCV2 majorly has predilection for the immune system of pigs by preferentially targeting the lymphoid tissues, leading to its depletion and histiocytic replacement in them which are the observable typical histological lesions [26, 91]. Pathological conditions could be exacerbated by immunostimulation or coinfections with other pathogens which occur as a result of immunosuppression and immunity reduction in the affected pigs [7, 90].

According to Segalés [26], the PCV2 infection's clinical scope and pathology have greatly increased over the years. Apart from the most popular and ravaging PMWS, other disease conditions and disorders which include reproductive failures which is usually characterized by abortions or stillbirths with foetuses having an observable necrotizing myocarditis have been observed in the field cases of PCV2 infection and have been reproduced experimentally [92, 93]. Moreover, a respiratory disease which is termed porcine respiratory disease complex (PRDC) which is known with respiratory distress has also been discovered in pigs infected with PCV2, with observable bronchiolitis with mononuclear infiltration of the lungs and interstitial pneumonia [94, 95]. The pathogen has equally been observed to be in connection with PDNS which is a disease that causes formation of skin lesions of red to purple colour in affected pigs. It is also characterized by glomerular and interstitial nephritis and vasculitis [96, 97], although it has not been experimentally reproduced in pigs infected by PCV2 [90]. The list also includes enteritis and proliferative and necrotizing pneumonia (PNP) [25, 98]. Another disease condition in which PCV2 was initially implicated is congenital tremor type A2 [99], which some subsequent research findings later exonerated from being the culprit etiologic agent [100, 101]. Nevertheless, in a latest research work, PCV2 antigen was again found in the brain tissue of newly born piglets having congenital tremor [102].

3.3.2. Multifactorial Status of PCVADs.

Though PCV2 had been confirmed to be the primary pathogen implicated in PCVAD, under experimental conditions, it has been established that infection with PCV2 solely in most cases does not cause overt clinical disease. Based on available information, it has been shown that several infectious cofactors and noninfectious conditions such as concurrent infection with other pathogens [103, 104], host genetic make-up [105], and management practices [106] are crucial for disease progression to PCVAD. Consequently, infections with PCV2 have been regarded as multifactorial at the instances of other underlying cofactors that exacerbate infection with the viral pathogens resulting in the clinical disease manifestations. Infectious cofactors that have been extensively studied till date consist of *Porcine parvovirus*, PPV [107–109], *Porcine reproductive and respiratory syndrome virus*, PRRS [110], *Swine influenza virus* SIV [111], *Torque teno virus* [71], *Swine hepatitis E virus*, HEV [112], *M. hyopneumoniae* [111, 113], *Salmonella* spp. [114], *E. coli* [115], and *Metastrongylus elongatus* [116]. The

noninfectious cofactors include the genetic background of the pig, high stocking density, and prevailing environmental conditions such as temperature fluctuation within the pen [106].

3.3.3. Transmission Modes of PCV2 Infection.

PCV2 is a pathogen with multidimensional spreading potentials. The rate at which the viral pathogen spreads brought about the analogy: "spreading like a wildfire" according to Meng [117] in a Guest Editorial Review. The spread of PCV2 can be viewed within the scope of international transmission through trading of pigs and pig products and also transmission among local herds. PCV2 has been confirmed to be transmitted through trading of live pigs with subclinical infection due to the subtle nature of the disease, which invariably calls for a more critical diagnostic check on imported animals or their products [5, 118]. There have been reported cases of transmission through selection of boars for breeding purposes and the importation of semen for the purpose of artificial insemination [119–121].

Spreading of PCV2 among local herds has been reported in various dimensions ranging from pig to pig [122, 123], man to pig [124], rodents to pig [125], insects to pig [126, 127], and pen environment to pig [128]. This becomes possible due to numerous routes of shedding the virus in cases of systemic infections, as observed in both natural and experimental conditions including oronasal secretions, faeces, urine, colostrum, milk, and semen from infected boar as earlier mentioned [129–132].

3.4. Diagnosis, Prevention, Control, and Treatment of PCV2 and Its Associated Diseases

3.4.1. General Diagnosis of PCV2.

As a complex disease of diverse clinical signs, accurate diagnosis of PCV2 infections is highly important in order to implement appropriate intervention strategy on affected herds [66]. Diagnosis of PCV2 infections could be done basically in two major ways. Firstly, on the basis of clinical disease manifestations, which could be regarded as tentative, and, secondly, based on the confirmatory detection of PCV2 antigen in lymphoid tissues and organs such as the liver, lungs, kidney, or intestine of an infected animal [89]. According to Gillespie et al. [89], for a farm to be tagged as experiencing PCVAD disease, percentages of clinical signs could be seen as follows: loss of weight (98.1%), diarrhea (77.2%), lymphadenopathy (44.8%), dyspnea (75.1%), central neurologic signs (39.6%), inappetence (90.4%), jaundice (37.1%), and death (96.8%). However, in a situation whereby a farm is experiencing subclinical infection, true status of such herd as regarded to PCV2 infection could be mistaken if based on clinical signs manifestation. This is because majority of clinically healthy pigs could be seropositive meaning subclinical infections [89].

PCV2 antigen or nucleic acid detection in samples from a swine herd is known as the golden standard suitable for the confirmatory diagnosis of PCVAD. This has been effectively achieved through PCR, immunohistochemistry (IHC), and in situ hybridization (ISH) [66, 133]. Other diagnostic tests

TABLE 2: Available commercial PCV2 vaccines and some of their features.

Vaccine	Antigen	Recommended usage	Manufacturer	Adjuvant
Circovac®	Inactivated PCV2a virus (whole virus)	Breeding sows (two doses at 5 weeks of age and 2 weeks ante -partum)/piglets	Merial, Lyon, France	Mineral oil
FosteraTM PCV	Killed chimeric PCV1-2a virus	One dose for piglets of three weeks old or above	Pfizer	SL-CD aqueous
Ingelvac CircoFLEX®	Capsid protein of PCV2a (recombinant)	One dose for piglets of three weeks of age or older	Boehringer Ingelheim Vetmedica Inc. Missouri, U.S.A.	Carbomer
Circumvent® PCV	Capsid protein of PCV2a (recombinant)	Two doses at 3 and 6 weeks of age of piglets/growers respectively	Intervet/SP (Merck)	Microsol Diluvac Forte® (MDF)
Porcilis® PCV	Capsid protein of PCV2a (recombinant)	One dose for piglets of three weeks of age or older	Schering-Plough (Merck)	Mineral oil

that have been developed and used in PCV2 detection in infected pigs include enzyme linked immunosorbent assay, immunofluorescence assay, IgM immune-peroxidase monolayer assay, serum virus neutralization assays, virus isolation, and electron microscopy [66, 134, 135].

3.4.2. Prevention, Control, and Treatment of PCV2 till Date. As a multifactorial disease which has been linked to both infectious and noninfectious factors, effective control of PCVAD can be solely achieved not only by vaccine applications but also by preventing triggering factors through improved swine management, control of coinfection, and change of genetic background of pigs through careful selection of boar for breeding. Though vaccination is traditionally considered as the most effective method for preventing viral diseases, it had been established that the protection period of vaccine against the disease is limited and that complete eradication of the virus has not be achieved through vaccination [136].

However, the currently available commercial PCV2 vaccines (Table 2), all of which are either an inactivated whole virus vaccine or subunit vaccine designed base on the immunogenic Cap protein of PCV2a, have shown effectiveness against clinical disease expression and enhanced major production parameters (mortality and average daily gain) in swine herds with PCV2 occurrence. While vaccine applications did not outrightly prevent infection with PCV2 nor restrict its spread, a reasonable reduction in the systemic viral loads and shedding had been observed, which invariably help in decreasing the load of the virus in the environment [137–139]. Although, animals under vaccination could still be infected with the virus, they generally do have lower viral loads compared to those not vaccinated. Thus, currently available vaccines applied most especially as a single-dose protocol do not give sterilizing immunity in swine herds [140].

Moreover, the introduction of the PCV2a vaccines has been observed to cause a corresponding world-wide shift in the prevalence of genotypes from PCV2a to 2b with attendant severe clinical manifestations in vaccinated herds [141]. Also, some reports on PCVAD cases have shown that a new variant

named mutant PCV2b (mPCV2b) was found in diseased pigs despite their prior vaccinations [142]. This has brought about serious concerns on possible emergence of PCV2 vaccine escape strains; however, it was observed that one of the current vaccines was effective against mPCV2b infection under experimental setup [143]. Nevertheless, it has been asserted that series of recent research findings concerning the increased PCV2 genetic diversity connotes that the available vaccines which are based on PCV2a may be inducing the observable selection pressure and possibly be the driving force behind the viral evolution [69], being pivoted on observable high nucleotide substitution rate earlier suggested for the continuous evolution of PCV2 and the emergence of novel PCV2 strains [144].

According to Constans et al. [69], some immune cells epitopes that were known to elicit immune response in the vaccine strain were not seen in the field strains, showing that there is a silent change in the antigenic profile of the strains as many nonconserved epitopes have been predicted to have immune cells functions. Furthermore, the substitutions in the epitopes have been ascertained to affect the immune response greatly, thereby causing immune escape [69]. Hence, many calls and recent research findings have raised support for a rational development of PCV2 vaccines to target evolving genotypes in order to increase the current threshold of protection against PCV2 and its associated diseases [69, 142, 145].

Based on recent laboratory findings of Peng et al. [146] there is a future possibility of producing effective commercial PCV2 antibodies and vaccines that could be based on nonvariable *rep* protein compared to the presently available ones that are based on variable *cap* protein of the virus. From the study, it was observed that the recombinant plasmids of *rep* gene that was constructed shows an efficient expression in the prokaryotic system and also the engineered proteins were immunogenic. Furthermore, the characterized polyclonal antiserum made with *rep* protein shown good reactivity and displayed considerable specificity against PCV2 in PK-15 cell line. Hence, the Rep protein seems to be having future potentials in PCV2 antibody and vaccine development [146].

The utility of commercially available PCV2 vaccines (both inactivated and subunit vaccines based on PCV2a genotype) has been proven over the years as they have shown effectiveness in decreasing mortality and increasing growth parameters in commercial swine herds [67]. There are unquestionable evidences from accumulated field data that confirms the efficacy of the commercial vaccines when production parameters such as average daily weight gain and economic gains in vaccinated pigs were compared with the unvaccinated pigs. In fact, cross-protection against other coinfecting agents is an additional advantage in the use of PCV2 vaccines [67, 147]. The good news is that, in countries where vaccination has been grossly employed, there has been an appreciable declination in the prevalence of PCV2 with good vaccination practices.

However, despite the huge successes recorded so far on PCV2 vaccines, it has been asserted that the protection period of a PCV2 vaccine against the disease is limited and that the virus could not be eradicated by a mass vaccination procedure when applied for a period of one year. This was because, after some months of stopping the intensive vaccination programme, there was a reemergence of PCV2 infection [136]. Although vaccination is recommended for healthy pigs, it is ineffective for pigs that are already infected with PCV2 [148]. In addition, the inherent potentials of vaccines to cause viral evolution [149], coupled with ineffectiveness of vaccines to prevent the multifactorial disease such as PCVAD, have necessitated urgent discovery and development of safe drugs as alternatives in a bid to eradicate or control PCV2 [150].

3.4.3. Promising Efforts on Ethnobotanicals. Recently, research efforts have been focused on developing antiviral drugs from natural compounds with promising outcomes. In a recent study in which twenty natural compounds isolated from traditional Chinese plants were evaluated for their antiviral activities against PCV2 in vitro, it was observed that Matrine (an alkaloid compound purified from the dried roots of *Sophora flavescens* Ait) and Scutellarin (a flavonoid compound from *Scutellaria barbata* D. Don) showed appreciable inhibition rates of 57 and 72.69%, respectively, against the virus out of all the tested compounds [148]. Furthermore, in a more recent study aimed at exploring the antiviral potential of Matrine against PRRSV and PCV2 concurrent infection in a porcine alveolar microphages (PAM) cell model, it was observed that the use of Matrine abated the proliferation of PRRSV and PCV2 effectively at twelve-hour postinfection period. This finding further necessitates the need for immediate exploration of natural products such as Matrine as antiviral agent against PCV2 in clinical settings [150].

In another related study which is aimed at investigating the antiviral activity of a phenylpropanoid dibenzylbutyrolactone lignan called Arctigenin (ACT), extracted from another Chinese traditional herb named *Arctium lappa* L. against PCV2 in vitro and in vivo, another promising result was obtained. It was observed that dosage of 15.6–62.5 μg/mL of ACT efficiently inhibit the thriving of PCV2 in PK-15 cells, while the intraperitoneal injection of 200 μg/kg of ACT into PCV2-challenged mice significantly inhibited PCV2 proliferation in the lungs, spleens, and inguinal lymph nodes of the mice, showing similar effect to ribavirin, an antiviral drug that was used as positive control, thereby demonstrating the effectiveness of ACT as an antiviral agent against PCV2 both in vitro and in vivo [151].

4. Global Status of PCV2 and Its Associated Diseases: Sub-Saharan Africa Scenario

4.1. PCV2 and Its PMWS: Is the Global Disease a Global Concern? Sequel to the first known outbreak and description of porcine multisystemic wasting syndrome, an important PCVAD in a very healthy, farrow-to-finish swine farm situated in Northeastern Saskatchewan, Western Canada, North America, in early 1990s [15, 152, 153], PMWS and other PCVADs have been subsequently seen in all regions of the world including many European countries such as Spain [21], France [154], Hungary [155], and United Kingdom [19, 36]; South America countries such as Brazil [156] and Uruguay [157]; Asian countries such as Korea [158] and China [159]; Oceania, Australia [160]; Caribbean, Cuba [161]; Middle East, Israel [162]; and African countries such as South Africa [119] and, recently, Uganda [53]. The ubiquitous status of *Porcine circovirus* and its numerous associated diseases has been said to be linked to the marketing of subclinically infected pigs vis-á-vis the choosing of such pigs for breeding programmes as the virus is known to be spread through semen from boars [5, 163].

Vidigal et al. [5] reported significant link between the routes of dispersal of PCV2 and international marketing of live pigs from obtained data, thereby showing how important the movements of livestock around the globe could be in the emergence and spread of new pathogens. Therefore, increase in the global trade of livestock and their products and increase in global livestock production as a result of the use of intensive animal rearing system have arguably contribute to the spread of infectious pathogens globally [5, 149, 164]. In addition to those mentioned facts and the multiple transmission routes earlier described for PCV2 coupled with the long-lasting viral life, the significance of world-wide proliferation of PCV2 in influencing the PMWS epidemics is indicated [27, 144, 165].

4.2. Incidence of Porcine circovirus Type 2 in Swine-Producing Countries of Sub-Saharan Africa

4.2.1. First Emergence of PCV2 in South African Swine Herds. Drew et al. [119] reported what seemed to be the first cases of PCV2 associated diseases in the region, which occurred in Gauteng Province, South Africa. The cases occurred in June 2001 on a large, well-managed breeding unit which serves as supplier of breeding stock to three member farms, separated by distances 100 and 500 km apart. The initial clinical manifestation observed in the pigs was PDNS which affects young pigs of two to three months old. In no distant time, the expression of clinical signs associated with PMWS became more evident, to the extent that by November 2001, the morbidity due to PMWS had increased to about 30 to 40% with mortality remaining below 10% [119].

Moreover, clinical manifestations of PMWS were also seen in approximately the same percentage of pigs of the same

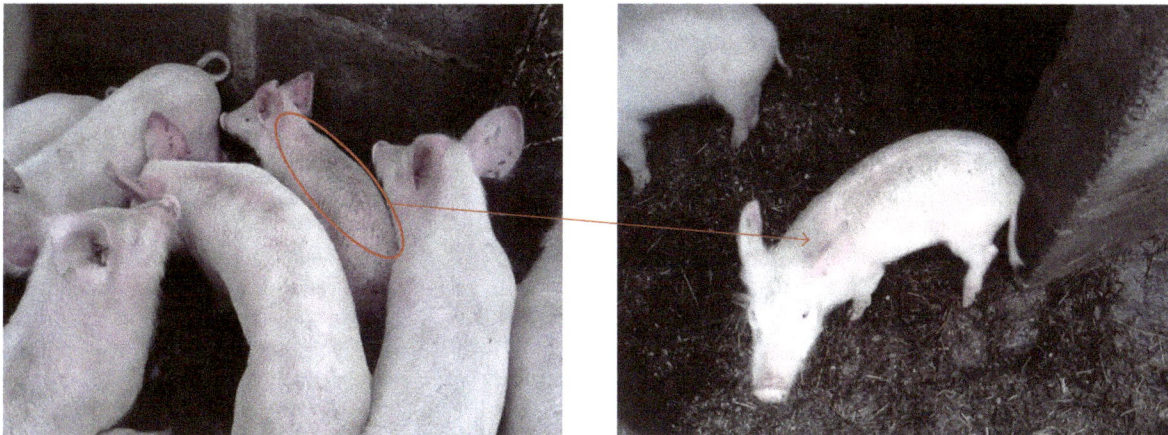

FIGURE 3: Wasting appearance of a pig with a notable respiratory distress within a herd of the same age at a farm in Lukhanji Local Municipality, Chris-Hani District, Eastern Cape, South Africa (Picture taken in April, 2016 during a sampling exercise).

ages bred on one of the member farms, specifically, the one situated about 100 km away from the main farm after the introduction of pigs from the main farm, on which the disease had first been noticed. However, tissues were collected from just two affected animals of about 12 to 15 weeks of age from each of the two premises and were submitted for histological, immunohistological, and molecular analysis. Tissues sections from the spleen, liver, brain, and heart of the four pigs did not show significant histopathology. It was observed that the lesions indicative of PMWS were concentrated in the precapsular, bronchial, and gastrohepatic lymph nodes. Also in many subcapsular areas in the lymph nodes, there were widespread areas of diffuse lymphocyte depletion with presence of multinucleate giant cells as evidence occasionally [119].

Furthermore, the molecular analysis of a 501-nucleotide fragments of the viral genome amplified from tissues samples of the reported cases revealed that they were identical to a PCV2 isolate from Iowa, USA, with GenBank Ascension number AF264039 [166], having just only two nucleotide substitutions from the USA isolate. The sequence obtained from a lymph node of a piglet from the main farm yielded the complete PCV2 genome (1768 base pairs) and was designated SAI, this is the only isolate deposited so far in the GenBank with ascension number AY325495 from South Africa and virtually in the entire sub-Saharan Africa. In their conclusion, Drew et al. [119] recommended for further molecular epidemiological studies to investigate PCV2 at other sites in South Africa. However till this time, little or no work has been done to that effect in South African pig population.

This assertion is further confirmed by more recent research work of Mokoele et al. [167] in which it was categorically stated that "though PCV2 may be an economically important disease in South Africa, to date, no specific surveillance has been conducted to validate the current status because the disease is thought to be ubiquitous in most countries." However, seeming negligence to know the health status of swine herds of the country as regarding the ubiquitous viral pathogen could pose a serious problem for the industry in a nearest future due to a recent observation during a field

trip which was part of our ongoing research work that is focused on determining the occurrence of some RNA and DNA viruses in swine herds of Eastern Cape Province South Africa; pigs with typical clinical manifestations of PMWS were seen (Figure 3), showing likelihood of existence of the viral pathogen in pig herds of the country.

In another study by An et al. [168], nucleotide sequences of 197 PCV2 strains submitted to GenBank nucleotide database at the National Center for Biotechnology Information (NCBI) from all over the world and 36 PCV2 strains obtained from PMWS and PDNS cases in Korean pigs over an 8-year period were used in grouping PCV2 into two groups (1 and 2) by phylogenetic tree analysis and multiple alignments of nucleotide sequences. In their study, it was observed that three countries, namely, South Africa, United Kingdom, and Thailand, were having just one PCV2 complete genome sequence each on GenBank as far back as then, indicating dearth of information on PCV2 from the three countries. They recommended further studies on PCV2 from the countries so that accurate documentation of PCV2 strains circulating in the three countries could be done. However till date, nothing has been done in South Africa as regarding the clarion call.

4.2.2. PCV2 in Ugandan Pigs. Recently, Ojok et al. [53] also reported on the molecular detection and characterization of PCV2 from pigs in Uganda, however with limitation of using a relatively small sample size ($n = 35$) like that of Drew et al. [119]. Only three cases of PCV2 were found in their study and they also recommended that further studies be conducted so as to fully understand the true prevalence of the virus in swine population of Uganda as well as their genetic diversity. The three PCV2 sequences in their study were observed to cluster with PCV2b genotype which was originally referred to as the European cluster or PCV2 group 1 in contrast to the South African strain which clustered with the PCV2a previously referred to as the North American strains or PCV2 group 2.

In a similar unpublished study conducted by Jonsson [169] aimed at investigating the disease transmission patterns in the livestock-wildlife interface in Uganda, being part of the Emerging Infectious Diseases (EID) surveillance programme conducted to study the prevalence of PCV2 in domestic pigs in Uganda, ninety-one domestic pigs around Murchison Falls national park were sampled and analysed. The sampled domestic pigs were all negative for PCV2a, while for PCV2b which is known to be genogroup mostly associated with PMWS, a point prevalence of 77% was reported. This is in support of the findings of Ojok et al. [53] that reported the presence of PCV2b genotype in a separate study on Ugandan pigs. The point prevalence of 77% for PCV2b in the study cannot be generalised to all of Ugandan pigs; this is because the sample selection was too small to arrive at such conclusion. As a result of this, more extensive studies were recommended by Jonsson [169], so as to obtain more accurate data on the prevalence of the PCV2b in Ugandan pigs.

4.2.3. PCV2 till Date in Cameroonian Pigs. The study of Ndze et al. [170] is another recent effort aimed at describing the occurrence and genetic diversity of selected DNA viruses belonging to different families, namely, Adenoviridae, Circoviridae, Anelloviridae, and Parvoviridae in Cameroonian pigs. However, only viruses belonging to the family Parvoviridae were detected, most especially those within the bocaviruses. In their remarks, they attributed their failure to detect other groups of viruses including *Circovirus* which is known to be ubiquitous to several possible factors including but not limited to short sampling period and low study sample number.

5. Conclusion

So far, the status of porcine circovirus type 2 is practically unknown in pigs of many swine-producing countries in sub-Saharan Africa. Moreover, countries where some research works have been done till date are having insufficient data that could enhance the detailed characterization of the viral genogroup that may likely be in circulation in swine herds of many countries within the region. There is, therefore, an urgent need for large scale molecular epidemiological studies on the virus and its associated diseases in the region, including origins of observed genogroups. This will help in facilitating adequate preventive and control measures against the pathogen through the establishment of effective vaccination regime that could help in combating this globally important and emerging porcine viral pathogen with huge economic implications in the global pig industry.

Conflicts of Interest

The authors declare that they have no conflicts of interest regarding the publication of this paper.

Acknowledgments

The authors acknowledge the National Research Foundation (NRF), South African Medical Research Council (SAMRC), and Govan Mbeki Research and Development Centre (GMRDC) of University of Fort Hare for their financial supports.

References

[1] FAO, *Pig Sector Kenya. FAO Animal Production and Health Livestock Country Reviews*, No. 3, FAO, Rome, Italy, 2012.

[2] S. Uddin Khan, K. R. Atanasova, W. S. Krueger, A. Ramirez, and G. C. Gray, "Epidemiology, geographical distribution, and economic consequences of swine zoonoses: a narrative review," *Emerging Microbes and Infections*, vol. 2, article e92, 2013.

[3] E. K. Ndyomugyenyi and J. Kyasimire, "Pig production in Kichwamba Sub-county, Rubirizi district, Uganda," *Livestock Research for Rural Development*, vol. 27, no. 10, 2015.

[4] M. M. Dione, E. A. Ouma, K. Roesel, J. Kungu, P. Lule, and D. Pezo, "Participatory assessment of animal health and husbandry practices in smallholder pig production systems in three high poverty districts in Uganda," *Preventive Veterinary Medicine*, vol. 117, no. 3-4, pp. 565–576, 2014.

[5] P. M. P. Vidigal, C. L. Mafra, F. M. F. Silva, J. L. R. Fietto, A. Silva Júnior, and M. R. Almeida, "Tripping over emerging pathogens around the world: a phylogeographical approach for determining the epidemiology of Porcine circovirus-2 (PCV-2), considering global trading," *Virus Research*, vol. 163, no. 1, pp. 320–327, 2012.

[6] P. Baekbo, C. S. Kristensen, and L. E. Larsen, "Porcine circovirus diseases: a review of PMWS," *Transboundary and Emerging Diseases*, vol. 59, no. 1, pp. 60–67, 2012.

[7] X. Wang, K. He, W. Wang et al., "Genetic variation of porcine circovirus type 2 isolate 201105ZJ," *Agricultural Science and Technology*, vol. 15, no. 11, pp. 1860–1864, 2014.

[8] C. Chae, "A review of porcine circovirus 2-associated syndromes and diseases," *Veterinary Journal*, vol. 169, no. 3, pp. 326–336, 2005.

[9] G. M. Allan, S. Kennedy, F. McNeilly et al., "Experimental reproduction of severe wasting disease by co-infection of pigs with porcine circovirus and porcine parvovirus," *Journal of Comparative Pathology*, vol. 121, no. 1, pp. 1–11, 1999.

[10] R. Anoopraj, T. K. Rajkhowa, S. Cherian et al., "Genetic characterisation and phylogenetic analysis of PCV2 isolates from India: indications for emergence of natural inter-genotypic recombinants," *Infection, Genetics and Evolution*, vol. 31, pp. 25–32, 2015.

[11] I. Tischer, R. Rasch, and G. Tochtermann, "Characterization of papovavirus-and picornavirus-like particles in permanent pig kidney cell lines," *ZBL.BAKT.REIHE A*, vol. 226, no. 2, pp. 153–167, 1974.

[12] I. Tischer, H. Gelderblom, W. Vettermann, and M. A. Koch, "A very small porcine virus with circular single-stranded DNA," *Nature*, vol. 295, no. 5844, pp. 64–66, 1982.

[13] G. M. Allan, F. McNeilly, J. P. Cassidy et al., "Pathogenesis of porcine circovirus; experimental infections of colostrum deprived piglets and examination of pig foetal material," *Veterinary Microbiology*, vol. 44, no. 1, pp. 49–64, 1995.

[14] I. Tischer, W. Mields, D. Wolff, M. Vagt, and W. Griem, "Studies on epidemiology and pathogenicity of porcine circovirus," *Archives of Virology*, vol. 91, no. 3-4, pp. 271–276, 1986.

[15] E. G. Clark, "Post-weaning multisystemic syndrome," in *Proceedings of the Western Canadian Association of Swine Practitioners Conference*, pp. 22–25, 1996.

[16] J. Harding, "Post-weaning multisystemic wasting syndrome (PMWS): preliminary epidemiology and clinical presentation," in *Proceedings of the Western Canadian Association of Swine Practitioners*, p. 21, 1996.

[17] J. Ellis, "Porcine circovirus: a historical perspective," *Veterinary Pathology*, vol. 51, no. 2, pp. 315–327, 2014.

[18] A. Bratanich, M. Lairmore, W. Heneine et al., "Lack of evidence of conserved lentiviral sequences in pigs with post weaning multisystemic wasting syndrome," *Canadian Journal of Veterinary Research*, vol. 63, no. 3, pp. 207–211, 1999.

[19] G. M. Allan, F. McNeilly, S. Kennedy et al., "Isolation of porcine circovirus-like viruses from pigs with a wasting disease in the USA and Europe," *Journal of Veterinary Diagnostic Investigation*, vol. 10, no. 1, pp. 3–10, 1998.

[20] J. C. S. Harding, E. G. Clark, J. H. Strokappe, P. I. Willson, and J. A. Ellis, "Postweaning multisystemic wasting syndrome: epidemiology and clinical presentation," *Journal of Swine Health and Production*, vol. 6, no. 6, pp. 249–254, 1998.

[21] J. Segalés, M. Sitjar, M. Domingo et al., "First report of post-weaning multisystemic wasting syndrome in pigs in Spain," *Veterinary Record*, vol. 141, no. 23, pp. 600–601, 1997.

[22] G. Allan, B. Meehan, D. Todd et al., "Novel porcine circoviruses from pigs with wasting disease syndromes," *The Veterinary Record*, vol. 142, no. 17, pp. 467–468, 1998.

[23] B. M. Meehan, F. McNeilly, D. Todd et al., "Characterization of novel circovirus DNAs associated with wasting syndromes in pigs," *Journal of General Virology*, vol. 79, no. 9, pp. 2171–2179, 1998.

[24] G. M. Allan, F. Mc Neilly, B. M. Meehan et al., "Isolation and characterisation of circoviruses from pigs with wasting syndromes in Spain, Denmark and Northern Ireland," *Veterinary Microbiology*, vol. 66, no. 2, pp. 115–123, 1999.

[25] J. Segalés, G. M. Allan, and M. Domingo, "Porcine circovirus diseases," *Animal health research reviews / Conference of Research Workers in Animal Diseases*, vol. 6, no. 2, pp. 119–142, 2005.

[26] J. Segalés, "Porcine circovirus type 2 (PCV2) infections: clinical signs, pathology and laboratory diagnosis," *Virus Research*, vol. 164, no. 1-2, pp. 10–19, 2012.

[27] N. Rose, T. Opriessnig, B. Grasland, and A. Jestin, "Epidemiology and transmission of porcine circovirus type 2 (PCV2)," *Virus Research*, vol. 164, no. 1-2, pp. 78–89, 2012.

[28] B. Jacobsen, L. Krueger, F. Seeliger, M. Bruegmann, J. Segalés, and W. Baumgaertner, "Retrospective study on the occurrence of porcine circovirus 2 infection and associated entities in Northern Germany," *Veterinary Microbiology*, vol. 138, no. 1-2, pp. 27–33, 2009.

[29] L. Grau-Roma, L. Fraile, and J. Segalés, "Recent advances in the epidemiology, diagnosis and control of diseases caused by porcine circovirus type 2," *Veterinary Journal*, vol. 187, no. 1, pp. 23–32, 2011.

[30] C. R. Pringle, "Virus taxonomy at the XIth International Congress of Virology, Sydney, Australia," *Archives of Virology*, vol. 144, no. 10, pp. 2065–2070, 1999.

[31] M. McNulty, J. Dale, P. Lukert, A. Mankertz, J. Randles, and D. Todd, "Circoviridae," in *Seventh Report of the International Committee on Taxonomy of Viruses*, M. H. V. van Regenmortel, C. M. Fauquet, D. H. L. Bishop et al., Eds., pp. 299–303, Academic Press, San Diego, Calif, USA, 2000.

[32] P. Biagini, M. Bendinelli, S. Hino et al., "Family circoviridae," in *Virus Taxonomy: Classification and Nomenclature of Viruses: Ninth Report of the International Committee on Taxonomy of Viruses*, A. M. Q. King, M. J. Adams, E. B. Carstens, and E. J. Lefkowitz, Eds., pp. 343–349, Academic Press, London, UK, 2012.

[33] B. M. Meehan, J. L. Creelan, M. Stewart McNulty, and D. Todd, "Sequence of porcine circovirus DNA: affinities with plant circoviruses," *Journal of General Virology*, vol. 78, pp. 221–227, 1997.

[34] F. D. Niagro, A. N. Forsthoefel, R. P. Lawther et al., "Beak and feather disease virus and porcine circovirus genomes: intermediates between the geminiviruses and plant circoviruses," *Archives of Virology*, vol. 143, no. 9, pp. 1723–1744, 1998.

[35] R. Sanchez, H. Nauwynck, and M. Pensaert, "Serological survey of porcine circovirus 2 antibodies in domestic and feral pig populations in Belgium," in *Proceedings of the Conference on ssDNA Viruses of Plants, Birds, Pigs and Primates Meeting*, p. 122, 2000.

[36] S. S. Grierson, D. P. King, T. Sandvik et al., "Detection and genetic typing of type 2 porcine circoviruses in archived pig tissues from the UK," *Archives of Virology*, vol. 149, no. 6, pp. 1171–1183, 2004.

[37] S. Krakowka, G. Allan, J. Ellis et al., "A nine-base nucleotide sequence in the porcine circovirus type 2 (PCV2) nucleocapsid gene determines viral replication and virulence," *Virus Research*, vol. 164, no. 1-2, pp. 90–99, 2012.

[38] I. W. Walker, C. A. Konoby, V. A. Jewhurst et al., "Development and application of a competitive enzyme linked immunosorbent assay for the detection of serum antibodies to porcine circovirus type 2," *Journal of Veterinary Diagnostic Investigation*, vol. 12, no. 5, pp. 400–405, 2000.

[39] R. Magar, P. Müller, and R. Larochelle, "Retrospective serological survey of antibodies to porcine circovirus type 1 and type 2," *Canadian Journal of Veterinary Research*, vol. 64, no. 3, pp. 184–186, 2000.

[40] G. M. Rodríguez-Arrioja, J. Segalés, C. Rosell et al., "Retrospective study on porcine circovirus type 2 infection in pigs from 1985 to 1997 in Spain," *Journal of veterinary medicine. B, Infectious diseases and veterinary public health*, vol. 50, no. 2, pp. 99–101, 2003.

[41] K. Rosario, M. Breitbart, B. Harrach et al., "Revisiting the taxonomy of the family Circoviridae: establishment of the genus Cyclovirus and removal of the genus Gyrovirus," *Archives of Virology*, pp. 1–17, 2017.

[42] E. Delwart and L. Li, "Rapidly expanding genetic diversity and host range of the *Circoviridae* viral family and other Rep encoding small circular ssDNA genomes," *Virus Research*, vol. 164, no. 1-2, pp. 114–121, 2012.

[43] L. Li, A. Kapoor, B. Slikas et al., "Multiple diverse circoviruses infect farm animals and are commonly found in human and chimpanzee feces," *Journal of Virology*, vol. 84, no. 4, pp. 1674–1682, 2010.

[44] I. Morozov, T. Sirinarumitr, S. D. Sorden et al., "Detection of a novel strain of porcine circovirus in pigs with postweaning multisystemic wasting syndrome," *Journal of Clinical Microbiology*, vol. 36, no. 9, pp. 2535–2541, 1998.

[45] A. Mankertz and B. Hillenbrand, "Analysis of transcription of porcine circovirus type 1," *Journal of General Virology*, vol. 83, no. 11, pp. 2743–2751, 2002.

[46] S.-L. Zhai, S.-N. Chen, Z.-H. Xu et al., "Porcine circovirus type 2 in China: an update on and insights to its prevalence and control," *Virology Journal*, vol. 11, article 88, 2014.

[47] A. Mankertz, J. Mankertz, K. Wolf, and H.-J. Buhk, "Identification of a protein essential for replication of porcine circovirus," *Journal of General Virology*, vol. 79, no. 2, pp. 381–384, 1998.

[48] P. Nawagitgul, I. Morozov, S. R. Bolin, P. A. Harms, S. D. Sorden, and P. S. Paul, "Open reading frame 2 of porcine circovirus type 2 encodes a major capsid protein," *Journal of General Virology*, vol. 81, no. 9, pp. 2281–2287, 2000.

[49] J. Liu, I. Chen, and J. Kwang, "Characterization of a previously unidentified viral protein in porcine circovirus type 2-infected cells and its role in virus-induced apoptosis," *Journal of Virology*, vol. 79, no. 13, pp. 8262–8274, 2005.

[50] J. Liu, I. Chen, Q. Du, H. Chua, and J. Kwang, "The ORF3 protein of porcine circovirus type 2 is involved in viral pathogenesis in vivo," *Journal of Virology*, vol. 80, no. 10, pp. 5065–5073, 2006.

[51] J. Gu, L. Wang, Y. Jin et al., "Characterization of specific antigenic epitopes and the nuclear export signal of the Porcine circovirus 2 ORF3 protein," *Veterinary Microbiology*, vol. 184, pp. 40–50, 2016.

[52] J. He, J. Cao, N. Zhou, Y. Jin, J. Wu, and J. Zhou, "Identification and functional analysis of the novel ORF4 protein encoded by porcine circovirus type 2," *Journal of Virology*, vol. 87, no. 3, pp. 1420–1429, 2013.

[53] L. Ojok, J. B. Okuni, C. Hohloch, W. Hecht, and M. Reinacher, "Detection and characterisation of porcine circovirus 2 from Ugandan pigs," *Indian Journal of Veterinary Pathology*, vol. 37, no. 1, pp. 77–80, 2013.

[54] A. L. Hamel, L. L. Lin, C. Sachvie, E. Grudeski, and G. P. Nayar, "PCR detection and characterization of type-2 porcine circovirus," *Canadian Journal of Veterinary Research*, vol. 64, no. 1, pp. 44–52, 2000.

[55] G. Franzo, M. Cortey, A. Olvera et al., "Revisiting the taxonomical classification of Porcine Circovirus type 2 (PCV2): still a real challenge," *Virology Journal*, vol. 12, article 131, 2015.

[56] L. J. Guo, Y. H. Lu, Y. W. Wei, L. P. Huang, and C. M. Liu, "Porcine circovirus type 2 (PCV2): genetic variation and newly emerging genotypes in China," *Virology Journal*, vol. 7, article 273, 2010.

[57] J. Segalés, A. Olvera, L. Grau-Roma et al., "PCV-2 genotype definition and nomenclature," *Veterinary Record*, vol. 162, no. 26, pp. 867–868, 2008.

[58] K. Dupont, E. O. Nielsen, P. Baekbo, and L. E. Larsen, "Genomic analysis of PCV2 isolates from Danish archives and a current PMWS case-control study supports a shift in genotypes with time," *Veterinary Microbiology*, vol. 128, no. 1-2, pp. 56–64, 2008.

[59] G. Franzo, M. Cortey, A. M. M. G. D. Castro et al., "Genetic characterisation of Porcine circovirus type 2 (PCV2) strains from feral pigs in the Brazilian Pantanal: an opportunity to reconstruct the history of PCV2 evolution," *Veterinary Microbiology*, vol. 178, no. 1-2, pp. 158–162, 2015.

[60] X. Liu, F.-X. Wang, H.-W. Zhu, N. Sun, and H. Wu, "Phylogenetic analysis of porcine circovirus type 2 (PCV2) isolates from China with high homology to PCV2c," *Archives of Virology*, vol. 161, no. 6, pp. 1591–1599, 2016.

[61] C. Xiao, K. M. Harmon, P. G. Halbur, and T. Opriessnig, "PCV2d-2 is the predominant type of PCV2 DNA in pig samples collected in the U.S. during 2014–2016," *Veterinary Microbiology*, vol. 197, pp. 72–77, 2016.

[62] T. Kwon, D. Lee, S. J. Yoo, S. H. Je, J. Y. Shin, and Y. S. Lyoo, "Genotypic diversity of porcine circovirus type 2 (PCV2) and genotype shift to PCV2d in Korean pig population," *Virus Research*, vol. 228, pp. 24–29, 2017.

[63] C.-T. Xiao, P. G. Halbur, and T. Opriessnig, "Global molecular genetic analysis of porcine circovirus type 2 (PCV2) sequences confirms the presence of four main PCV2 genotypes and reveals a rapid increase of PCV2d," *Journal of General Virology*, vol. 96, no. 7, pp. 1830–1841, 2015.

[64] C. Chae, "An emerging porcine circovirus type 2b mutant (mPCV2b) originally known as PCV2d," *Veterinary Journal*, vol. 203, no. 1, pp. 6–9, 2015.

[65] M. Cortey, A. Olvera, L. Grau-Roma, and J. Segalés, "Further comments on porcine circovirus type 2 (PCV2) genotype definition and nomenclature," *Veterinary Microbiology*, vol. 149, no. 3-4, pp. 522–523, 2011.

[66] T. Opriessnig, X. J. Meng, and P. G. Halbur, "Porcine circovirus type 2-associated disease: update on current terminology, clinical manifestations, pathogenesis, diagnosis, and intervention strategies," *Journal of Veterinary Diagnostic Investigation*, vol. 19, no. 6, pp. 591–615, 2007.

[67] N. M. Beach and X.-J. Meng, "Efficacy and future prospects of commercially available and experimental vaccines against porcine circovirus type 2 (PCV2)," *Virus Research*, vol. 164, no. 1-2, pp. 33–42, 2012.

[68] G. M. Allan, F. McNeilly, M. McMenamy et al., "Temporal distribution of porcine circovirus 2 genogroups recovered from postweaning multisystemic wasting syndrome-affected and -nonaffected farms in Ireland and Northern Ireland," *Journal of Veterinary Diagnostic Investigation*, vol. 19, no. 6, pp. 668–673, 2007.

[69] M. Constans, M. Ssemadaali, O. Kolyvushko, and S. Ramamoorthy, "Antigenic determinants of possible vaccine escape by porcine circovirus subtype 2b viruses," *Bioinformatics and Biology Insights*, vol. 9, pp. 1–12, 2015.

[70] M. Cortey, E. Pileri, M. Sibila et al., "Genotypic shift of porcine circovirus type 2 from PCV-2a to PCV-2b in Spain from 1985 to 2008," *Veterinary Journal*, vol. 187, no. 3, pp. 363–368, 2011.

[71] C. A. Gagnon, D. Tremblay, P. Tijssen, M.-H. Venne, A. Houde, and S. M. Elahi, "The emergence of porcine circovirus 2b genotype (PCV-2b) in swine in Canada," *Canadian Veterinary Journal*, vol. 48, no. 8, pp. 811–819, 2007.

[72] L. Huang, Y. Wang, Y. Wei et al., "Capsid proteins from PCV2a genotype confer greater protection against a PCV2b strain than those from PCV2b genotype in pigs: evidence for PCV2b strains becoming more predominant than PCV2a strains from 2000 to 2010s," *Applied Microbiology and Biotechnology*, vol. 100, no. 13, pp. 5933–5943, 2016.

[73] T. Opriessnig, S. Ramamoorthy, D. M. Madson et al., "Differences in virulence among porcine circovirus type 2 isolates are unrelated to cluster type 2a or 2b and prior infection provides heterologous protection," *Journal of General Virology*, vol. 89, no. 10, pp. 2482–2491, 2008.

[74] K. M. Lager, P. C. Gauger, A. L. Vincent, T. Opriessnig, M. E. Kehrli Jr., and A. K. Cheung, "Mortality in pigs given porcine circovirus type 2 subgroup 1 and 2 viruses derived from DNA clones," *Veterinary Record*, vol. 161, no. 12, pp. 428–429, 2007.

[75] A. Tomás, L. T. Fernandes, O. Valero, and J. Segalés, "A meta-analysis on experimental infections with porcine circovirus type 2 (PCV2)," *Veterinary Microbiology*, vol. 132, no. 3-4, pp. 260–273, 2008.

[76] D. J. Lefebvre, S. Costers, J. Van Doorsselaere, G. Misinzo, P. L. Delputte, and H. J. Nauwynck, "Antigenic differences among porcine circovirus type 2 strains, as demonstrated by the use of monoclonal antibodies," *Journal of General Virology*, vol. 89, no. 1, pp. 177–187, 2008.

[77] S.-B. Shang, Y.-L. Jin, X.-T. Jiang et al., "Fine mapping of antigenic epitopes on capsid proteins of porcine circovirus, and antigenic phenotype of porcine circovirus Type 2," *Molecular Immunology*, vol. 46, no. 3, pp. 327–334, 2009.

[78] A. K. Cheung, K. M. Lager, O. I. Kohutyuk et al., "Detection of two porcine circovirus type 2 genotypic groups in United States swine herds," *Archives of Virology*, vol. 152, no. 5, pp. 1035–1044, 2007.

[79] A. Olvera, M. Cortey, and J. Segalés, "Molecular evolution of porcine circovirus type 2 genomes: phylogeny and clonality," *Virology*, vol. 357, no. 2, pp. 175–185, 2007.

[80] L. Guo, Y. Fu, Y. Wang et al., "A porcine circovirus type 2 (PCV2) mutant with 234 amino acids in Capsid protein showed more virulence in vivo, compared with classical PCV2a/b strain," *PLoS ONE*, vol. 7, no. 7, Article ID e41463, 2012.

[81] T. Opriessnig, C.-T. Xiao, P. F. Gerber, and P. G. Halbur, "Emergence of a novel mutant PCV2b variant associated with clinical PCVAD in two vaccinated pig farms in the U.S. concurrently infected with PPV2," *Veterinary Microbiology*, vol. 163, no. 1-2, pp. 177–183, 2013.

[82] C.-T. Xiao, P. G. Halbur, and T. Opriessnig, "Complete genome sequence of a novel porcine circovirus type 2b variant present in cases of vaccine failures in the United States," *Journal of Virology*, vol. 86, no. 22, pp. 12469–12469, 2012.

[83] H. W. Seo, J. Lee, K. Han, C. Park, and C. Chae, "Comparative analyses of humoral and cell-mediated immune responses upon vaccination with different commercially available single-dose porcine circovirus type 2 vaccines," *Research in Veterinary Science*, vol. 97, no. 1, pp. 38–42, 2014.

[84] R. L. Salgado, P. M. Vidigal, L. F. de Souza et al., "Identification of an emergent porcine circovirus-2 in vaccinated pigs from a brazilian farm during a postweaning multisystemic wasting syndrome outbreak," *Genome Announcements*, vol. 2, no. 2, 2014.

[85] N. Ramos, S. Mirazo, G. Castro, and J. Arbiza, "First identification of Porcine Circovirus Type 2b mutant in pigs from Uruguay," *Infection, Genetics and Evolution*, vol. 33, pp. 320–323, 2015.

[86] M. Eddicks, R. Fux, F. Szikora et al., "Detection of a new cluster of porcine circovirus type 2b strains in domestic pigs in Germany," *Veterinary Microbiology*, vol. 176, no. 3-4, pp. 337–343, 2015.

[87] G. Reiner, R. Hofmeister, and H. Willems, "Genetic variability of porcine circovirus 2 (PCV2) field isolates from vaccinated and non-vaccinated pig herds in Germany," *Veterinary Microbiology*, vol. 180, no. 1-2, pp. 41–48, 2015.

[88] N. E. McKeown, T. Opriessnig, P. Thomas et al., "Effects of porcine circovirus type 2 (PCV2) maternal antibodies on experimental infection of piglets with PCV2," *Clinical and Diagnostic Laboratory Immunology*, vol. 12, no. 11, pp. 1347–1351, 2005.

[89] J. Gillespie, T. Opriessnig, X. J. Meng, K. Pelzer, and V. Buechner-Maxwell, "Porcine circovirus type 2 and porcine circovirus-associated disease," *Journal of Veterinary Internal Medicine*, vol. 23, no. 6, pp. 1151–1163, 2009.

[90] X.-J. Meng, "Porcine circovirus type 2 (PCV2): pathogenesis and interaction with the immune system," *Annual Review of Animal Biosciences*, vol. 1, pp. 43–64, 2013.

[91] C. Chae, "Porcine circovirus type 2 and its associated diseases in Korea," *Virus Research*, vol. 164, no. 1-2, pp. 107–113, 2012.

[92] J.-S. Park, J. Kim, Y. Ha et al., "Birth abnormalities in pregnant sows infected intranasally with porcine circovirus 2," *Journal of Comparative Pathology*, vol. 132, no. 2-3, pp. 139–144, 2005.

[93] C. Salogni, M. Lazzaro, E. Giacomini et al., "Infectious agents identified in aborted swine fetuses in a high-density breeding area: A Three-Year Study," *Journal of Veterinary Diagnostic Investigation*, vol. 28, no. 5, pp. 550–554, 2016.

[94] P. A. Harms, S. D. Sorden, P. G. Halbur et al., "Experimental reproduction of severe disease in CD/CD pigs concurrently infected with type 2 porcine circovirus and porcine reproductive and respiratory syndrome virus," *Veterinary Pathology*, vol. 38, no. 5, pp. 528–539, 2001.

[95] J. Kim, H.-K. Chung, and C. Chae, "Association of porcine circovirus 2 with porcine respiratory disease complex," *Veterinary Journal*, vol. 166, no. 3, pp. 251–256, 2003.

[96] C. Rosell, J. Segalés, J. A. Ramos-Vara et al., "Identification of porcine circovirus in tissues of pigs with porcine dermatitis and nephropathy syndrome," *Veterinary Record*, vol. 146, no. 2, pp. 40–43, 2000.

[97] G. J. Wellenberg, N. Stockhofe-Zurwieden, M. F. De Jong, W. J. A. Boersma, and A. R. W. Elbers, "Excessive porcine circovirus type 2 antibody titres may trigger the development of porcine dermatitis and nephropathy syndrome: A Case-Control Study," *Veterinary Microbiology*, vol. 99, no. 3-4, pp. 203–214, 2004.

[98] J. Kim, Y. Ha, K. Jung, C. Choi, and C. Chae, "Enteritis associated with porcine circovirus 2 in pigs," *Canadian Journal of Veterinary Research*, vol. 68, no. 3, pp. 218–221, 2004.

[99] G. W. Stevenson, M. Kiupel, S. K. Mittal, J. Choi, K. S. Latimer, and C. L. Kanitz, "Tissue distribution and genetic typing of porcine circoviruses in pigs with naturally occurring congenital tremors," *Journal of Veterinary Diagnostic Investigation*, vol. 13, no. 1, pp. 57–62, 2001.

[100] Y. Ha, K. Jung, and C. Chae, "Lack of evidence of porcine circovirus type 1 and type 2 infection in piglets with congenital tremors in Korea," *Veterinary Record*, vol. 156, no. 12, pp. 383–384, 2005.

[101] S. Kennedy, J. Segalés, A. Rovira et al., "Absence of evidence of porcine circovirus infection in piglets with congenital tremors," *Journal of Veterinary Diagnostic Investigation*, vol. 15, no. 2, pp. 151–156, 2003.

[102] P. Tummaruk and P. Pearodwong, "Porcine circovirus type 2 expression in the brain of neonatal piglets with congenital tremor," *Comparative Clinical Pathology*, vol. 25, no. 4, pp. 727–732, 2016.

[103] F. Hasslung, P. Wallgren, A.-S. Ladekjær-Hansen et al., "Experimental reproduction of postweaning multisystemic wasting syndrome (PMWS) in pigs in Sweden and Denmark with a Swedish isolate of porcine circovirus type 2," *Veterinary Microbiology*, vol. 106, no. 1-2, pp. 49–60, 2005.

[104] T. Opriessnig and P. G. Halbur, "Concurrent infections are important for expression of porcine circovirus associated disease," *Virus Research*, vol. 164, no. 1-2, pp. 20–32, 2012.

[105] Y. Li, H. Liu, P. Wang et al., "RNA-seq analysis reveals genes underlying different disease responses to porcine circovirus type 2 in pigs," *PLoS ONE*, vol. 11, no. 5, Article ID e0155502, 2016.

[106] R. Patterson, A. Nevel, A. V. Diaz et al., "Exposure to environmental stressors result in increased viral load and further reduction of production parameters in pigs experimentally infected with PCV2b," *Veterinary Microbiology*, vol. 177, no. 3-4, pp. 261–269, 2015.

[107] S. Kennedy, D. Moffett, F. McNeilly et al., "Reproduction of lesions of postweaning multisystemic wasting syndrome by infection of conventional pigs with porcine circovirus type 2 alone or in combination with porcine parvovirus," *Journal of Comparative Pathology*, vol. 122, no. 1, pp. 9–24, 2000.

[108] B. Lukač, A. Knežević, N. Milić et al., "Molecular detection of PCV2 and PPV in pigs in Republic of Srpska, Bosnia and Herzegovina," *Acta Veterinaria*, vol. 66, no. 1, pp. 51–60, 2016.

[109] J. Sun, L. Huang, Y. Wei et al., "Prevalence of emerging porcine parvoviruses and their co-infections with porcine circovirus type 2 in China," *Archives of Virology*, vol. 160, no. 5, pp. 1339–1344, 2015.

[110] G. M. Allan, F. McNeilly, J. Ellis et al., "Experimental infection of colostrum deprived piglets with porcine circovirus 2 (PCV2) and porcine reproductive and respiratory syndrome virus (PRRSV) potentiates PCV2 replication," *Archives of Virology*, vol. 145, no. 11, pp. 2421–2429, 2000.

[111] P. M. Dorr, R. B. Baker, G. W. Almond, S. R. Wayne, and W. A. Gebreyes, "Epidemiologic assessment of porcine circovirus type 2 coinfection with other pathogens in swine," *Journal of the American Veterinary Medical Association*, vol. 230, no. 2, pp. 244–250, 2007.

[112] Y. Yang, R. Shi, R. She et al., "Fatal disease associated with Swine Hepatitis E virus and Porcine circovirus 2 co-infection in four weaned pigs in China," *BMC Veterinary Research*, vol. 11, no. 1, article 77, 2015.

[113] T. Opriessnig, E. L. Thacker, S. Yu, M. Fenaux, X.-J. Meng, and P. G. Halbur, "Experimental reproduction of postweaning multisystemic wasting syndrome in pigs by dual infection with Mycoplasma hyopneumoniae and porcine circovirus type 2," *Veterinary Pathology*, vol. 41, no. 6, pp. 624–640, 2004.

[114] Y. Ha, K. Jung, K. Kim, C. Choi, and C. Chae, "Outbreak of salmonellosis in pigs with postweaning multisystemic wasting syndrome," *Veterinary Record*, vol. 156, no. 18, pp. 583–584, 2005.

[115] C. E. Dewey, W. T. Johnston, L. Gould, and T. L. Whiting, "Postweaning mortality in Manitoba swine," *Canadian Journal of Veterinary Research*, vol. 70, no. 3, pp. 161–167, 2006.

[116] G. Marruchella, B. Paoletti, R. Speranza, and G. Di Guardo, "Fatal bronchopneumonia in a *Metastrongylus elongatus* and Porcine circovirus type 2 co-infected pig," *Research in Veterinary Science*, vol. 93, no. 1, pp. 310–312, 2012.

[117] X.-J. Meng, "Spread like a wildfire—the omnipresence of porcine circovirus type 2 (PCV2) and its ever-expanding association with diseases in pigs," *Virus Research*, vol. 164, no. 1-2, pp. 1–3, 2012.

[118] G. Franzo, C. M. Tucciarone, G. Dotto, A. Gigli, L. Ceglie, and M. Drigo, "International trades, local spread and viral evolution: the case of porcine circovirus type 2 (PCV2) strains heterogeneity in Italy," *Infection, Genetics and Evolution*, vol. 32, pp. 409–415, 2015.

[119] T. W. Drew, S. S. Grierson, D. P. King et al., "Genetic similarity between porcine circovirus type 2 isolated from the first reported case of PMWS in South Africa and North American isolates," *Veterinary Record*, vol. 155, no. 5, pp. 149–151, 2004.

[120] V. R. Monger, J. A. Stegeman, G. Koop, K. Dukpa, T. Tenzin, and W. L. A. Loeffen, "Seroprevalence and associated risk factors of important pig viral diseases in Bhutan," *Preventive Veterinary Medicine*, vol. 117, no. 1, pp. 222–232, 2014.

[121] N. Rose, G. Larour, G. Le Diguerher et al., "Risk factors for porcine post-weaning multisystemic wasting syndrome (PMWS) in 149 French farrow-to-finish herds," *Preventive Veterinary Medicine*, vol. 61, no. 3, pp. 209–225, 2003.

[122] K. Dupont, C. K. Hjulsager, C. S. Kristensen, P. Baekbo, and L. E. Larsen, "Transmission of different variants of PCV2 and viral dynamics in a research facility with pigs mingled from PMWS-affected herds and non-affected herds," *Veterinary Microbiology*, vol. 139, no. 3-4, pp. 219–226, 2009.

[123] H. Shen, C. Wang, D. M. Madson, and T. Opriessnig, "High prevalence of porcine circovirus viremia in newborn piglets in five clinically normal swine breeding herds in North America," *Preventive Veterinary Medicine*, vol. 97, no. 3-4, pp. 228–236, 2010.

[124] P. Alarcon, M. Velasova, A. Mastin, A. Nevel, K. D. C. Stärk, and B. Wieland, "Farm level risk factors associated with severity of post-weaning multi-systemic wasting syndrome," *Preventive Veterinary Medicine*, vol. 101, no. 3-4, pp. 182–191, 2011.

[125] M. Lőrincz, Á. Cságola, I. Biksi, L. Szeredi, Á. Dán, and T. Tuboly, "Detection of porcine circovirus in rodents—short communication," *Acta Veterinaria Hungarica*, vol. 58, no. 2, pp. 265–268, 2010.

[126] R. Blunt, S. McOrist, J. McKillen, I. McNair, T. Jiang, and K. Mellits, "House fly vector for porcine circovirus 2b on commercial pig farms," *Veterinary Microbiology*, vol. 149, no. 3-4, pp. 452–455, 2011.

[127] X. Yang, L. Hou, J. Ye, Q. He, and S. Cao, "Detection of porcine circovirus type 2 (PCV2) in mosquitoes from pig farms by PCR," *Pakistan Veterinary Journal*, vol. 32, no. 1, pp. 134–135, 2012.

[128] D. Verreault, V. Létourneau, L. Gendron, D. Massé, C. A. Gagnon, and C. Duchaine, "Airborne porcine circovirus in Canadian swine confinement buildings," *Veterinary Microbiology*, vol. 141, no. 3-4, pp. 224–230, 2010.

[129] M.-T. Chiou, C.-Y. Yang, T.-C. Chang, C. Chen, C.-F. Lin, and L.-J. Ye, "Shedding pattern and serological profile of porcine circovirus type 2 infection in cesarean-derived, colostrum-deprived and farm-raised pigs," *Journal of Veterinary Medical Science*, vol. 73, no. 4, pp. 521–525, 2011.

[130] A. R. Patterson, D. M. Madson, P. G. Halbur, and T. Opriessnig, "Shedding and infection dynamics of porcine circovirus type 2 (PCV2) after natural exposure," *Veterinary Microbiology*, vol. 149, no. 1-2, pp. 225–229, 2011.

[131] A. R. Patterson, S. Ramamoorthy, D. M. Madson, X. J. Meng, P. G. Halbur, and T. Opriessnig, "Shedding and infection dynamics of porcine circovirus type 2 (PCV2) after experimental infection," *Veterinary Microbiology*, vol. 149, no. 1-2, pp. 91–98, 2011.

[132] J. Segalés, M. Calsamiglia, A. Olvera, M. Sibila, L. Badiella, and M. Domingo, "Quantification of porcine circovirus type 2 (PCV2) DNA in serum and tonsillar, nasal, tracheo-bronchial, urinary and faecal swabs of pigs with and without postweaning multisystemic wasting syndrome (PMWS)," *Veterinary Microbiology*, vol. 111, no. 3-4, pp. 223–229, 2005.

[133] I. Shibata, Y. Okuda, S. Yazawa et al., "PCR detection of Porcine circovirus type 2 DNA in whole blood, serum, oropharyngeal swab, nasal swab, and feces from experimentally infected pigs and field cases," *Journal of Veterinary Medical Science*, vol. 65, no. 3, pp. 405–408, 2003.

[134] C. Liu, T. Ihara, T. Nunoya, and S. Ueda, "Development of an ELISA based on the baculovirus-expressed capsid protein of porcine circovirus type 2 as antigen," *Journal of Veterinary Medical Science*, vol. 66, no. 3, pp. 237–242, 2004.

[135] M. Sibila, M. Calsamiglia, J. Segales et al., "Use of a polymerase chain reaction assay and an ELISA to monitor porcine circovirus type 2 infection in pigs from farms with and without postweaning multisystemic wasting syndrome," *American Journal of Veterinary Research*, vol. 65, no. 1, pp. 88–92, 2004.

[136] H. Feng, G. Blanco, J. Segalés, and M. Sibila, "Can Porcine circovirus type 2 (PCV2) infection be eradicated by mass vaccination?" *Veterinary Microbiology*, vol. 172, no. 1-2, pp. 92–99, 2014.

[137] L. Fraile, M. Sibila, M. Nofrarías et al., "Effect of sow and piglet porcine circovirus type 2 (PCV2) vaccination on piglet mortality, viraemia, antibody titre and production parameters," *Veterinary Microbiology*, vol. 161, no. 1-2, pp. 229–234, 2012.

[138] P. F. Gerber, F. M. Garrocho, Â. M. Q. Lana, and Z. I. P. Lobato, "Serum antibodies and shedding of infectious porcine circovirus 2 into colostrum and milk of vaccinated and unvaccinated naturally infected sows," *Veterinary Journal*, vol. 188, no. 2, pp. 240–242, 2011.

[139] J. Segalés, A. Urniza, A. Alegre et al., "A genetically engineered chimeric vaccine against porcine circovirus type 2 (PCV2) improves clinical, pathological and virological outcomes in postweaning multisystemic wasting syndrome affected farms," *Vaccine*, vol. 27, no. 52, pp. 7313–7321, 2009.

[140] T. Kekarainen, K. McCullough, M. Fort, C. Fossum, J. Segalés, and G. M. Allan, "Immune responses and vaccine-induced immunity against Porcine circovirus type 2," *Veterinary Immunology and Immunopathology*, vol. 136, no. 3-4, pp. 185–193, 2010.

[141] S. Carman, H. Y. Cai, J. DeLay et al., "The emergence of a new strain of porcine circovirus-2 in Ontario and Quebec swine and its association with severe porcine circovirus associated disease—2004-2006," *Canadian Journal of Veterinary Research*, vol. 72, no. 3, pp. 259–268, 2008.

[142] T. Opriessnig, K. O'Neill, P. F. Gerber et al., "A PCV2 vaccine based on genotype 2b is more effective than a 2a-based vaccine to protect against PCV2b or combined PCV2a/2b viremia in pigs with concurrent PCV2, PRRSV and PPV infection," *Vaccine*, vol. 31, no. 3, pp. 487–494, 2013.

[143] T. Opriessnig, C. T. Xiao, P. F. Gerber, and P. G. Halbur, "Identification of recently described porcine parvoviruses in archived North American samples from 1996 and association with porcine circovirus associated disease," *Veterinary Microbiology*, vol. 173, no. 1-2, pp. 9–16, 2014.

[144] C. Firth, M. A. Charleston, S. Duffy, B. Shapiro, and E. C. Holmes, "Insights into the evolutionary history of an emerging livestock pathogen: porcine circovirus 2," *Journal of Virology*, vol. 83, no. 24, pp. 12813–12821, 2009.

[145] M. A. Ssemadaali, M. Ilha, and S. Ramamoorthy, "Genetic diversity of porcine circovirus type 2 and implications for detection and control," *Research in Veterinary Science*, vol. 103, pp. 179–186, 2015.

[146] Z. Peng, T. Ma, D. Pang et al., "Expression, purification and antibody preparation of PCV2 Rep and ORF3 proteins," *International Journal of Biological Macromolecules*, vol. 86, pp. 277–281, 2016.

[147] Z. Afghah, B. Webb, X. Meng, and S. Ramamoorthy, "Ten years of PCV2 vaccines and vaccination: is eradication a possibility?" *Veterinary Microbiology*, 2016.

[148] N. Sun, T. Yu, J.-X. Zhao et al., "Antiviral activities of natural compounds derived from traditional chinese medicines against porcine circovirus type 2 (PCV2)," *Biotechnology and Bioprocess Engineering*, vol. 20, no. 1, pp. 180–187, 2015.

[149] J. Segalés, T. Kekarainen, and M. Cortey, "The natural history of porcine circovirus type 2: from an inoffensive virus to a devastating swine disease?" *Veterinary Microbiology*, vol. 165, no. 1-2, pp. 13–20, 2013.

[150] N. Sun, P. Sun, H. Lv et al., "Matrine displayed antiviral activity in porcine alveolar macrophages co-infected by porcine reproductive and respiratory syndrome virus and porcine circovirus type 2," *Scientific Reports*, vol. 6, Article ID 24401, 2016.

[151] J. Chen, W. Li, E. Jin et al., "The antiviral activity of arctigenin in traditional Chinese medicine on porcine circovirus type 2," *Research in Veterinary Science*, vol. 106, pp. 159–164, 2016.

[152] J. Ellis, L. Hassard, E. Clark et al., "Isolation of circovirus from lesions of pigs with postweaning multisystemic wasting syndrome," *Canadian Veterinary Journal*, vol. 39, no. 1, pp. 44–51, 1998.

[153] J. C. Harding and E. Clark, "Recognizing and diagnosing postweaning multisystemic wasting syndrome (PMWS)," *Journal of Swine Health Production*, vol. 5, pp. 201–203, 1997.

[154] P. LeCann, E. Albina, F. Madec, R. Cariolet, and A. Jestin, "Piglet wasting disease," *The Veterinary Record*, vol. 141, no. 25, p. 660, 1997.

[155] Á. Dán, T. Molnár, I. Biksi, R. Glávits, M. Shaheim, and B. Harrach, "Characterisation of Hungarian porcine circovirus 2 genomes associated with PMWS and PDNS cases," *Acta Veterinaria Hungarica*, vol. 51, no. 4, pp. 551–562, 2003.

[156] A. M. Martins Gomes De Castro, A. Cortez, M. B. Heinemann, P. E. Brandão, and L. J. Richtzenhain, "Genetic diversity of Brazilian strains of porcine circovirus type 2 (PCV-2) revealed by analysis of the cap gene (ORF-2)," *Archives of Virology*, vol. 152, no. 8, pp. 1435–1445, 2007.

[157] N. Ramos, S. Mirazo, G. Castro, and J. Arbiza, "Detection and molecular characterization of porcine circovirus type 2 (PCV2) from piglets with exudative epidermitis in Uruguay," *Research in Veterinary Science*, vol. 93, no. 2, pp. 1042–1045, 2012.

[158] K.-S. Choi and J.-S. Chae, "Genetic characterization of porcine circovirus type 2 in Republic of Korea," *Research in Veterinary Science*, vol. 84, no. 3, pp. 497–501, 2008.

[159] Z.-Z. Yang, J.-B. Shuai, X.-J. Dai, and W.-H. Fang, "A survey on porcine circovirus type 2 infection and phylogenetic analysis of its ORF2 gene in Hangzhou, Zhejiang Province, China," *Journal of Zhejiang University: Science B*, vol. 9, no. 2, pp. 148–153, 2008.

[160] W. R. Raye, *An investigation into the status of porcine circovirus in Australia [Ph.D. thesis]*, Murdoch University, Perth, Australia, 2004.

[161] L. J. Pérez, H. Díaz de Arce, M. I. Percedo, P. Domínguez, and M. T. Frías, "First report of porcine circovirus type 2 infections in Cuba," *Research in Veterinary Science*, vol. 88, no. 3, pp. 528–530, 2010.

[162] S. P. Pozzi, H. Yadin, J. Lavi, M. Pacciarini, and L. Alborali, "Porcine circovirus type 2 (PCV2) infection of pigs in Israel: clinical presentation, diagnosis and virus identification," *Israel Journal of Veterinary Medicine*, vol. 63, no. 4, pp. 122–125, 2008.

[163] F. Schmoll, C. Lang, A. S. Steinrigl, K. Schulze, and J. Kauffold, "Prevalence of PCV2 in Austrian and German boars and semen used for artificial insemination," *Theriogenology*, vol. 69, no. 7, pp. 814–821, 2008.

[164] D. Tilman, K. G. Cassman, P. A. Matson, R. Naylor, and S. Polasky, "Agricultural sustainability and intensive production practices," *Nature*, vol. 418, no. 6898, pp. 671–677, 2002.

[165] A. R. Patterson and T. Opriessnig, "Epidemiology and horizontal transmission of porcine circovirus type 2 (PCV2)," *Animal*

Health Research Reviews / Conference of Research Workers in Animal Diseases, vol. 11, no. 2, pp. 217–234, 2010.

[166] M. Fenaux, P. G. Halbur, M. Gill, T. E. Toth, and X.-J. Meng, "Genetic characterization of type 2 porcine circovirus (PCV-2) from pigs with postweaning multisystemic wasting syndrome in different geographic regions of North America and development of a differential PCR-restriction fragment length polymorphism assay to detect and differentiate between infections with PCV-1 and PCV-2," *Journal of Clinical Microbiology*, vol. 38, no. 7, pp. 2494–2503, 2000.

[167] J. M. Mokoele, L. Janse van Rensburg, S. van Lochem et al., "Overview of the perceived risk of transboundary pig diseases in South Africa," *Journal of the South African Veterinary Association*, vol. 86, no. 1, article 1197, 2015.

[168] D.-J. An, I.-S. Roh, D.-S. Song, C.-K. Park, and B.-K. Park, "Phylogenetic characterization of porcine circovirus type 2 in PMWS and PDNS Korean pigs between 1999 and 2006," *Virus Research*, vol. 129, no. 2, pp. 115–122, 2007.

[169] L. Jonsson, *Emerging infectious diseases: using PCV2 as a model of disease transmission dynamics at the livestock-wildlife interface in Uganda [Dissertation]*, Fakulteten för Veterinärmedicin och Husdjursvetenskap, Institutionen för Biomedicin och Veterinär Folkhälsovetenskap, Sveriges Lantbruksuniversitet, Uppsala, Sweden, 2013, http://stud.epsilon.slu.se/5278/7/jonsson_l_130130.pdf.

[170] V. N. Ndze, D. Cadar, A. Cságola et al., "Detection of novel porcine bocaviruses in fecal samples of asymptomatic pigs in Cameroon," *Infection, Genetics and Evolution*, vol. 17, pp. 277–282, 2013.

8

Pathogenesis and Diagnostic Approaches of Avian Infectious Bronchitis

Faruku Bande,[1,2] **Siti Suri Arshad,**[1] **Abdul Rahman Omar,**[1,3] **Mohd Hair Bejo,**[1,3] **Muhammad Salisu Abubakar,**[1] **and Yusuf Abba**[1]

[1]*Department of Veterinary Pathology and Microbiology, Faculty of Veterinary Medicine, Universiti Putra Malaysia (UPM), 43400 Serdang, Selangor, Malaysia*
[2]*Department of Veterinary Services, Ministry of Animal Health and Fisheries Development, PMB 2109, Usman Faruk Secretariat, Sokoto 840221, Sokoto State, Nigeria*
[3]*Laboratory of Vaccine and Immunotherapeutics, Institute of Bioscience, Universiti Putra Malaysia (UPM), 43400 Serdang, Selangor, Malaysia*

Correspondence should be addressed to Siti Suri Arshad; suri@upm.edu.my

Academic Editor: Stefan Pöhlmann

Infectious bronchitis (IB) is one of the major economically important poultry diseases distributed worldwide. It is caused by infectious bronchitis virus (IBV) and affects both galliform and nongalliform birds. Its economic impact includes decreased egg production and poor egg quality in layers, stunted growth, poor carcass weight, and mortality in broiler chickens. Although primarily affecting the respiratory tract, IBV demonstrates a wide range of tissues tropism, including the renal and reproductive systems. Thus, disease outcome may be influenced by the organ or tissue involved as well as pathotypes or strain of the infecting virus. Knowledge on the epidemiology of the prevalent IBV strains in a particular region is therefore important to guide control and preventions. Meanwhile previous diagnostic methods such as serology and virus isolations are less sensitive and time consuming, respectively; current methods, such as reverse transcription polymerase chain reaction (RT-PCR), Restriction Fragment Length Polymorphism (RFLP), and sequencing, offer highly sensitive, rapid, and accurate diagnostic results, thus enabling the genotyping of new viral strains within the shortest possible time. This review discusses aspects on pathogenesis and diagnostic methods for IBV infection.

1. Introduction

Infectious bronchitis (IB) causes significant economic losses to the poultry industry worldwide [1, 2]. The disease was first identified in North Dakota, USA, when Schalk and Hawn reported a new respiratory disease in young chickens [3]. Since then, IBV has been recognized widely, especially in countries with large commercial poultry populations. Apart from respiratory infections, IB affects the kidney and reproductive tract, causing renal dysfunction and decreased egg production, respectively. Although the disease first was believed to occur primarily in young chickens, however, chickens of all age are also susceptible [1].

2. Aetiology and Molecular Biology

Infectious bronchitis is caused by infectious bronchitis virus (IBV), a single stranded positive sense, enveloped RNA virus of 27–32 kb length [4]. The virus has been classified under the *Gammacoronavirus* genus in the family Coronaviridae, order Nidovirales. Like other members of coronavirus family, the IBV genome is composed of structural and nonstructural proteins. Structural proteins include the spike [S] glycoprotein, envelope [E], matrix [M], and nucleocapsid [N]. These proteins together play different roles in viral attachment, replication, and inducing clinical disease. Of major structural proteins, the M protein is the most abundant transmembrane protein, which play vital role in coronavirus assembly through interaction with viral ribonucleocapsid and spike glycoprotein [5, 6]. IBV E protein is, however, scant and contains highly hydrophobic transmembrane N-terminal and cytoplasmic C-terminal domains. Studies have shown that the E protein is localized to the Golgi complex in IBV infected cells and is integrally associated with viral envelope formation, assembly, budding, ion channel activity, and apoptosis [7, 8]. Similar to other coronaviruses, the phosphorylated 409 amino acid of IBV-N protein is highly conserved between amino acid residues 238 and 293 [9]. IBV-N protein binds with the genomic RNA to form a helical ribonucleoprotein complex (RNP), thus aiding transcription, replication, translation, and packaging of the viral genome during replication [10]. The S1 portion of the spike glycoprotein plays important role in the attachment and entry of the virus into the cell via sialic acid receptors and has been considered as the determinant for viral diversity and immune protection [11]. This protein has been targeted for genotypic characterization as well as recombinant IBV serotypes vaccines [6, 12, 13].

3. Pathogenesis

Infectious bronchitis virus infects primarily the respiratory system. However, some variants and several field isolates affect the reproductive, renal, and digestive systems of chickens. Disease pathogenesis differs according to the system involved, as well as the strain of the virus [1].

3.1. Host Susceptibility. Although domestic fowl (*Gallus gallus*) and pheasant (*Phasianus* spp.) are considered to be natural hosts for IBV [14], other IBV-like coronaviruses have been identified in nondomestic avian species including pheasant, peafowl, turkey, teal, geese, pigeon, penguins quail, duck, and Amazon parrot [15–18]. Antigenic similarities between turkey coronavirus (TCoV) and avian infectious bronchitis virus (AIBV) have also been demonstrated [19]. Antibodies to IBV have been demonstrated in humans with close contact to poultry, but the virus has not been reported to cause human clinical disease [20].

3.2. Age and Breed Predisposition. Chickens of all ages and breed types are susceptible to IBV infection, but the extent and severity of the disease is pronounced in young chicks, compared to adults. Similarly, resistance to infection was suggested to increase with increasing age [21]. Experimental evidence suggests that line C white leghorn chickens are more resistant to M41 IBV challenge, compared to line 151, although both lines had similar virus shedding rate [22, 23], perhaps influenced by genetic polymorphism in the chicken major histocompatibility complex (MHC), as observed between B^*15, B^*13, or B^*21 chicken haplotypes [24].

3.3. Receptor and Entry. The IBV receptor-binding domain (RBD) in the S1-spike plays a major role in attachment of the virus to host cells [25, 26]. Thus, variation in the S1 glycoprotein partly determines tissue tropism and virulence [27, 28]. IBV affects trachea, kidney, and reproductive tract through interaction of S1 glycoproteins RBD (AAs 19–69 in M41) with α-2,3-sialic acid receptors on the surface of the cells [29, 30]. In addition to the sialic acid receptor, attenuated Baudette-IBV strain has been shown to interact with a putative heparan sulfate- (HS-) binding site that might contribute to its wide host range [31]. Following viral attachment, conformational changes occurring in the S1 glycoprotein mediate the membrane fusion activity of the S2 carboxylic acid terminal of the spike glycoprotein [1]. Subsequently, IBV enters the cell and releases its nucleocapsid into the cell's cytoplasm, thus triggering replication, virus budding, and release [32].

3.4. Infection and Transmission. The virus is transmitted via the respiratory secretions, as well as faecal droplets from infected poultry. Contaminated objects and utensils may aid transmission and spread of the virus from one flock to another. Evidence of virus was shown in trachea, kidney, and Bursa of Fabricius 24 hrs following aerosol transmission [33]. The nature of IBV persistence remains to be elucidated; however, detection of the virus in the caecal tonsils (up to 14 weeks) and from faeces (20 weeks) after infection might suggest a role of faecal shedding in viral transmission and persistence [34].

3.5. Incubation Period. Generally the short incubation period for IBV varies with infective dose and route of infection. For example, while infection via the tracheal route may take a course as short as 18 hours, ocular inoculation leads to an incubation period of 36 hours [33].

3.6. Clinical Course and Manifestations. In the host, initial infection occurs at epithelia of Harderian gland, trachea, lungs, and air sacs. The virus then moves to the kidney and urogenital tract, to establish systemic infection [33, 35]. In this regard, the severity and clinical features of IB depend on the organ or system involved. Infection of the respiratory system may result in clinical signs such as gasping, sneezing, tracheal rales, listlessness, and nasal discharges. Affected birds appeared listless and dull with ruffled feathers (Figure 1). Other signs may include weight loss and huddling of birds together under a common heat source [33].

Other clinical outcomes associated with IB infection include frothy conjunctivitis, profuse lacrimation, oedema, and cellulitis of periorbital tissues. Infected birds may also appear lethargic, with evidence of dyspnoea and reluctance to move [36]. Nephropathogenic IBV strains are most described in broiler-type chickens. Clinical signs include depression, wet droppings, and excessive water intake. Infection of reproductive tract is associated with lesions of the oviduct, leading to decreased egg production and quality. Eggs may appear misshapen, rough-shelled, or soft with watery egg yolk (Figure 2). Unless effective measures are instituted, decline in egg production does not return to normal laying, thus contributing to high economic loss [1, 37].

3.7. Gross and Histopathology. Pathological changes observed grossly at necropsy include congestion and oedema of

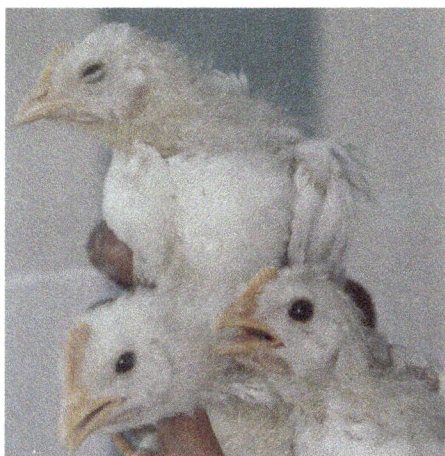

FIGURE 1: Dullness exhibited in chickens infected following experimental infection with IBV (courtesy: Siti Suri Arshad).

tracheal mucosa and extrapulmonary bronchi (Figure 3) [38, 39].

Histopathological changes include loss of cilia, oedema, rounding and sloughing of epithelial cells, and infiltration by lymphocytes (Figure 4). Presence of Russell bodies in Harderian cells has been observed following infection with H120 IBV serotype [40].

Nephropathogenic IBV strains cause nephritis characterized by swelling and congestion of the kidney (Figure 5), sometimes with pallor of ureters that contain urate deposits. Coinfection with bacterial pathogens such as E. coli may lead to a more complex outcome, usually associated with high morbidity and mortality. Similarly, infection with nephropathogenic IBV strains may result in pale, swollen, and mottled kidneys [39, 41]. Histological findings include interstitial nephritis, tubular degeneration, and infiltration by heterophils. In some cases, necrotic and dilated tubules are filled with urates and casts [33]. Experimental studies have shown that IBV-T-strain causes necrosis of the proximal convoluted tubule and distension of distal convoluted tubule. In addition, necrotic foci, heterophils, and lymphocytes are observed in the interstitial spaces. Oedema of Bowman's capsule and granulocytic infiltration has been reported in the collecting ducts and spheroids [42, 43].

When the reproductive system is affected, there may be nonpatent and hypoglandular oviduct, especially in severely affected chickens [43, 44]. Large accumulation of yolk fluid may be seen in the abdominal cavity (Figure 6), often associated with bacterial infection in laying hens [45, 46]. Cystic oviduct has also been observed in young layers following infection with certain IBV strains (Figure 7).

3.8. Morbidity and Mortality. Morbidity due to IBV infection can reach up to 100%. Mortality rate may range from 25 to 30% in young chicks but may increase to 80% as a result of factors that are host-associated (age, immune status), virus-associated (strain, pathogenicity, virulence, and tissue tropism), or environmental (cold and heat stresses, dust, and

presence of ammonia). Secondary bacterial infections (*E. coli*) or coinfection with immunosuppressive viruses such as Marek's disease virus, infectious bursal disease virus (IBDV) [33, 47, 48], may worsen the outcomes of IBV infection. Generally, nephropathogenic IBV strain causes high mortality, compared with strains infecting only the respiratory or reproductive systems [49].

4. Diagnosis

Conventional and more advanced methods have been used for the diagnosis of IBV infection. The choice of one test over another is guided by type of sample, availability of test materials and facilities, test reporting time, purpose of the test, and whether the test is carried out in the field or at the laboratory. Selected testing procedures are discussed below.

4.1. Serology. In the past, serological assays such as virus neutralization (VN) and haemagglutination inhibition (HI) were used widely for detecting and serotyping IBV strains. These tests also have been used to measure flock protection following vaccination [50, 51]. Serotype-specific antibodies usually are detected using HI, even though the HI test is less reliable [51]. On the other hand, ELISA assays are more sensitive and easily applied for field use and in monitoring antibody response following vaccination or exposure. However, emergence of different IBV serotypes that do not cross-react with commonly available antisera generally made serological tests less applicable and nonconclusive in classifying new or emerging IBV isolates [52, 53].

4.2. Virus Isolation and Identification. Virus isolation has been the gold standard for the diagnosis of IBV [54, 55]. Taking samples during early onset of the disease and ensuring the right sampling techniques are important keys for successful isolation of IBV. To support successful virus isolation from swabs, recommended to place swab sample in buffered solutions of media or PBS before transporting them to the laboratory. If tissue samples are to be collected, recommended tissues are trachea, kidney, proventriculus, tonsil, and oviduct. Tissue samples must be collected aseptically from scarified chickens or immediately upon death, placed in sterile, tightly sealed plastic specimen bags, and transported to the laboratory on ice for further processing [56]. The stringent technique requirements and factors, such as the time required for several passages of virus in egg or cell culture, limit the use of virus isolation as a diagnostic method of choice for IBV infection. Notwithstanding, different laboratories use various isolation methods, as described below.

4.2.1. Embryonated Chicken Egg. Most IBV strains grow well when inoculated into the allantoic cavity of a 9–11-day-old chicken embryo. Clinical samples from tracheal swab, broth, or tissue homogenate (10% w/v) are inoculated into the allantoic cavity of specific pathogen-free eggs and incubated at 34–37°C, after inoculation. Eggs are candled daily to monitor embryo viability; death within 24 hrs is considered nonspecific. After 48–72 hrs, allantoic fluid (AF) is harvested from

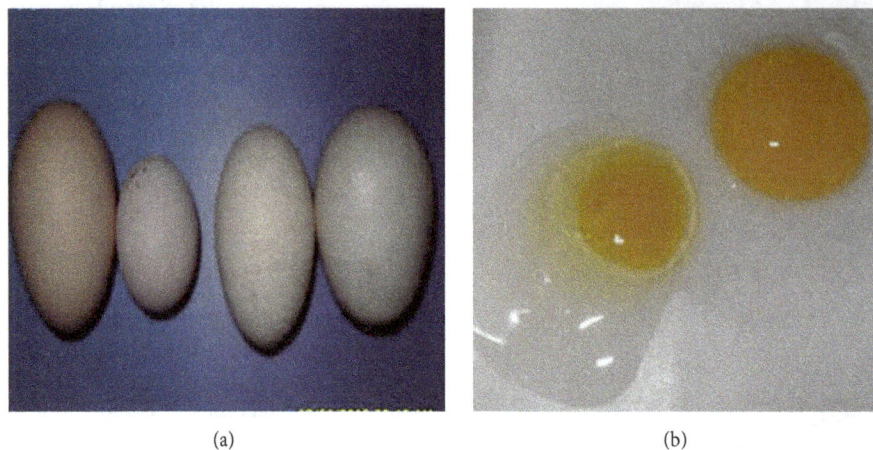

(a)   (b)

FIGURE 2: Irregularity in the shape and sizes of eggs from natural IBV infected breeder chickens (a). Watery albumen from IBV infected chicken ((b) left) compared to normal egg ((b) right).

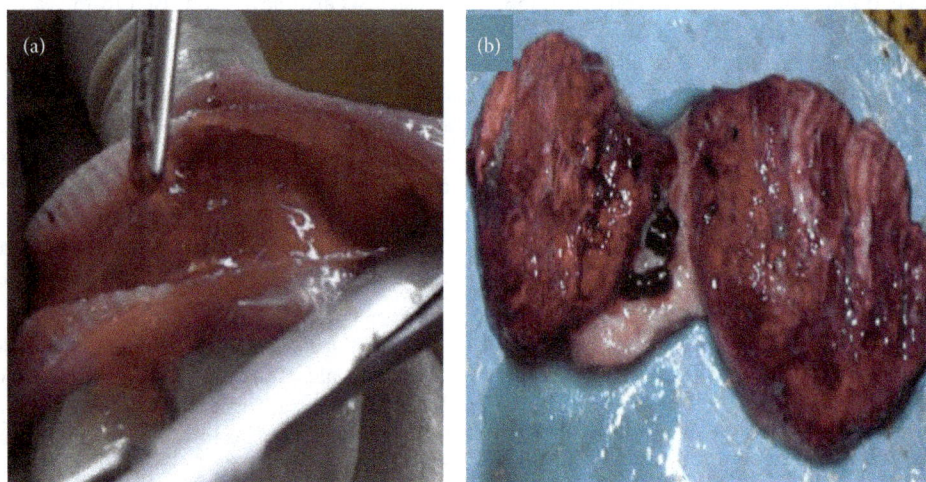

FIGURE 3: Gross lesions observed on respiratory organs of chicken naturally infected with IBV. Presence of mucoid secretion, congestion, and hyperaemia in the trachea (a); mild focal areas of lung consolidation (b).

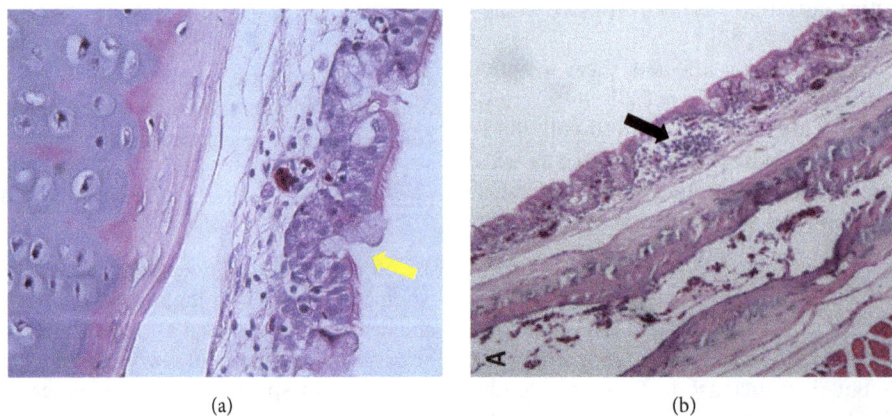

(a)   (b)

FIGURE 4: Histopathological changes in the trachea of naturally IBV infected chicken. Note: the marked infiltration of lymphocytes within the epithelia (black arrow (b)) and evidence of mucosal secretions of goblet cells (yellow arrow (a)).

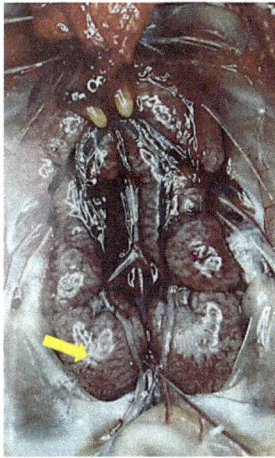

FIGURE 5: Gross lesions in kidney of chicken following experimental infection with a nephropathogenic infectious bronchitis virus. Note: swelling and congestion of the kidney (arrow) (courtesy: Siti Suri Arshad).

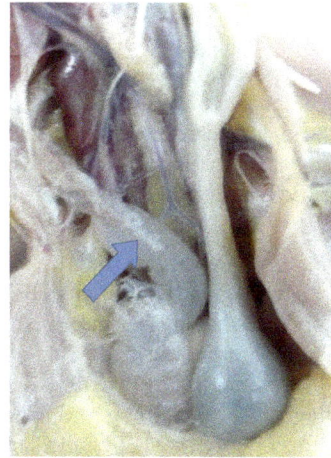

FIGURE 7: Cystic oviduct in 11-week-old chicken experimentally infected with a CR88 infectious bronchitis virus strain. Note the distention of the entire oviduct and fluid accumulation (arrow).

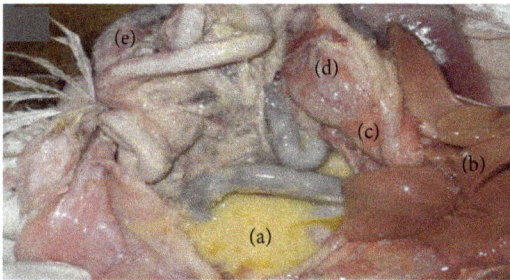

FIGURE 6: Chicken showing natural IBV infection. Accumulation of egg yolk in abdominal cavity (a); slightly enlarged, pale, friable liver (b) and multiple petechial haemorrhages on the serosal surfaces of proventriculus (c), gizzard (d), and small intestine (e).

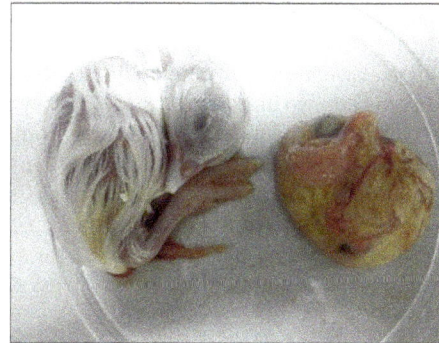

FIGURE 8: Embryo development at 17 days old following inoculations with IBV-CR88 strain. Note evidence of dwarfism and curling of the toes in IBV infected embryo (right) compared to a noninfected control embryo (left).

representative eggs that were chilled overnight and tested for the presence of IBV using serological tests or RT-PCR assay. Sometimes the allantoic fluid needs to be subjected to several passages to allow the virus to adapt and replicate to high titre, thus increasing the period that is needed to obtain results. The latter may vary among viral strains [54]. After 5–7 days, inoculated eggs are opened and observed for characteristic IB lesions such as curling and dwarfism of the infected embryo (Figure 8). It is important to note that such findings are suggestive, but not pathognomonic [57].

4.2.2. Cell Cultures. Isolation of IBV has been attempted in various primary and secondary cells, such as chicken embryo kidney fibroblast and Vero cells, respectively [58, 59]. Infected cultures are characterized by rounding, development of syncytia, and subsequent detachment from the surface of the plate [59]. A major limitation of cell culture methods for IBV isolation is that not all strains of IBV are easily adapted in cell culture. Even for some cell culture adaptable IBV (M41, Iowa 97, and NZ) strains, growth of the virus often requires primary isolation in embryonated eggs and several passages,

prior to adaptation. In some cases, attempts to grow IBV in various cell lines either failed or resulted in very low viral titre [58].

4.2.3. Organ Cultures. Tracheal organ culture (TOC) can be used to propagate both embryo-adapted and non-embryo-adapted IBV strains. TOC is prepared from tracheal rings of 20-day-old chicken embryo. The tracheal rings are maintained in a roller bottle and infected with IBV-suspected samples. The culture is observed microscopically for evidence of ciliostasis under light microscope. Complete impairment of ciliary activity usually is considered as a positive culture [60]. Successful growth of IBV has been demonstrated in organ cultures derived from kidney, intestine, proventriculus, and oviduct. However, susceptibility of these organs to IBV can be influenced by the strain of the virus and the amount of virus presence in the sample (infective dose). While a study suggested the universality of using kidney, bursa, and proventriculus in growing IBV, a poor result was obtained when IBV was propagated in cultures derived from different intestinal segments [61]. An advantage of this method includes easy titration and serotyping of IBV, since no virus adaptation is required [62]. Possible constraints include lack of affinity of some IBV strain for some organ cells and difficulty in differentiating ciliostasis arising from other viruses, such as Newcastle disease virus and avian adenovirus [33].

4.3. Electron Microscopy. Electron microscopy provides a direct means of detecting and identifying IBV in biological samples based on morphological characteristics of coronavirus. Positive cultures are confirmed based on the presence of coronavirus-like pleomorphic structures with spike projections, following negative staining with phosphotungstic acid (Figure 9). Importantly, the shape and diameter (120 nm) of the virus are taken into consideration when making diagnostic judgements. Apart from the negative staining method, transmission electron microscopy (TEM) is also a useful tool which enables the visualization of virus-like particles in infected cells [59, 63]. However, this method is often applied to understand viral attachment and entry into the cell but is not a specific diagnostic test [35].

4.4. Immunohistochemistry. Immunoperoxidase and immunofluorescenc are two important histochemistry methods for detection and confirmation of IBV antigen from infected tissue and/or cells. These methods work based on antigen-antibody reactions [64, 65]. Immunoperoxidase methods such as the avidin-biotin complex (ABC) have been used successfully to localize IBV antigen in tissue samples [66]. Likewise, indirect immunofluorescent assay is the most frequently used fluorescent technique [66, 67].

4.5. Molecular Diagnostic Assays. In view of their increased sensitivity and reduced reporting time, molecular methods, such as Reverse Transcriptase Polymerase Chain Reaction (RT-PCR), real-time PCR, Restriction Fragment Length Polymorphism (RFLP), and genome sequencing, have nearly replaced conventional serology and virus cultivation methods of IBV diagnosis [68, 69].

4.5.1. RT-PCR Methods. This approach uses viral RNA, amplified either directly (one-step RT-PCR) or following cDNA synthesis (two-step RT-PCR). An RT-PCR assay was designed and introduced in 1991 for detecting the IBV-S2 gene [70]. Subsequently, general and serotype-specific RT-PCR assays were designed to target different regions and/or fragments (Figure 10) in the IBV viral genome [71–73]. The UTR and N-gene-based RT-PCR are used for universal detection, because of the conserved nature of the target region in many IBV serotypes [68, 71]. A pan-coronavirus primer, targeting a conserved region of different coronavirus isolates, could also be used in one-step RT-PCR amplification of IBV strains [55]. However, amplification and sequencing of the S1 gene provide a reliable means for genotypic classification of new IBV strains [74]. A serotype-specific PCR assay has been designed to enable differentiation of Massachusetts, Connecticut, Arkansas, and Delaware field isolates [73].

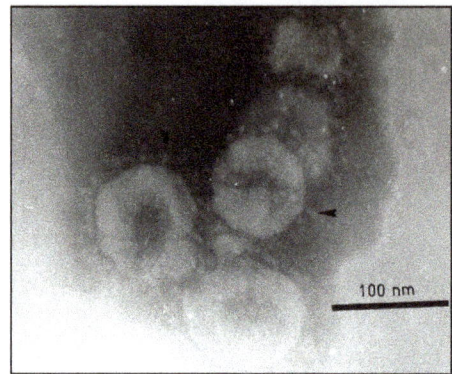

FIGURE 9: Negative staining electron microscope showing spherical shape of virus with typical spike projections (arrow) surrounding the virion of avian infectious bronchitis virus (courtesy: Siti Suri Arshad).

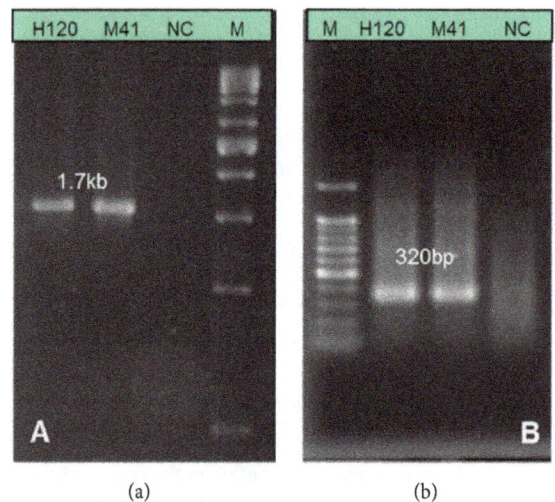

FIGURE 10: Electropherogram showing 1.7 kb RT-PCR amplified S1 genes from vaccine (H120) and virulent (M41) IBV strains (a) compared to a 320 bp RT-PCR amplified N-gene (b) of H120 and M41 IBV serotypes. Lane M = 1 kb molecular ladder (a) and 100 bp ladder (b); lane NC: negative control (no template control).

4.5.2. Restriction Fragment Length Polymorphism (RFLP). This is an IBV genotyping method carried out to differentiate different known strains of IBV and to identify new variants following RT-PCR amplification [75]. Full-length sequence of IBV S1 glycoprotein could be targeted for amplification and enzymes analysis [72, 76]. RFLP allows differentiation of various known IBV strains, based on their unique electrophoresis banding patterns defined by restriction enzyme digestion [72, 77]. The assay was found to be comparable with traditional virus neutralization assay, although some strains such as the Gray and JMK strains were reportedly difficult to differentiate using arrays of restriction enzymes, thus limiting the universal application of this method [72].

4.5.3. Real-Time RT-PCR and Other Forms of PCR Assays. For increased test sensitivity and specificity, real-time RT-PCR

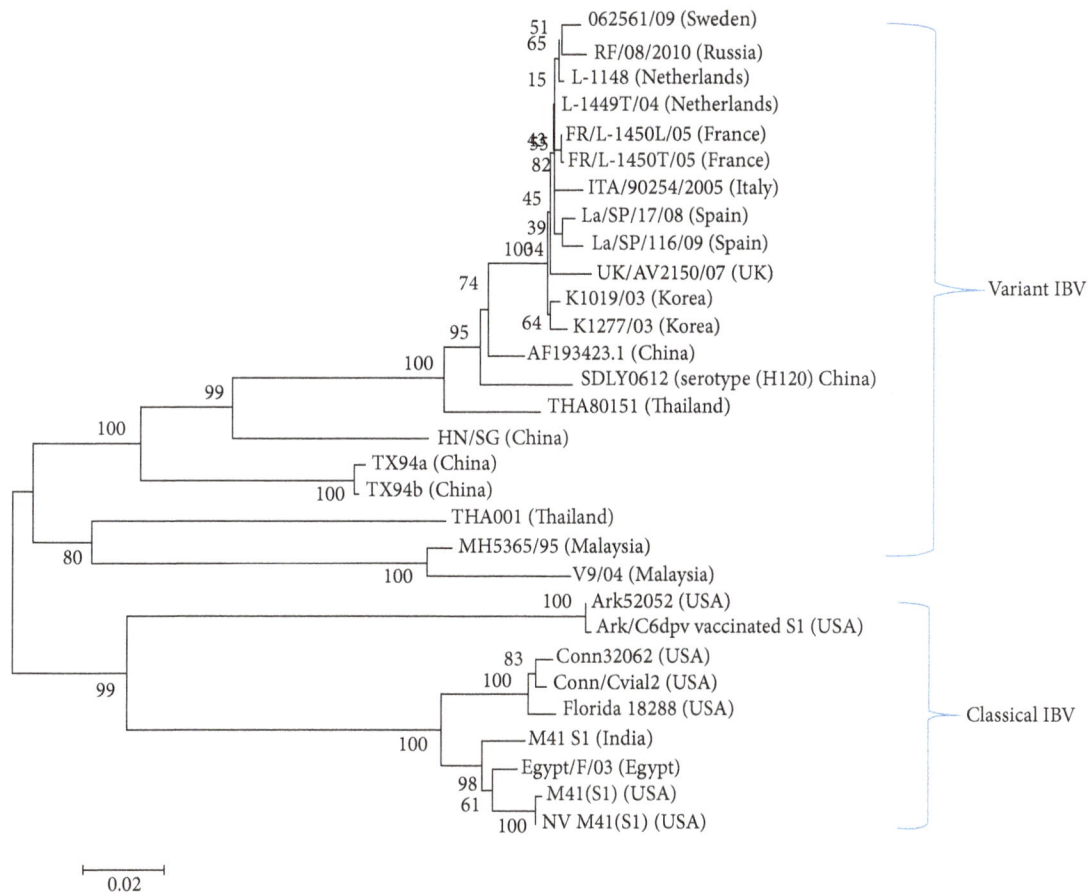

FIGURE 11: Neighbour joining phylogenetic analysis based on nucleotide acid sequence of S1-spike gene of classical and variant IBV strains identified in different countries. The tree was drawn with MEGA5 software using 1000 bootstrap replicates.

assays [78, 79] have been introduced for detecting IBV. Apart from detection, it is possible to quantify IBV viral load from tissue and/or clinical samples by real-time RT-PCR assays based on viral copy number or fold changes [80, 81]. Likewise, differentiation of Massachusetts from non-Massachusetts is possible by real-time RT-PCR assay targeting S1 glycoprotein gene [79, 82]. Recently, a high resolution melt curve analysis (HRM) was also developed to allow differentiation of field from vaccine IBV strains as well as for rapid and sensitive detection of recombinant variants [83, 84]. Meir et al. [85] reported that real-time RT-PCR was comparable to virus isolation and one or two times more sensitive in detecting M41 IBV than ordinary N-gene and S1 gene specific RT-PCR assays. On the other hand, real-time RT-PCR was tenfold more sensitive compared to virus isolation and 30- or 40-fold compared to N-gene or S1 gene-based RT-PCR, respectively. The authors, however, reported variations in sensitivity when either N-gene or S1 genes were targeted as well as when different samples are used for viral amplification. Other forms of PCR methods used in detecting IBV include nested PCR [68]; multiplex PCR [86]; and reverse transcription loop-mediated isothermal amplification (RT-LAMP) [87]. While these methods are more sensitive than standard RT-PCR, they are more expensive as well and might be beyond the financial capacity of many producers.

4.5.4. Sequence and Phylogenetic Analyses. For genotyping, S1 gene usually is amplified using RT-PCR, sequenced, and subjected to bioinformatics analyses [88, 89]. Following S1 gene sequencing, isolates are characterized through bioinformatics analyses based on their phylogenetic relatedness with reference sequences available in sequence databases such as the NCBI, EMBL, and DDBJ (Figure 11). Lack of method standardization among laboratories, particularly with respect to the S1 gene segment length that is used in phylogenetic analysis, limits genotyping to some extent. Currently, molecular methods such as next generation sequencing (NGS) have been introduced to sequence whole genomes within limited periods of time, though this approach has been used only in the laboratory.

5. Differential Diagnosis

Several respiratory diseases, such as Newcastle disease (ND), infectious laryngotracheitis, infectious coryza, avian metapneumovirus (aMPV), and avian influenza (AI), may produce clinical signs similar to avian infectious bronchitis. However, certain clinical features, including neurological signs and diarrhoea in ND, high mortality in AI, and pronounced head swelling in coryza, are uncommon in IBV infection and thus may be used in ruling out or arriving at narrowed tentative differential list [33, 90].

6. Conclusion

Ever since the first identification of IBV in 1930s, the poultry industry has suffered a growing number of emerging IBV serotypes. Importantly, the newly evolved strains have been favoured by selection pressure, mutation, and/or recombinations, thus allowing them to avoid detection, evade host immune response, and cause diverse pathological outcomes. Lack of effective diagnostic methods and vaccines that could easily tackle the menace caused by multiple IBV serotypes is partly blamed for the serious economic losses as results of infectious bronchitis disease. Conventional detection assays such as virus neutralization and virus isolation have been used extensively, but, due to lack of sensitivity and specificity of serological assays and laborious nature of virus isolation methods, these assays have gradually been replaced by the new sensitive and specific assays such as RT-PCR, RFLP, and qRT-PCR that enable rapid genotyping and identification of new IBV strains. However, there is a need for standardization across laboratories with respect to the type and length of target gene to be considered for genotyping so as to ensure common understanding of genotype distributions in order to guide vaccine selection for prevention and control.

Authors' Contribution

Faruku Bande conceived the idea, collected and studied published papers, drafted the review paper, and made all uncited photos from cases handled in his Ph.D. work available. Siti Suri Arshad, Abdul Rahman Omar, Mohd Hair Bejo, Yusuf Abba, and Muhammad Salisu Abubakar all participated in conceptualization of the idea, study design, review, and editing of paper. Siti Suri Arshad provided photos used in Figures 1, 5, and 9. All authors have read and agreed with submission of final paper to the journal.

Acknowledgments

The authors would like to thank the Universiti Putra Malaysia and Ministry of Science, Technology and Innovation (MOSTI), Project no. 02-01-04-SF1070 for funding supports. Dennis F. Lawler also provided paper-editing assistance.

References

[1] D. Cavanagh, "Coronavirus avian infectious bronchitis virus," *Veterinary Research*, vol. 38, no. 2, pp. 281–297, 2007.

[2] S. S. Arshad, "Infectious bronchitis," in *Diseases of Poultry in South East Asia*, M. Zamri-Saad, Ed., pp. 199–206, Universiti Putra Malaysia Press, Serdang, Malaysia, 2006.

[3] A. Schalk and M. Hawn, "An apparently new respiratory disease of baby chicks," *Journal of the American Veterinary Medical Association*, vol. 78, pp. 413–422, 1931.

[4] M. M. Lai and D. Cavanagh, "The molecular biology of coronaviruses," *Advances in Virus Research*, vol. 48, pp. 1–100, 1997.

[5] C. A. M. de Haan, H. Vennema, and P. J. M. Rottier, "Assembly of the coronavirus envelope: homotypic interactions between the M proteins," *Journal of Virology*, vol. 74, no. 11, pp. 4967–4978, 2000.

[6] F. Bande, S. S. Arshad, M. Hair Bejo, H. Moeini, and A. R. Omar, "Progress and challenges toward the development of vaccines against avian infectious bronchitis," *Journal of Immunology Research*, vol. 2015, Article ID 424860, 12 pages, 2015, 10.1155/2015/424860.

[7] E. Corse and C. E. Machamer, "The cytoplasmic tails of infectious bronchitis virus E and M proteins mediate their interaction," *Virology*, vol. 312, no. 1, pp. 25–34, 2003.

[8] L. Wilson, P. Gage, and G. Ewart, "Hexamethylene amiloride blocks E protein ion channels and inhibits coronavirus replication," *Virology*, vol. 353, no. 2, pp. 294–306, 2006.

[9] A. K. Williams, W. Li, L. W. Sneed, and E. W. Collisson, "Comparative analyses of the nucleocapsid genes of several strains of infectious bronchitis virus and other coronaviruses," *Virus Research*, vol. 25, no. 3, pp. 213–222, 1992.

[10] J. Jayaram, S. Youn, and E. W. Collisson, "The virion N protein of infectious bronchitis virus is more phosphorylated than the N protein from infected cell lysates," *Virology*, vol. 339, no. 1, pp. 127–135, 2005.

[11] M. W. Jackwood, D. Hall, and A. Handel, "Molecular evolution and emergence of avian gammacoronaviruses," *Infection, Genetics and Evolution*, vol. 12, no. 6, pp. 1305–1311, 2012.

[12] Z. J. Wei, P. Wei, M. L. Mo, M. Li, T. C. Wei, and K. R. Li, "Genetic variation of S1 gene hypervariable region I of infectious bronchitis viruses isolated in different periods in Guangxi," *Chinese Journal of Virology*, vol. 24, no. 2, pp. 126–132, 2008.

[13] X.-M. Shi, Y. Zhao, H.-B. Gao et al., "Evaluation of recombinant fowlpox virus expressing infectious bronchitis virus S1 gene and chicken interferon-7 gene for immune protection against heterologous strains," *Vaccine*, vol. 29, no. 8, pp. 1576–1582, 2011.

[14] D. Cavanagh, K. Mawditt, D. D. B. Welchman, P. Britton, and R. E. Gough, "Coronaviruses from pheasants (Phasianus colchicus) are genetically closely related to coronaviruses of domestic fowl (infectious bronchitis virus) and turkeys," *Avian Pathology*, vol. 31, no. 1, pp. 81–93, 2002.

[15] S. Dea and P. Tijssen, "Detection of turkey enteric coronavirus by enzyme-linked immunosorbent assay and differentiation from other coronaviruses," *American Journal of Veterinary Research*, vol. 50, no. 2, pp. 226–231, 1989.

[16] C. M. Jonassen, T. Kofstad, I.-L. Larsen et al., "Molecular identification and characterization of novel coronaviruses infecting graylag geese (*Anser anser*), feral pigeons (*Columbia livia*) and mallards (*Anas platyrhynchos*)," *Journal of General Virology*, vol. 86, no. 6, pp. 1597–1607, 2005.

[17] D. Cavanagh, "*Coronaviridae*: a review of coronaviruses and toroviruses," in *Coronaviruses with Special Emphasis on First Insights Concerning SARS*, pp. 1–54, Birkhäuser, Basel, Switzerland, 2005.

[18] E. Circella, A. Camarda, V. Martella, G. Bruni, A. Lavazza, and C. Buonavoglia, "Coronavirus associated with an enteric

syndrome on a quail farm," *Avian Pathology*, vol. 36, no. 3, pp. 251–258, 2007.

[19] J. S. Guy, "Turkey coronavirus is more closely related to avian infectious bronchitis virus than to mammalian coronaviruses: a review," *Avian Pathology*, vol. 29, no. 3, pp. 207–212, 2000.

[20] L. T. Miller and V. J. Yates, "Neutralization of infectious bronchitis virus human sera," *American Journal of Epidemiology*, vol. 88, no. 3, pp. 406–409, 1968.

[21] R. A. Crinion and M. S. Hofstad, "Pathogenicity of four serotypes of avian infectious bronchitis virus for the oviduct of young chickens of various ages," *Avian Diseases*, vol. 16, no. 2, pp. 351–363, 1972.

[22] K. Otsuki, M. Huggins, and J. K. Cook, "Comparison of the susceptibility to avian infectious bronchitis virus infection of two inbred lines of white leghorn chickens," *Avian Pathology*, vol. 19, no. 3, pp. 467–475, 1990.

[23] N. Bumstead, "Genetic resistance to avian viruses," *OIE Revue Scientifique et Technique*, vol. 17, no. 1, pp. 249–255, 1998.

[24] L. D. Bacon, D. B. Hunter, H. M. Zhang, K. Brand, and R. Etches, "Retrospective evidence that the MHC (B haplotype) of chickens influences genetic resistance to attenuated infectious bronchitis vaccine strains in chickens," *Avian Pathology*, vol. 33, no. 6, pp. 605–609, 2004.

[25] G. J. Babcock, D. J. Esshaki, W. D. Thomas Jr., and D. M. Ambrosino, "Amino acids 270 to 510 of the severe acute respiratory syndrome coronavirus spike protein are required for interaction with receptor," *Journal of Virology*, vol. 78, no. 9, pp. 4552–4560, 2004.

[26] N. Promkuntod, R. E. W. van Eijndhoven, G. de Vrieze, A. Gröne, and M. H. Verheije, "Mapping of the receptor-binding domain and amino acids critical for attachment in the spike protein of avian coronavirus infectious bronchitis virus," *Virology*, vol. 448, pp. 26–32, 2014.

[27] R. Casais, B. Dove, D. Cavanagh, and P. Britton, "Recombinant avian infectious bronchitis virus expressing a heterologous spike gene demonstrates that the spike protein is a determinant of cell tropism," *Journal of Virology*, vol. 77, no. 16, pp. 9084–9089, 2003.

[28] D. E. Wentworth and K. V. Holmes, *Coronavirus Binding and Entry. Coronaviruses: Molecular and Cellular Biology*, Caister Academic Press, Norfolk, UK, 2007.

[29] C. Winter, C. Schwegmann-Weßels, D. Cavanagh, U. Neumann, and G. Herrler, "Sialic acid is a receptor determinant for infection of cells by avian infectious bronchitis virus," *Journal of General Virology*, vol. 87, no. 5, pp. 1209–1216, 2006.

[30] K. Shahwan, M. Hesse, A.-K. Mork, G. Herrler, and C. Winter, "Sialic acid binding properties of soluble coronavirus spike (S1) proteins: differences between infectious bronchitis virus and transmissible gastroenteritis virus," *Viruses*, vol. 5, no. 8, pp. 1924–1933, 2013.

[31] I. G. Madu, V. C. Chu, H. Lee, A. D. Regan, B. E. Bauman, and G. R. Whittaker, "Heparan sulfate is a selective attachment factor for the avian coronavirus infectious bronchitis virus Beaudette," *Avian Diseases*, vol. 51, no. 1, pp. 45–51, 2007.

[32] V. C. Chu, L. J. McElroy, V. Chu, B. E. Bauman, and G. R. Whittaker, "The avian coronavirus infectious bronchitis virus undergoes direct low-pH-dependent fusion activation during entry into host cells," *Journal of Virology*, vol. 80, no. 7, pp. 3180–3188, 2006.

[33] D. Cavanagh and J. Gelb, "Infectious bronchitis," in *Diseases of Poultry*, pp. 117–135, Wiley-Blackwell, 12th edition, 2008.

[34] D. J. Alexander and R. E. Gough, "Isolation of avian infectious bronchitis virus from experimentally infected chickens," *Research in Veterinary Science*, vol. 23, no. 3, pp. 344–347, 1977.

[35] S. Arshad, K. Al-Salihi, and M. Noordin, "Ultrastructural pathology of trachea in chicken experimentally infected with infectious bronchitis Virus-MH-5365/95," *Annals of Microscopy*, vol. 3, pp. 43–47, 2002.

[36] C. Terregino, A. Toffan, M. Serena Beato et al., "Pathogenicity of a QX strain of infectious bronchitis virus in specific pathogen free and commercial broiler chickens, and evaluation of protection induced by a vaccination programme based on the Ma5 and 4/91 serotypes," *Avian Pathology*, vol. 37, no. 5, pp. 487–493, 2008.

[37] R. W. Winterfield, H. L. Thacker, and S. F. Badylak, "Effects of subtype variations in the Holland strain of infectious bronchitis virus when applied as a vaccine," *Poultry Science*, vol. 63, no. 2, pp. 246–250, 1984.

[38] D. A. Purcell and J. B. McFerran, "The histopathology of infectious bronchitis in the domestic fowl," *Research in Veterinary Science*, vol. 13, no. 2, pp. 116–122, 1972.

[39] Z. Boroomand, K. Asasi, and A. Mohammadi, "Pathogenesis and tissue distribution of avian infectious bronchitis virus isolate IRFIBV32 (793/B serotype) in experimentally infected broiler chickens," *The Scientific World Journal*, vol. 2012, Article ID 402537, 6 pages, 2012.

[40] H. Toro, V. Godoy, J. Larenas, E. Reyes, and E. F. Kaleta, "Avian infectious bronchitis: viral persistence in the harderian gland and histological changes after eyedrop vaccination," *Avian Diseases*, vol. 40, no. 1, pp. 114–120, 1996.

[41] F. Cong, X. Liu, Z. Han, Y. Shao, X. Kong, and S. Liu, "Transcriptome analysis of chicken kidney tissues following coronavirus avian infectious bronchitis virus infection," *BMC Genomics*, vol. 14, no. 1, article 743, 2013.

[42] K. K. Chousalkar, J. R. Roberts, and R. Reece, "Histopathology of two serotypes of infectious bronchitis virus in laying hens vaccinated in the rearing phase," *Poultry Science*, vol. 86, no. 1, pp. 59–62, 2007.

[43] K. K. Chousalkar and J. R. Roberts, "Ultrastructural study of infectious bronchitis virus infection in infundibulum and magnum of commercial laying hens," *Veterinary Microbiology*, vol. 122, no. 3-4, pp. 223–236, 2007.

[44] K. K. Chousalkar, J. R. Roberts, and R. Reece, "Comparative histopathology of two serotypes of infectious bronchitis virus (T and N1/88) in laying hens and cockerels," *Poultry Science*, vol. 86, no. 1, pp. 50–58, 2007.

[45] R. W. Winterfield and S. B. Hitchner, "Etiology of an infectious nephritis-nephrosis syndrome of chickens," *American Journal of Veterinary Research*, vol. 23, pp. 1273–1279, 1962.

[46] J. J. de Wit, J. Nieuwenhuisen-van Wilgen, A. Hoogkamer, H. vande Sande, G. J. Zuidam, and T. H. F. Fabri, "Induction of cystic oviducts and protection against early challenge with infectious bronchitis virus serotype D388 (genotype QX) by maternally derived antibodies and by early vaccination," *Avian Pathology*, vol. 40, no. 5, pp. 463–471, 2011.

[47] M. P. Ariaans, M. G. R. Matthijs, D. van Haarlem et al., "The role of phagocytic cells in enhanced susceptibility of broilers to colibacillosis after infectious bronchitis virus infection," *Veterinary Immunology and Immunopathology*, vol. 123, no. 3-4, pp. 240–250, 2008.

[48] R. A. Gallardo, V. L. van Santen, and H. Toro, "Effects of chicken anaemia virus and infectious bursal disease virus-induced

immunodeficiency on infectious bronchitis virus replication and genotypic drift," *Avian Pathology*, vol. 41, no. 5, pp. 451–458, 2012.

[49] J. Ignjatovic, D. F. Ashton, R. Reece, P. Scott, and P. Hooper, "Pathogenicity of Australian strains of avian infectious bronchitis virus," *Journal of Comparative Pathology*, vol. 126, no. 2-3, pp. 115–123, 2002.

[50] D. King and D. Cavanagh, "Infectious bronchitis," *Diseases of Poultry*, vol. 9, pp. 471–484, 1991.

[51] OIE, *Avian Infectious Bronchitis*, chapter 2. 3. 2., 2008.

[52] D. Cavanagh, P. J. Davis, and J. K. Cook, "Infectious bronchitis virus: evidence for recombination within the Massachusetts serotype," *Avian Pathology*, vol. 21, no. 3, pp. 401–408, 1992.

[53] A. Kant, G. Koch, D. J. Van Roozelaar, J. G. Kusters, F. A. J. Poelwijk, and B. A. M. Van der Zeijst, "Location of antigenic sites defined by neutralizing monoclonal antibodies on the S1 avian infectious bronchitis virus glycopolypeptide," *Journal of General Virology*, vol. 73, no. 3, pp. 591–596, 1992.

[54] F. Beaudette and C. Hudson, "Cultivation of the virus of infectious bronchitis," *Journal of the American Veterinary Medical Association*, vol. 90, pp. 51–60, 1937.

[55] C. B. Stephensen, D. B. Casebolt, and N. N. Gangopadhyay, "Phylogenetic analysis of a highly conserved region of the polymerase gene from 11 coronaviruses and development of a consensus polymerase chain reaction assay," *Virus Research*, vol. 60, no. 2, pp. 181–189, 1999.

[56] J. Gelb Jr., W. A. Nix, and S. D. Gellman, "Infectious bronchitis virus antibodies in tears and their relationship to immunity," *Avian Diseases*, vol. 42, no. 2, pp. 364–374, 1998.

[57] L. N. Loomis, C. H. Cunningham, M. L. Gray, and F. Thorp Jr., "Pathology of the chicken embryo infected with infectious bronchitis virus," *American Journal of Veterinary Research*, vol. 11, no. 40, pp. 245–251, 1950.

[58] K. Otsuki, H. Yamamoto, and M. Tsubokura, "Studies on avian infectious bronchitis virus (IBV)—I. Resistance of IBV to chemical and physical treatments," *Archives of Virology*, vol. 60, no. 1, pp. 25–32, 1979.

[59] S. S. Arshad, *A study on two malaysian isolates of infectious bronchitis virus [Ph.D. thesis]*, Universiti Pertanian Malaysia, 1993.

[60] B. V. Jones and R. M. Hennion, "The preparation of chicken tracheal organ cultures for virus isolation, propagation, and titration," *Methods in Molecular Biology*, vol. 454, pp. 103–107, 2008.

[61] P. S. Bhattacharjee and R. C. Jones, "Susceptibility of organ cultures from chicken tissues for strains of infectious bronchitis virus isolated from the intestine," *Avian Pathology*, vol. 26, no. 3, pp. 553–563, 1997.

[62] M. Armesto, S. Evans, D. Cavanagh, A.-B. Abu-Median, S. Keep, and P. Britton, "A recombinant Avian infectious bronchitis virus expressing a heterologous spike gene belonging to the 4/91 serotype," *PLoS ONE*, vol. 6, no. 8, Article ID e24352, 2011.

[63] S. Patterson and R. W. Bingham, "Electron microscope observations on the entry of avian infectious bronchitis virus into susceptible cells," *Archives of Virology*, vol. 52, no. 3, pp. 191–200, 1976.

[64] A. Bezuidenhout, S. P. Mondal, and E. L. Buckles, "Histopathological and immunohistochemical study of air sac lesions induced by two strains of infectious bronchitis virus," *Journal of Comparative Pathology*, vol. 145, no. 4, pp. 319–326, 2011.

[65] S. S. Arshad and K. A. Al-Salihi, "Immunohistochemical detection of infectious bronchitis virus antigen in chicken respiratory and kidney tissues," in *Proceedings of the 12th Federation of Asian Veterinary Associations Congress/14th Veterinary Association Malaysia Scientific Congress*, p. 51, August 2002.

[66] A. S. Abdel-Moneim, P. Zlotowski, J. Veits, G. M. Keil, and J. P. Teifke, "Immunohistochemistry for detection of avian infectious bronchitis virus strain M41 in the proventriculus and nervous system of experimentally infected chicken embryos," *Virology Journal*, vol. 6, article 15, 2009.

[67] K. Yagyu and S. Ohta, "Detection of infectious bronchitis virus antigen from experimentally infected chickens by indirect immunofluorescent assay with monoclonal antibody," *Avian Diseases*, vol. 34, no. 2, pp. 246–252, 1990.

[68] A. Adzhar, K. Shaw, P. Britton, and D. Cavanagh, "Universal oligonucleotides for the detection of infectious bronchitis virus by the polymerase chain reaction," *Avian Pathology*, vol. 25, no. 4, pp. 817–836, 1996.

[69] A. Adzhar, R. E. Gough, D. Haydon, K. Shaw, P. Britton, and D. Cavanagh, "Molecular analysis of the 793/B serotype of infectious bronchitis virus in Great Britain," *Avian Pathology*, vol. 26, no. 3, pp. 625–640, 1997.

[70] Z. Lin, A. Kato, Y. Kudou, K. Umeda, and S. Ueda, "Typing of recent infectious bronchitis virus isolates causing nephritis in chicken," *Archives of Virology*, vol. 120, no. 1-2, pp. 145–149, 1991.

[71] K. A. Zwaagstra, B. A. M. van der Zeijst, and J. G. Kusters, "Rapid detection and identification of avian infectious bronchitis virus," *Journal of Clinical Microbiology*, vol. 30, no. 1, pp. 79–84, 1992.

[72] H. M. Kwon, M. W. Jackwood, and J. Gelb Jr., "Differentiation of infectious bronchitis virus serotypes using polymerase chain reaction and restriction fragment length polymorphism analysis," *Avian Diseases*, vol. 37, no. 1, pp. 194–202, 1993.

[73] C. L. Keeler Jr., K. L. Reed, W. A. Nix, and J. Gelb Jr., "Serotype identification of avian infectious bronchitis virus by RT-PCR of the peplomer (S-1) gene," *Avian Diseases*, vol. 42, no. 2, pp. 275–284, 1998.

[74] J. G. Zhu, H. D. Qian, Y. L. Zhang, X. G. Hua, and Z. L. Wu, "Analysis of similarity of the S1 gene in infectious bronchitis virus (IBV) isolates in Shanghai, China," *Archivos de Medicina Veterinaria*, vol. 39, no. 3, pp. 223–228, 2007.

[75] Z. Lin, A. Kato, Y. Kudou, and S. Ueda, "A new typing method for the avian infectious bronchitis virus using polymerase chain reaction and restriction enzyme fragment length polymorphism," *Archives of Virology*, vol. 116, no. 1–4, pp. 19–31, 1991.

[76] K. Mardani, A. H. Noormohammadi, J. Ignatovic, and G. F. Browning, "Typing infectious bronchitis virus strains using reverse transcription-polymerase chain reaction and restriction fragment length polymorphism analysis to compare the 3' 7.5 kb of their genomes," *Avian Pathology*, vol. 35, no. 1, pp. 63–69, 2006.

[77] M. D. F. S. Montassier, L. Brentano, H. J. Montassier, and L. J. Richtzenhain, "Genetic grouping of avian infectious bronchitis virus isolated in Brazil based on RT-PCR/RFLP analysis of the S1 gene," *Pesquisa Veterinaria Brasileira*, vol. 28, no. 3, pp. 190–194, 2008.

[78] K. K. Chousalkar, B. F. Cheetham, and J. R. Roberts, "LNA probe-based real-time RT-PCR for the detection of infectious bronchitis virus from the oviduct of unvaccinated and vaccinated laying hens," *Journal of Virological Methods*, vol. 155, no. 1, pp. 67–71, 2009.

[79] A. M. Acevedo, C. L. Perera, A. Vega et al., "A duplex SYBR Green I-based real-time RT-PCR assay for the simultaneous detection and differentiation of Massachusetts and non-Massachusetts serotypes of infectious bronchitis virus," *Molecular and Cellular Probes*, vol. 27, no. 5-6, pp. 184–192, 2013.

[80] M. W. Jackwood, D. A. Hilt, and S. A. Callison, "Detection of infectious bronchitis virus by real-time reverse transcriptase-polymerase chain reaction and identification of a quasispecies in the Beaudette strain," *Avian Diseases*, vol. 47, no. 3, pp. 718–724, 2003.

[81] S. A. Callison, D. A. Hilt, T. O. Boynton et al., "Development and evaluation of a real-time Taqman RT-PCR assay for the detection of infectious bronchitis virus from infected chickens," *Journal of Virological Methods*, vol. 138, no. 1-2, pp. 60–65, 2006.

[82] R. M. Jones, R. J. Ellis, W. J. Cox et al., "Development and validation of RT-PCR tests for the detection and S1 genotyping of infectious bronchitis virus and other closely related gammacoronaviruses within clinical samples," *Transboundary and Emerging Diseases*, vol. 58, no. 5, pp. 411–420, 2011.

[83] K. Hewson, A. H. Noormohammadi, J. M. Devlin, K. Mardani, and J. Ignjatovic, "Rapid detection and non-subjective characterisation of infectious bronchitis virus isolates using high-resolution melt curve analysis and a mathematical model," *Archives of Virology*, vol. 154, no. 4, pp. 649–660, 2009.

[84] K. A. Hewson, G. F. Browning, J. M. Devlin, J. Ignjatovic, and A. H. Noormohammadi, "Application of high-resolution melt curve analysis for classification of infectious bronchitis viruses in field specimens," *Australian Veterinary Journal*, vol. 88, no. 10, pp. 408–413, 2010.

[85] R. Meir, O. Maharat, Y. Farnushi, and L. Simanov, "Development of a real-time TaqMan® RT-PCR assay for the detection of infectious bronchitis virus in chickens, and comparison of RT-PCR and virus isolation," *Journal of Virological Methods*, vol. 163, no. 2, pp. 190–194, 2010.

[86] H.-W. Chen and C.-H. Wang, "A multiplex reverse transcriptase-PCR assay for the genotyping of avian infectious bronchitis viruses," *Avian Diseases*, vol. 54, no. 1, pp. 104–108, 2010.

[87] H.-T. Chen, J. Zhang, Y.-P. Ma et al., "Reverse transcription loop-mediated isothermal amplification for the rapid detection of infectious bronchitis virus in infected chicken tissues," *Molecular and Cellular Probes*, vol. 24, no. 2, pp. 104–106, 2010.

[88] Z. M. Zulperi, A. R. Omar, and S. S. Arshad, "Sequence and phylogenetic analysis of S1, S2, M, and N genes of infectious bronchitis virus isolates from Malaysia," *Virus Genes*, vol. 38, no. 3, pp. 383–391, 2009.

[89] S. H. Abro, L. H. M. Renström, K. Ullman et al., "Emergence of novel strains of avian infectious bronchitis virus in Sweden," *Veterinary Microbiology*, vol. 155, no. 2–4, pp. 237–246, 2012.

[90] R. Droual and P. Woolcock, "Swollen head syndrome associated with *E. coli* and infectious bronchitis virus in the Central Valley of California," *Avian Pathology*, vol. 23, no. 4, pp. 733–742, 1994.

9

Adapted Lethality: What We can Learn from Guinea Pig-Adapted Ebola Virus Infection Model

S. V. Cheresiz,[1,2] E. A. Semenova,[1,2] and A. A. Chepurnov[3]

[1]Department of Medicine, Novosibirsk State University, Pirogova Street 2, 630090 Novosibirsk-90, Russia
[2]Institute of Internal and Preventive Medicine, Bogatkova Street 175/1, 630089 Novosibirsk-89, Russia
[3]Institute of Clinical Immunology, Yadrincevskaya Street 14, 630047 Novosibirsk-47, Russia

Correspondence should be addressed to A. A. Chepurnov; alexa.che.purnov@gmail.com

Academic Editor: Jih-Hui Lin

Establishment of small animal models of Ebola virus (EBOV) infection is important both for the study of genetic determinants involved in the complex pathology of EBOV disease and for the preliminary screening of antivirals, production of therapeutic heterologic immunoglobulins, and experimental vaccine development. Since the wild-type EBOV is avirulent in rodents, the adaptation series of passages in these animals are required for the virulence/lethality to emerge in these models. Here, we provide an overview of our several adaptation series in guinea pigs, which resulted in the establishment of guinea pig-adapted EBOV (GPA-EBOV) variants different in their characteristics, while uniformly lethal for the infected animals, and compare the virologic, genetic, pathomorphologic, and immunologic findings with those obtained in the adaptation experiments of the other research groups.

1. Introduction

Several animal models for Ebola virus infection have been established in rodents and nonhuman primates (NHPs). The NHPs, including rhesus and cynomolgus macaques, are best suited for pathogenesis, treatment, and vaccine studies, since only they can be lethally infected by nonadapted EBOV strains with the resulting pathology closely resembling the human EBOV disease [1]. However, due to ethical, practical, and expense reasons, small animal models of EBOV infection were developed including guinea pig, mouse, and, recently, Syrian hamster models [2]. Those are established by a serial passage required for virus adaptation, since the wild-type EBOV is avirulent or causes a nonlethal disease in rodents. Although even the lethal adapted EBOV infection in rodents is different in many aspects from the disease in primates, the important similarities in the courses of both infections make small animal models useful, especially, in the study of genetic determinants of EBOV disease and in antiviral screening [1].

In primates, the pathogenesis of EBOV infection is associated with the viral replication in several major cell targets accompanied with immune dysregulation and coagulopathies. Viral reproduction in primary targets, the mononuclear phagocytes of spleen and lymph nodes, is followed by a massive replication in the liver, mostly, in macrophages and hepatocytes, and the virus spread to the other organs and tissues (adrenals, kidneys, reproductive organs, and lungs). A bystander lymphocyte apoptosis by an unknown mechanism is proposed to be the cause of severe lymphopenia occurring in EBOV infection. Inhibition of IFN-mediated response mediated by viral proteins VP24 and VP35 blocks the innate antiviral defense. Vascular damage either occurring directly, due to lytic virus reproduction in the endothelial cells, or induced indirectly by the effects of proinflammatory cytokines on the vascular wall is an important factor of pathogenesis. The mechanisms of coagulation dysfunctions, such as disseminated intravascular coagulation (DIC) and hemorrhages, as well as thrombopenia occurring in primate EBOV infection, are still to be investigated in more detail [3].

In guinea pigs, the lethal EBOV variants are established through the sequential passages (4–8 times) of an originally wild-type virus, in which, first, incomplete and, further, complete lethality in the groups of inoculated animals are acquired [4–7]. The guinea pig-adapted EBOV is causing a lethal infection with minor manifestations in the first 4-5 days and a subsequent rapid development of a highly febrile condition resulting in the animal death on days 8–11. First detected in lymph node macrophages as early as 24 h p/i, the virus spreads to the spleen and liver on day 2 and to the other organs and tissues further on. The virus spread can be accompanied with a progressive rise of tissue virus titers (from 1.7 to 4.8–6.4 $\log_{10}$ PFU/g in different tissues including spleen, liver, adrenals, lungs, kidneys, and pancreas) on days 1–9 of the infection, and the peak viremia in blood is reached on day 7 with ~10^5 PFU/mL [7]. However, in two of our adaptation experiments, an only modest [8] or even zero increase in virus titer [9] between the nonlethal and lethal adapted EBOV was occurring. A prolongation of the prothrombin time (PT) and the partial thromboplastin time (aPTT) is observed in the infected animals [1].

While resembling the course of EBOV infection in primates in many aspects, the EBOV disease in rodents has some important differences. Fever and maculopapular rash, which are the typical signs of infection in primates, are both not present in mice infected with mouse-adapted Ebola virus (MA-EBOV) [10]. In guinea pigs infected with guinea pig-adapted Ebola virus (GPA-EBOV), only fever, but not the rash, is present [5, 7]. Unlike in mice and similarly to Syrian hamster, lethal EBOV infection in guinea pigs induces serious coagulation abnormalities including the drop of platelets and an increase in coagulation time; however, fibrin depositions and disseminated intravascular coagulation (DIC) are not readily observed in these animals [2, 7, 11]. Occurrence of hemorrhages in EBOV disease in guinea pigs is still disputable: some researchers report that death of animals is not accompanied by the visible signs of hemorrhage [6]; however, we regularly observed typical hemorrhagic foci in the liver of, at least, part of the animals infected with GPA-EBOV in our experiments [12]. Despite the severe lymphopenia in the course of GPA-EBOV infection, lymphocyte bystander apoptosis, which is an important feature of infection in primates and mice, is not generally observed in guinea pigs [7].

Here, we present a comprehensive overview of the virologic, pathomorphologic, and hematologic data obtained in the EBOV adaptation experiments in guinea pigs (including four passage series performed in our laboratory) and discuss the value of those findings obtained in the rodent models for the general understanding of pathology of EBOV infection.

2. Establishment of Guinea Pig-Adapted Lethal Strains of Ebola Virus and the Study of Their Virulence and Virologic Characteristics

Serial passage of different viruses in animals or cell cultures can result in the selection of mutants with different reproduction characteristics and either higher or lower virulence, as compared to the original wild-type virus [13, 14]. Adult guinea pigs inoculated with the wild-type EBOV isolated from primates typically develop a nonlethal mild febrile or even asymptomatic disease. However, it has been previously shown that young guinea pigs may occasionally develop a lethal EBOV infection, and the serial passage of EBOV causes a substantial increase in lethality in these animals [4, 15]. In this review paper, we summarize our own data on the establishment of four independent adaptation series in guinea pigs using the original stocks of EBOV subtype Zaire, strain Mayinga, differing in their passage history [5, 8, 9, 11], and compare them with those from other labs where the EBOV adaptation series were successfully performed [6, 7, 10].

The original EBOV, strain Mayinga, stock of the first adaptation series (8mc) was passaged 24 times in Vero E6 cell line prior to the guinea pig adaptation experiments [5], while the stock of the second series (K-5) was passaged twice in NHPs (green monkeys) followed by 15 passages in human lung L68 cells [9]. In the third series (GLA), the wild-type EBOV, strain Mayinga, was passaged twice in NHPs and further multiplied in Vero cell culture [11]. The fourth series (GPA-P7) was started with an individual clone of strain Mayinga EBOV, which was obtained by triple-cloning/passaging in Vero cells and was confirmed to cause no lethal disease prior to its adaptation to guinea pigs. This virus clone further used for the inoculation of animals was designated as the precursor of guinea pig-adapted EBOV (pre-GPA clone) [8].

At first passage of 8mc adaptation series [5], a group of animals (we used the groups of 6 animals in all our adaptation experiments) was inoculated with virus derived from a liver homogenate of a rhesus macaque lethally infected by Mayinga strain of EBOV and passaged 24 times in Vero E6 cells. In some animals, a nonlethal febrile condition developed with the body temperature rising up to 40°C. The liver homogenates of the animals, which demonstrated high-grade fevers and higher levels of liver virus titer, were used for the next passage inoculation. With each passage, the febrile temperature was increasing (from 39.8–40.0°C at earlier passages to 41.5–42.0°C at later passages), as was the liver virus titer, which showed the overall growth from $2.9 \pm 0.4 \log_{10}$ PFU/mL to $5.5 \pm 0.7 \log_{10}$ PFU/mL (as determined by plaque forming assay in Vero cells). The first lethal outcomes were detected at passage 3, and the lethality and infectivity of the adapting virus isolate were gradually increasing until passage 8. In guinea pigs inoculated with the virus isolates of late passage 8, the fever occurred at days 4–7 and represented a double-peaked pattern with the second peak at days 11–13. Fever episodes were associated with the maximum levels of tissue virus titers. The adapted virus strain was designated EBOV-8mc, and several clones were derived from it and proved to have similar features as the noncloned EBOV-8mc virus itself [5].

As mentioned above, the original EBOV stock of K-5 series was passaged twice in NHPs and further 15 times in L68 cell culture prior to its adaptation to guinea pig, and its infectivity and virulence were evolving in the passage series. The biological titer of the virus harvest in PFU decreased from the first to third passage and then began to increase, reaching its plateau by passage 12 and further remaining stable. However, the virus infectivity in guinea pigs was unchanged throughout the L68 passages. Following the cell culture passages, the virus cloning was performed, and the biological titer (in PFU) of the intermediate virus stock (after passage 15, stock designation Ch-15) and the three obtained clones were shown to be equal. When adaptation to guinea pigs was started, clone 2 turned out to cause no febrile reaction, and virus isolation from blood samples of inoculated animals failed. However, clone 1 caused a rise in the rectal temperature in guinea pigs up to 40.5–41.8°C after the first passage, affecting up to 100% of animals. Beginning from the fourth passage, lethal outcomes were recorded. After the fifth passage, the virus became highly lethal for guinea pigs. The virus presence in the blood was recorded at a titer of $3.5 \log_{10}$ PFU/mL at passage 1 and did not change throughout the passage series. The resulting virus strain was designated K-5 [9].

In the third passage series, GLA [11], the animals inoculated at passage 1 developed a low-grade (below 40°C) fever, which showed a double-peak pattern with the peaks at days 7 and 20. A low amount of virus ($1.62 \log_{10}$ PFU/mL) could only be detected in the serum after the virus concentration by centrifugation, while no virus could be isolated from the whole blood. The tissue virus titers were detectable at $1.6 \log_{10}$ PFU/mL (in liver) and $3.22 \log_{10}$ PFU/mL (in peritoneal exudates). The first lethal outcomes were detected at passage 2 (on day 10), concomitant with the increase of serum and tissue virus titers to $4.2 \log_{10}$ PFU/mL. Interestingly, the second peak of fever was not observed in the surviving animals. At passage 3, the adapting EBOV became fully lethal to the guinea pigs with all animals dying between days 5 and 7, and the serum and tissue virus titers stabilized at the levels of $3.0–4.0 \log_{10}$ PFU/mL. The GPA-EBOV strain obtained in this series was used for a comprehensive analysis of pathomorphologic, hematologic, immunologic, and coagulation patterns of EBOV disease in guinea pigs.

In the last series, GPA-P7 [8], the precursor pre-GPA clone was obtained by a triple passage of original Mayinga EBOV in Vero cells and subsequent cloning. In the course of adaptation series, at each passage, one animal that displayed the most pronounced temperature response by day 7 p/i was used as a donor of the virus for the next passage. At all passages, the fever onset in the infected animals was recorded on day 4 p/i. The duration of fever episodes increased from passage to passage (from 6 days at passages 1-2 to 10–12 days in the surviving animals at passages 5-6). By day 7 p/i, the animals of all passages displayed a low level of viremia, which was not increasing throughout the passage series. The ability of virus to reproduce in the liver of infected animals was not changing significantly, as well. In the first two passages, EBOV induced a mild disease in guinea pigs with an increase in temperature to 40.0–40.4°C on days 4–9 p/i and eventual recovery. The first lethal outcome was recorded at passage 3, at day 15 p/i. No lethal outcomes were recorded at passage 4, while two lethal outcomes (40% lethality) were recorded at passage 4. Further on, the lethality increased, while the time of survival decreased. At passage 6, 80% lethality was observed, and, finally, at passage 7, full lethality of infection was acquired. The survival time in this fully lethal EBOV infection averaged 11.6 days. In lethal infections, the animals rapidly lost weight, displayed anorexia, and

developed impaired motor coordination, especially in the terminal stage. Two-three days before death, guinea pigs had diarrhea and the signs of intestinal hemorrhage were observed. This highly lethal EBOV variant obtained by the 7-passage adaptation of pre-GPA clone was designated GPA-P7 [8].

Our several attempts were made to adapt two original Mayinga strain EBOV stocks (of adaptation series 8mc and K-5) to adult ICR mice, using the same approach as the adaptation series to guinea pigs. All attempts to adapt the K-5 virus stock failed; however, using high doses of the first EBOV stock, we obtained a paradoxical variant of EBO. This passage series in adult ICR mice caused no lethal cases but resulted in the increasing virus titer in the liver reaching 5.55×10^{11} PFU/mL at later passages. Of note, the EBOV titers in the liver even at the first passage reached 3.5×10^9 PFU/mL on day 11. This mouse-adapted virus variant was named D-5 [9].

All adaptation series and the designations of all original and derivative viral stocks are provided in Figure 1.

The guinea pig-adapted EBOV strains, 8mc, K-5, GLA, and GPA-P7, as well as two other adapted variants obtained by the other research groups [6, 7], thus, represent the virus variants, which appear to be very similar in their virulence and lethality (despite the number of passages needed to acquire the full-scale pathogenicity), while strikingly different in the serum and tissue virus titers in the course of adaptation. Two of our adaptation series, 8mc and GLA, and the two series reported by others [6, 7] represent a 2-3-order-of-magnitude growth of tissue virus titers (in PFU) accompanying the development of strain virulence for guinea pigs, while in the other two, K-5 and GPA-P7, no or slight virus titer increase has been observed despite the acquisition of full lethality to the animals [5, 8, 9]. The adaptation series [5–7, 11], in which an increase in the virus titers in the liver or spleen has been observed (Table 1), prompted the hypothesis that the development of high virulence/lethality of the adapted virus variants could be due to the increasing virus replication in the infected tissues. However, the establishment of K-5 and GPA-P7 virus stocks, which do not show any significant increase in virus titers, while demonstrating high lethality to the animals, does not support this hypothesis. Similarly, a proposed link between the increasing rate of virus replication and the development of lethality in the adaptation of Mayinga EBOV strain to mice [10] is contradicted by our data on the mouse-adapted D-5 variant demonstrating the extraordinary high tissue virus titers, while lacking any pathogenicity in ICR mice [9]. It seems, therefore, that an increase in virus reproduction may not be the central determinant of EBOV virulence evolution in the course of virus adaptation to different animal models.

3. Study of the Genetic Determinants of Virulence/Lethality in Guinea Pig-Adapted EBOV Variants

The information on the genetic markers of EBOV virulence is important for the understanding of EBOV infection

TABLE 1: Comparison of lethality, virus reproduction, and the time to adaptation (# of passages) in different adaptation series.

Adaptation series	8mc [5]	K-5 [9]	GLA [11]	GPA-P7 [8]	[6]	[7]	D-5 [9]	[10]
Original virus stock	Mayinga, ZEBOV	Mayinga, ZEBOV	Mayinga, ZEBOV	Mayinga, ZEBOV	Mayinga, ZEBOV	Mayinga, ZEBOV	Mayinga, ZEBOV	Mayinga, ZEBOV
Preadaptation history	Vero E6 cell line passages	NHPs + L68 cell line passages	NHPs + Vero cell line passages	Individual clone, obtained from infected Vero cells	Vero E6 cell line passages	—	—	—
Adaptation to	Guinea pig	Guinea pig	Guinea pig	Guinea pig	Guinea pig	Guinea pig	Mouse	Mouse
Adapted virus lethality	100%	100%	100%	100%	80%	100%	0%	100%
Number of passages to full lethality	8	5	3	7	7	4	5	9
Increase in virus titer (nonadapted nonlethal versus adapted lethal, $\log_{10}$ PFU/mL)	2.9/5.5 Liver	3.5/3.5 Plasma	0.0/4.2 Plasma 1.62/4.2 Liver 3.22/4.2 Peritoneal exudate	6.3/7.0	2.9/5.0	2.1/5.2 Plasma 1.7/(4.8–6.4) In different tissues	9.5/11.7	4.2/7.8

Note: all virus titers in our adaptation series 8mc, K-5, GLA, GPA-P7, and D-5 were determined on day 6 p/i.

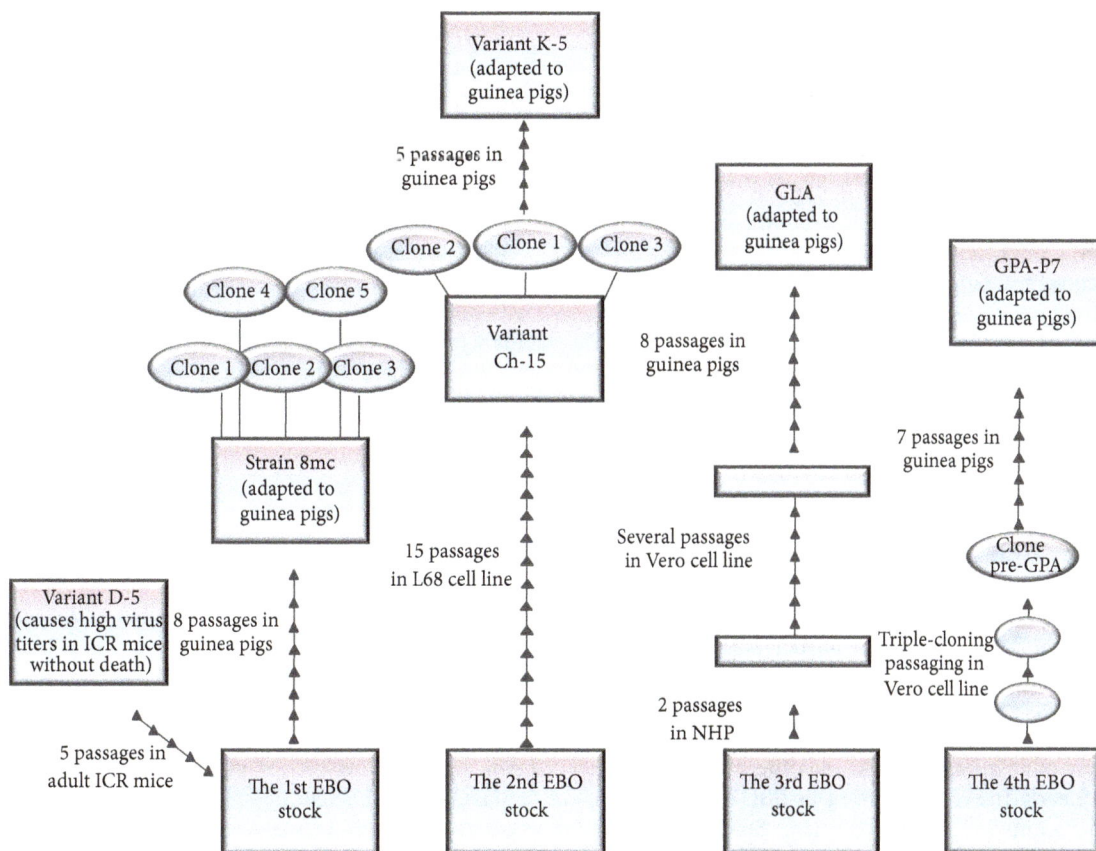

FIGURE 1: Adaptation series of wild-type Mayinga strain EBOV to guinea pigs and mice resulting in the establishment of 8mc, K-5, GLA, and GPA-P7 lethal guinea pig-adapted virus variants and a paradoxical high-titer, avirulent mouse-adapted virus variant D-5.

pathogenesis, as well as for the development of vaccines and antivirals. Since some new mutations (as compared to the wild-type virus stocks) can occur *de novo* and some rare mutations can be amplified and fixed in the adapted virus stocks in the process of adaptation, comparison of genetic changes in adapted lethal and preadaptation nonlethal EBOV genomes and matching of those to the virulence of different EBOV variants can yield invaluable information on the genetic determinants of virulence/lethality.

In our first adaptation series, 8mc, a detailed analysis of nucleotide sequences of the EBOV genomes of the original and guinea pig-adapted virus stocks revealed several changes in genome regions encoding for the five viral proteins [9, 16]. The 8mc clones showed, in total, eight common sequence changes compared to the original first EBO stock. Two silent base changes were found in the ORF encoding NP protein, which are, obviously, not affecting the NP function, while another base change in NP gene leads to a conservative amino acid substitution Phe→Leu(648), also unlikely to affect the virulence. No base changes were found in vp35 and vp40 genes. A single uridine insertion at the gene-editing site of viral glycoprotein (GP) gene and an amino acid substitution Asp→Gly(397) were found in three of five 8mc clones; however, all five clones were similar in their pathogenicity for guinea pigs, despite the significant change of GP expression pattern caused by the former mutation. A single base change in the 3′ noncoding region of vp30 gene also seems irrelevant to the acquisition of virus pathogenicity in the course of adaptation.

Contrarily to the above mutations, at least some of the three nucleotide changes in the coding region of vp24 gene, which led to amino acid substitutions Met→Ile(71), Leu→Pro(147), and Thr→Ile(187), may be linked to the adaptation process, since the gel mobility of 8mc-EBOV VP24 is lower than its wild-type counterpart, suggesting a major structural rearrangement of this protein and, probably, the crucial role for VP24 in the adaptation process.

A conservative amino acid substitution Thr→Ala(820) in L gene, similarly to Phe→Leu(648) substitution in NP gene, does not seem to be responsible for virus virulence. However, since both are found in all five EBOV-8mc clones, they may have a supportive role in the increase in virulence [16].

A comparative nucleotide sequence analysis of the virus variants of the second adaptation series (K-5) reveals two single nucleotide substitutions in vp24 ORF in the adapted virus strain K-5 (as compared to the original second EBOV stock), which lead to the amino acid substitutions Asp→Gly(165) and His→Tyr(186) [17]. Since the former is present in the initial virus variant Ch-15 used for adaptation in guinea pigs, it has, obviously, been introduced during passaging in NHPs or L68 cells and seems irrelevant to the development of pathogenicity of an adapted virus. The other vp24 mutation is found at nearly the same location in EBOV variant K-5, as in another guinea pig-adapted variant, 8mc, obtained in the first passage series, thus, supporting the hypothesis of a possible involvement of this protein in the host adaptation and increase in pathogenicity [16].

To further evaluate the contribution of genetic differences present in guinea pig-adapted EBOV variants in the virus

virulence, two different approaches were employed. The first one was another adaptation series started with a cloned EBOV stock (pre-GPA), in which the genetic events occurring were determined at every passage and compared to the pathogenic reactions in guinea pigs reflecting the emerging EBOV virulence [8]. The other study was using the reverse genetic approach and was focused on the effects of individual mutations of EBOV-8mc variant and their combinations on EBOV virulence [18].

In the former study, the GPA-P7 adapted strain genome was found to differ from the genome of the pre-GPA clone by 17 nucleotide changes. No genetic differences were found in the terminal untranslated regions of the GPA-P7 genome (3′-leader and 5′-trailer). The nucleotide sequence of the GPA-P7 NP gene contained 12 nucleotide substitutions, 8 of those being synonymous and 4 leading to amino acid changes in the encoded NP protein (Leu→Pro(544), Asn→Ser(566), Ser→Pro(598), and Asn→Asp(663)). Three substitutions leading to amino acid changes were detected in the nucleotide sequence of the GPA-P7 VP24 gene (Met→Ile(71), Leu→Pro(147), and Arg→Leu(154)). The L gene (encoding the RNA-dependent RNA polymerase) of GPA-P7 contained two nucleotide substitutions, one synonymous and one nonsynonymous, the latter resulting in amino acid change (Val→Ile(236)) [8].

Correlation of the mutations in GPA-P7 with the time of their occurrence (passage number) and the emerging virus pathogenicity in guinea pigs allows one to evaluate their roles in the virulence. Of 17 nucleotide substitutions that distinguish between GPA-P7 and the pre-GPA clone, 12 occurred as early as the first passage (GPA-P1 variant). These 12 substitutions comprise nine synonymous (eight in NP gene and one in L gene) and three nonsynonymous substitutions resulting in 3 amino acid changes in NP gene (Leu→Pro(544), Ser→Pro(598), and Asn→Asp(663)). Those mutations were considered not related to the emerging EBOV virulence, since they occurred before the acquisition of lethality. Two other mutations emerged at passage 3, leading to the amino acid changes Asn→Ser(566) in NP protein and Leu→Pro(147) in VP24 protein. Of note, the first lethal outcome in this series was recorded at passage 3, although no lethal outcomes among the infected animals were recorded at passage 4. Those two loci remained heterogenous until the substitutions were fixed in the genome of the GPA-P5 variant (at passage 5) representing increased virulence for guinea pigs and causing the disease with 40% lethality (2 lethal outcomes of five observed animals). At passage 6, a mutation in the VP24 gene sequence, G10557A, occurred resulting in amino acid change Met→Ile(71). This passage was accompanied by a further increase in EBOV virulence for guinea pigs, appearing as an 80% lethal disease (four lethal outcomes between days 10 and 12 out of 5 animals). At passage 7, a nucleotide substitution G10805U, resulting in an amino acid change Arg→Leu(154), was fixed in the VP24 gene sequence, and a heterogeneous site (G12286A, Val→Ile(236)) appeared in the L gene sequence. Emergence of these mutations correlated with a further increase in EBOV pathogenicity for guinea pigs, which manifested as 100% lethality (between days 8 and 12). Thus, only the three amino acid changes in VP24 protein (positions 147, 71, and 154), one change in NP protein (position 566), and one change in L-polymerase (position 236) may have an essential contribution to the gradually emerging virulence of EBOV in the course of GPA-P7 series [8]. Of interest, two identical mutations in VP24 (positions 71 and 147) were discovered in the abovementioned 8mc adapted virus strain [16].

In the latter study [18], recombinant viruses carrying various combinations of wild-type and guinea pig-adapted genes were generated by reverse genetic approach and their contribution to the EBOV virulence in guinea pigs was evaluated. The membrane-associated protein VP24 was shown to play a critical role in EBOV pathogenesis, and amino acid changes in VP24 were shown essential and sufficient to confer EBOV virulence in guinea pigs. Indeed, recombinant virus stocks carrying only those 8mc mutations harbored in VP24 gene are causing a uniformed lethality in guinea pigs. Inoculation of animals with the viruses carrying NP and/or L gene mutations did not show any sign of the disease except for the death of two guinea pigs in the group infected with recombinant virus carrying a mutation in NP gene (rEBOV-NP/8mc, F648L). Sequence analysis of virus from the blood of those dead animals revealed the additional amino acid substitution L26F in the VP24. Inoculation of guinea pigs with virus from such animals resulted in their uniform death. To evaluate the role of this mutation in the virulence of guinea pig-adapted EBOV, a recombinant virus was generated that differed from the wild-type virus by a single mutation in VP24, rEBOV-VP24/L26F. Strikingly, all animals infected with rEBOV-VP24/L26F developed signs of EBOV disease approximately 4 days p/i. Importantly, no additional mutations were found in the viruses recovered from guinea pigs inoculated with this recombinant virus, suggesting that adaptive mutations in VP24 are necessary and sufficient for an increase in EBOV virulence in guinea pigs. The "8mc" mutation in NP (Phe→Leu(648)) is not strictly required for the increase in pathogenicity but seems to lead to the accelerated selection of EBOV variant, in which a single mutation in VP24 was able to confer lethality [18].

Of interest, a similar major contribution of VP24 mutations in the EBOV adaptation to mice has been observed, with the requirement for the supportive mutations in NP [19]. The role of VP24 and NP proteins in the virulence of mouse-adapted EBOV strain, however, correlated with their ability to evade IFN-I-triggered antiviral responses. The guinea pig-adapted and wild-type EBOV VP24, on the contrary, were similar in their ability to block IFN-I-stimulated response [18], which underlines the importance of different animal-adapted EBOV models in the dissection of a complex phenotype of EBOV disease.

A summary of all genetic determinants revealed in the guinea pig adaptation series of EBOV is provided in Table 2.

4. Pathomorphological Findings in EBOV-Infected Guinea Pigs

Ebola virus infection in primates is associated with diffuse parenchymal necrosis in the liver without marked inflammatory changes [20]. Unlike that, Ryabchikova and colleagues

report the occurrence of granulomatous lesions in the liver to be the hallmark of the wild-type EBOV infection in guinea pigs [6]. Those granulomas are proposed to play an important role in virus clearance. Granuloma-like foci consisting of the monocytes, macrophages, and neutrophils appear at day 5 p/i and increase in size and number thereafter. No involvement of hepatocytes was observed in this study until days 7-8, when some of the perifocal hepatocytes demonstrate lipid droplet accumulation and destruction of organoids. The other organs were only slightly involved, except for the spleen and lymph nodes, in which some signs of immunosuppression (decreased number of mitoses, lack of plasma cell formation, and destruction of stroma cells and macrophages) were found. Virus reproduction occurred in the mononuclear phagocytes of the liver only at later stages of infection (on day 7) and was observed as the presence of viral nucleocapsids and specific membranous structures in the infected cells. Most of the infected macrophages were located in the granuloma-like foci and contained virions, which appeared eroded with their nucleoids indistinct. No reproduction of wild-type virus was detected in the other organs [21].

In our study, we were able to observe the dynamics of pathomorphologic changes in wild-type EBOV infection in guinea pigs [12], which was somewhat different from the pattern described above. Electron microscopy revealed the occurrence of EBO virions in the dilated Disse spaces as early as 24 h p/i. Simultaneously, a developing inflammatory reaction in the periphery of liver acini was observed with ballooning degeneration of hepatocytes showing disorganization of organelles (swollen mitochondria) and necrotic foci containing phagocyting macrophages and virus particles (Figure 2(a)). However, no virus replication centers were observed in the macrophages. By day 5, the necrobiotic changes are progressing and involve the major part of liver parenchyma with the often occurrence of necrotic hepatocytes, numerous hemorrhages in the swollen subendothelial space, and centers of virus replication in the necrotic foci, although with only few virus particles visible (Figure 2(b)). By day 7 of infection, however, the progression of necrobiotic changes ceases, and the tissue structure stabilizes. At this time, macrophages with numerous osmiophilic inclusions, nuclei containing viroplasm, and numerous virions in their neighborhood are seen (Figure 2(c)). The major difference from the course of wild-type EBOV infection in guinea pigs observed by Ryabchikova et al. [6] was the presence of damaged hepatocytes at days 5-7 p/i.

The gradual emergence of EBOV virulence to guinea pigs in a series of passages is reflected in the changes of pathomorphological pattern of the infection. At early passages (1–3), only quantitative differences in the numbers of activated and infected liver macrophages were observed. The pathomorphological pattern of infection changes at passage 4, with greater numbers of liver macrophages involved, as well as the virus reproduction first detected in hepatocytes. However, only the formation of nucleocapsids, not the proper virus budding, occurs in hepatocytes at this stage, making it unclear whether the infection in these cells is productive. In general, the liver lesions are more severe than at earlier

TABLE 2: Genetic changes occurring in different adaptation series and reverse genetics experiments and their relevance to the development of GPA-EBOV virulence/lethality.

Viral ORF	Nucleotide position	Amino acid substitution	Relevance to adaptation	Comment
EBOV-8mc adaptation series				
NP	1852	None	No	Synonymous
	2410	None	No	Synonymous
	2411	Phe → Leu(648)	Unlikely	Conservative, may play a supportive role in adaptation
GP	6924 (insertion)	Frameshift	No	Clones with or without those GP mutations do not differ from each other in their pathogenicity in guinea pigs
	7228	Asp → Gly(397)	No	
VP30	9595	None	No	Located in 3′-untranslated region
VP24	10557	Met → Ile(71)	Probably	At least, one of those three VP24 mutations induces major structural rearrangements in EBOV-8mc VP24, which are presented as gel mobility shift in electrophoresis
	10784	Leu → Pro(147)	Probably	
	10904	Thr → Ile(187)	Probably	
L	14038	Thr → Ala(820)	Unlikely	Conservative, may play a supportive role in adaptation
EBOV-5K adaptation series				
VP24	10838	Asp → Gly(165)	No	Is acquired in the course of passage in NHPs or L68 cells, prior to adaptation
	10907	His → Tyr(186)	Probably	Acquired during adaptation, lies close to EBOV-8mc VP24 Thr → Ile(187)
EBOV-GPA-P7 series				
	1781	Asn → His(438)	No	Is found in nonadapted pre-GPA clone
	2043	Arg → Lys(525)	No	Is found in nonadapted pre-GPA clone
	2092	None	No	Synonymous
	2100	Leu → Arg(544)	No	Occurred at passage 1 after pre-GPA, before the acquisition of lethality
	2164	None	No	Synonymous
	2166	Asn → Ser(566)	Probably	Occurred at passage 3, when the first lethal outcome was recorded, heterogenous site until fixed at passage 5, concomitant with 40% lethality
NP	2188	None	No	Synonymous
	2191	None	No	Synonymous
	2209	None	No	Synonymous
	2222	None	No	Synonymous
	2233	None	No	Synonymous
	2260	None	No	Synonymous
	2261	Ser → Pro(598)	No	Occurred at passage 1 after pre-GPA, before the acquisition of lethality
	2409	Ser → Phe(647)	No	Is found in nonadapted pre-GPA clone
	2456	Asp → Asn(663)	No	Occurred at passage 1 after pre-GPA, before the acquisition of lethality
VP40	5576	None	No	Synonymous
	5597	None	No	Synonymous
VP24	10557	Met → Ile(71)	Probably	Occurred at passage 6, concomitant with lethality increase to 80%
	10784	Leu → Pro(147)	Probably	Occurred at passage 3, when the first lethal outcome was recorded, heterogenous site until fixed at passage 5, concomitant with 40% lethality
	10805	Arg → Leu(154)	Probably	Occurred at passage 7, concomitant with full lethality
L	12286	Val → Ile(236)	Probably	Occurred at passage 7, concomitant with full lethality
	16821	None	No	Synonymous
Reverse genetics of EBOV-8mc mutations				
VP24	10422	Leu → Phe(26)	Definitely	Derived from the blood of an animal, which died after inoculation with a nonlethal recombinant rEBOV-NP/8mc, F648L virus. When introduced into an otherwise wild-type Zaire EBOV genome by reverse genetics, this mutation alone confers full lethality to guinea pigs

(a) Activated macrophage (MP) with phagosomes and polymorphous virus particles (Vpt) in the necrotic focus of the liver. Day 1 p/i

(b) Necrotic focus in the liver, day 5 p/i. Arrows show the virus replication centers in the cell debris

(c) Cell fragment with osmiophilic inclusions (arrows), virus particles (Vpt), and viroplasm (Vpl) in the nucleus. Day 7 p/i

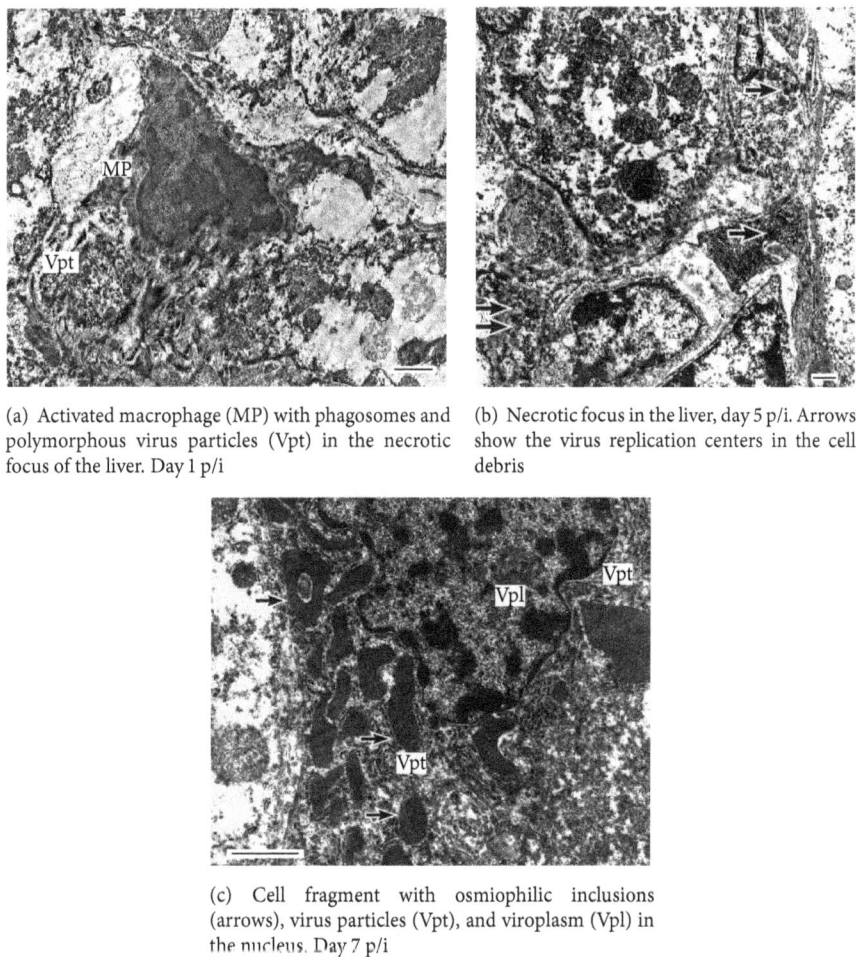

FIGURE 2: Wild-type EBOV nonlethal infection in guinea pigs. Electron microscopy of the liver.

passages, and the signs of spleen and kidney involvement become evident. All observed morphological changes gradually become more prominent at passages 5-6, with liver focal lesions becoming widespread and number of infected cells and virions increasing. With the acquisition of full lethality of the adapted virus to guinea pigs (passage 8), the hepatic tissue becomes filled with infected hepatocytes and macrophages with intracellular nucleocapsids, as well as numerous virions. Some cells contain structurally abnormal viroplasm and nucleocapsids. Areas of liver necrosis containing lysed hepatocytes, macrophages, and virions become all-pervading. Other organs and tissues show greater severity of lesions, as well [21].

In GPA-EBOV-infected guinea pigs, we, similarly, observed the necrotic hepatocytes (Figure 3(a)) and virus particles in subendothelial space (Figure 3(b)) as early as 24 h p/i [12]. On day 2, the tissue destruction is more prominent, with multiple hemorrhages and necrotic foci containing numerous virus particles, fibrin deposits, and macrophages (Figure 3(c)). The centrilobular hepatocytes, typically, show the signs of ballooning dystrophy, while the perilobular hepatocytes become necrotic and contain virus particles (Figure 3(d)). This pattern indicates a progression of liver

damage on day 2. By day 5, the necrotic process involves the central parts of acini where numerous necrotic foci with fibrin impregnation (Figure 3(e)) and Kupffer cells with viroplasm and virus particles (Figure 3(f)) are detected. At day 7, the pronounced and overall destruction of liver tissue of animals infected with GPA-EBOV is visible with large areas of necrosis involving both stromal and parenchymal cells (Figure 3(g)). Those necrotic lesions contain actively phagocyting macrophages with small and large phagosomes, viroplasm, and virus particles (Figure 3(h)), as well as hepatocytes containing numerous viruses (Figure 3(i)). Also, by this time, the liver lesions involve massive hemorrhages resulting in the occurrence of new areas of inflammation and the generalization of liver injury. We believe that the lethality in GPA-EBOV-infected guinea pigs is, thus, due to the triggering damage by the virus and the subsequent involvement of different areas of the liver resulting from the inflammatory reaction [12].

Day-by-day dynamics of pathomorphologic changes occurring in the GPA-infected guinea pigs illustrated by Connolly and colleagues [7] is in a good agreement with structural changes described above. In animals infected with the adapted, fully lethal EBOV variant, the viral RNA and

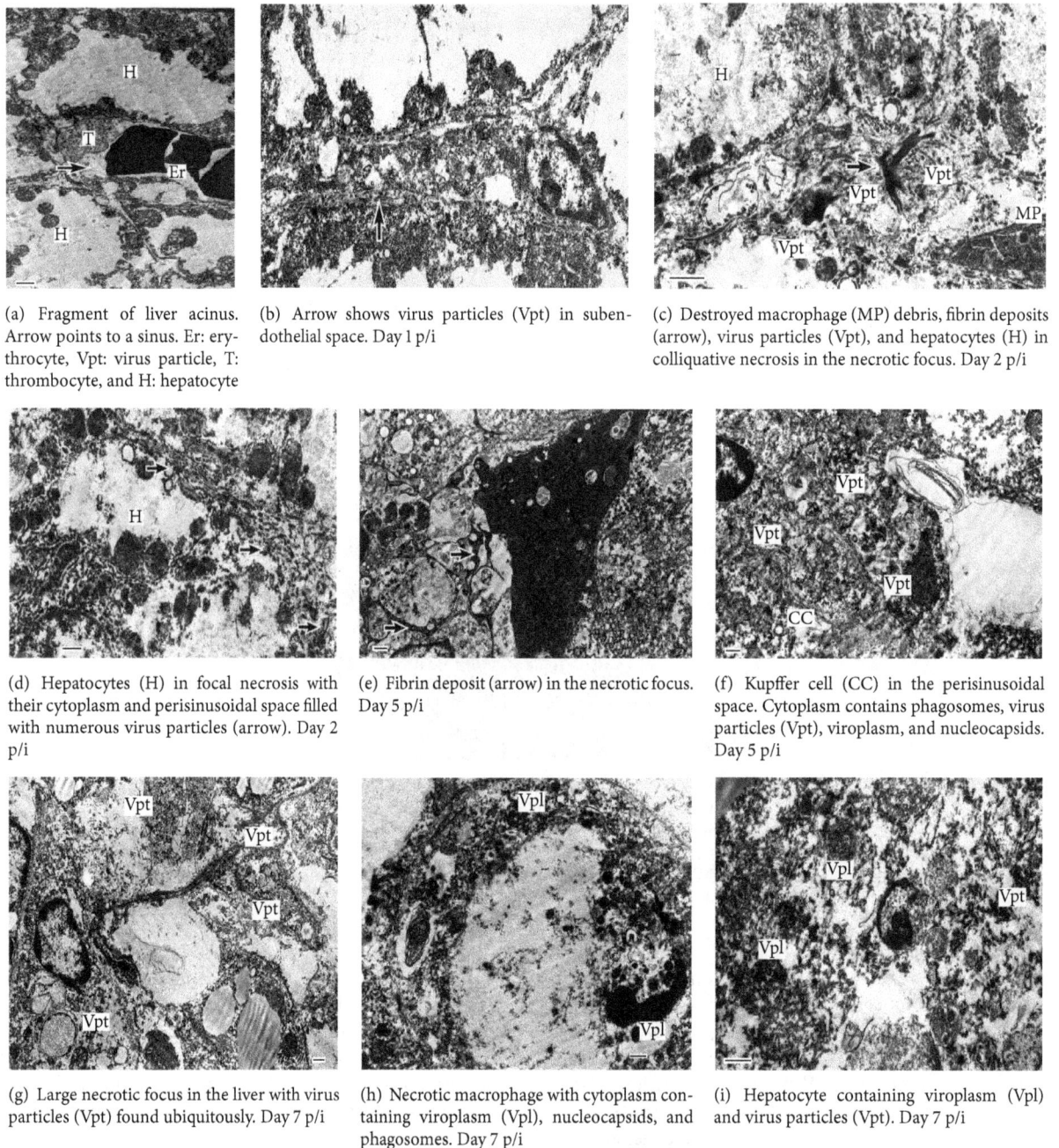

(a) Fragment of liver acinus. Arrow points to a sinus. Er: erythrocyte, Vpt: virus particle, T: thrombocyte, and H: hepatocyte

(b) Arrow shows virus particles (Vpt) in subendothelial space. Day 1 p/i

(c) Destroyed macrophage (MP) debris, fibrin deposits (arrow), virus particles (Vpt), and hepatocytes (H) in colliquative necrosis in the necrotic focus. Day 2 p/i

(d) Hepatocytes (H) in focal necrosis with their cytoplasm and perisinusoidal space filled with numerous virus particles (arrow). Day 2 p/i

(e) Fibrin deposit (arrow) in the necrotic focus. Day 5 p/i

(f) Kupffer cell (CC) in the perisinusoidal space. Cytoplasm contains phagosomes, virus particles (Vpt), viroplasm, and nucleocapsids. Day 5 p/i

(g) Large necrotic focus in the liver with virus particles (Vpt) found ubiquitously. Day 7 p/i

(h) Necrotic macrophage with cytoplasm containing viroplasm (Vpl), nucleocapsids, and phagosomes. Day 7 p/i

(i) Hepatocyte containing viroplasm (Vpl) and virus particles (Vpt). Day 7 p/i

FIGURE 3: GPA-EBOV lethal infection in guinea pigs. Electron microscopy of the liver.

antigens are detected in the lymph node macrophages as early as 24 h p/i. The number of infected macrophages, in which the typical EBOV intracytoplasmic inclusions representing viral nucleocapsids are seen by electron microscopy, increases 4–20-fold by 48 h p/i, confirming an ongoing productive infection. From day 3, a developing multifocal lymphoid necrosis and the depletion of lymph nodes of different localization are observed, which progressed by days 7–9. Ultrastructurally, the sinuses contain necrotic cellular debris, infected macrophages, and free virions, while no evidence of EBOV-infected lymphocytes in the lymph nodes is found.

In the spleen, the occurrence of single-cell necrosis in the red pulp is seen at day 2 p/i, progressing into a more extensive necrosis of both splenic white and red pulp and the depletion of hematopoietic elements in the red pulp by day 4. All signs of productive infection (viral antigens, RNA, and intracytoplasmic inclusions) are detected in the red pulp macrophages and the antigen-presenting cells (dendritic and reticular cells) of some white pulp follicles. The spread of infection is associated with numerous circulating monocytes and tissue macrophages containing EBOV inclusions, with some of infected cells already showing budding virions and clusters of virions along their plasma membrane. In the liver, small foci of hepatocellular necrosis occur at days 2-3 p/i with EBOV-staining hepatocytes and Kupffer cells seen. On day 4, the ongoing infection in the liver spreads to the hepatocytes surrounding the necrotic foci and Kupffer cells, since they also begin to contain viral cytoplasmic inclusions. Most of these foci stain EBOV RNA- and antigen-positive, and the sinuses are filled with antigen-positive debris. Free virions in the Disse spaces and virus capsid inclusions are found in Kupffer cells at day 5. Later, at day 7, some periportal fibroblast-like cells become involved in the infection and stained EBOV-positive. The occurrence of the virion-containing fibrin depositions in subendothelial spaces and virus particles in subepithelial connective tissue of the bile ducts (both as free virions and cytoplasmic viral inclusions in degenerate fibroblasts), probably, marks the onset of a systemic spread of infection from the liver at day 9. In fact, at later stages of infection, involvement of different organs and tissues, as well as cellular targets, is observed: gastrointestinal fibroblasts and macrophages, adrenal cortical cells and fibroblasts, bladder epithelium, interstitial and alveolar macrophages, the occasional fibroblasts and endothelial cell of pulmonary venules in the lungs, and so forth [7, 21].

An independent morphological study of the wild-type and guinea pig-adapted EBOV infection reveals an inability of the nonadapted virus to reproduce in its primary target, the macrophages [18]. Peritoneal guinea pig macrophages infected *in vitro* by the recombinant virus obtained by reverse genetics and carrying the adaptive mutations in VP24 identical to those occurring in the 8mc adaptation series show characteristic inclusion bodies containing viral nucleocapsids. Contrarily, no typical viral nucleocapsids but only massive protein inclusions were found in the cells infected by the wild-type virus, which correlated with the lack of infectious virus release from those cells. This data suggested an efficient block of wild-type EBOV infection already in the primary target cells, probably, at the stage of VP24-mediated nucleocapsid assembly/budding [18].

Thus, the morphologic patterns of wild-type and adapted EBOV infection in guinea pigs are suggestive of the inability of the virus to establish productive infection in macrophages and, particularly, in hepatocytes. Failure to massively produce infectious wild-type EBO virions may result in the host defense successfully blocking further virus spread by locking the infection in granuloma-like inflammation foci with a subsequent virus clearance. The adaptive mutations in the EBOV genome can restore the ability of a virus to reproduce in its major targets, macrophages and hepatocytes, thus, facilitating systemic virus spread in the infected animals that results in high virulence. On the other hand, this mechanism of adaptation would present itself as the increase of blood and liver virus titers in the adapted virus-infected animals, as compared to those inoculated with the wild-type virus, which is not the case for two adaptation series, K-5 and GPA-P7. There should be, therefore, an alternative mechanism of virulence increase during adaptation, which is relevant to those series. A morphological study of K-5 and GPA-P7 virus infections, which has not been done as yet, and its comparison with the morphological patterns of infection described earlier would, thus, be of interest.

5. Hematologic, Immunologic, and Coagulation Shifts in the Guinea Pig Infections by Wild-Type and Adapted Virus

Wild-type EBOV infection causes serious hematologic aberrations in its natural hosts including leukocytosis due to marked neutrophilia and, frequently, lymphopenia in terminally ill primates. Thrombocytopenia develops in acutely ill human patients and experimentally infected primates experiencing hemorrhagic syndrome. Unlike that, both neutrophilia and lymphopenia can be observed in EBOV-infected guinea pigs as early as day 2 p/i and are progressing over the course of the disease. According to some reports, the scale of those hematological shifts in individual infected animals can be as great as a >3.5-fold increase in the number of neutrophils and >3.0-fold drop in the number of lymphocytes. This finding appears intriguing, since lymphocytes are not infected by EBOV *in vivo* despite the progression of lymphoid necrosis, and they are resistant to infections by different EBOV strains *in vitro* [7]. The bystander lymphocyte apoptosis, an important feature of EBOV infection in primates and mice, has not been determined in guinea pigs infected with adapted EBOV, as well [2]. The mechanisms of lymphoid necrosis and depletion occurring both in primates and in guinea pigs remain unclear but are, probably, caused by the events resulting from a massive macrophage infection and changing the microenvironment of lymphoid tissue. Severe thrombocytopenia (>14-fold, as compared to the preinfection levels) develops later, on day 7 of infection (two days before death at day 9), resembling the loss of platelets in terminally ill primates [7].

It appears, though, that the leukocyte counts should be taken with care, since a wide-range variation of different leukocyte types between the animals and their experimental groups is natural to guinea pigs (cf. neutrophil/lymphocyte percentage in the reported group, 21/77, to the data from one of our adaptation series, 57/38 [11]). Therefore, the analysis of dynamics of hematologic indices at different passages of adaptation and its correlation with the clinical course of EBOV disease appears to be more valid.

In one of our adaptation series, GLA, we specifically aimed to study the evolution of different blood indices in the course of adaptation [11]. In this experiment, the leukocyte counts remained stable throughout passages 1–3, demonstrating a significant 3-fold decrease at next passage 4, remaining at this lower level throughout the further adaptation. This passage was also notable for the first occurrence of eosinophils in blood samples and an abrupt (~8-fold), although transient, increase in monocyte and plasmacyte counts, which returned to baseline values at the next passage. Also, the amount of neutrophils dropped by 20% at this passage (transiently, to recover at passage 5), while the percentage of young, atypical, and large, probably activated, lymphocytes showed a transient increase at passage 4 (also to return to the baseline values at passage 5). Interestingly,

TABLE 3: Serum and peritoneal TNF activity in EBOV-infected guinea pigs and rabbits.

Virus	Guinea pigs		Rabbits
	Mayinga (wild-type)	8mc, guinea pig-adapted	Mayinga (wild-type)
TNF activity, serum (U/mL)	3.4 ± 0.1 (day 7)	2.5 ± 0.16 (day 7)	104 ± 36 (day 3) 471 ± 137 (day 5) 1398 ± 909 (day 9)
Virus titer, serum (PFU)	10^3	$10^4 - 10^5$	Nondetectable
TNF activity, peritoneal (U/mL)	Nondetectable	Nondetectable	15.3 ± 2.1 (days 5–9)
Virus titer, peritoneal (PFU)	$10^2 - 10^3$	$10^2 - 10^3$	Nondetectable

these changes followed the acquirement of full lethality by the adapting EBOV at passage 3 [11].

The percentage of young thrombocytes demonstrated a 3-fold increase at passage 2 and an overall 12-fold increase by passage 6. The total thrombocyte count remained stable until it fell abruptly (2-fold) at passage 6. The occurrence of young thrombocytes at early passages, before the fully lethal EBOV has been selected, indicates the important shifts in the thrombocytic hemostasis, which resulted in a progressive loss of platelets observed in the next passages.

An interesting finding was the change of erythrocyte morphology in the EBOV adaptation. The percentage of normal red blood cells was progressively decreasing at every passage concomitant with the occurrence of echinocytes and erythrocytes with inclusions, which suggests the exit of immature erythrocytes from the bone marrow, apparently, to compensate for the deficiency of red blood cells in the organism. The occurrence of echinocytes in the peripheral blood has been noticed in the acute viral hepatitis and some other viral and inflammatory diseases [22]; however, the involvement of erythrocytes into the EBOV infection has never been reported earlier.

The shifts of the peripheral blood counts were accompanied by the changes in bone marrow composition, firstly, by the increase in the number of blast cells as early as passage 2, reaching its peak of 65 pro mille by passage 5 but further dropping. This may indicate compensatory activation of bone marrow function with subsequent exhaustion. Megakaryocyte counts started growing at passage 2 and reached their peak at passage 5, clearly reflecting the upward dynamics of young thrombocytes.

Finally, the phagocytic function of neutrophils was progressively decreasing from passage 2, although the number of neutrophils was variable at different passages. Contrarily, the phagocytic function of peritoneal macrophages was remaining stable for 6 passages and then dropping abruptly [11, 23].

Although many of the hematologic indices were fluctuating in the passage series or changing at later passages (which allowed ruling out their causative role in the emerging lethality of adapting EBOV), some were evidently concomitant with the increasing pathogenicity or even appearing prior to the acquiring of full lethality by the adapted virus. Those include the increase of the percentage of young thrombocytes along with the growing number of blast cells and megakaryocytes and the decrease of phagocytic activity of neutrophils,

all commencing as early as passage 2, alongside the significant growth of blood and tissue virus titer and the occurrence of the first lethal cases in the inoculated animals. It is, thus, tempting to hypothesize that the evolving wild-type EBOV acquires new characteristics triggering those early responses in hematologic parameters [11]. Those key parameters were also changing consistently in our other adaptation series, GPA-7, although it was rather different from the above GLA experiment, since the virus titer was not growing in the passage series and the full lethality has been acquired later, at passage 5 versus passage 3 for GLA series [8]. However, the decreasing phagocytic activity of neutrophils was also an early response appearing at passage 2, and the trend of accumulation of atypical lymphocytes in the course of adaptation was evident, probably, due to the progressing apoptotic and necrotic processes.

A rather intriguing immunologic finding was the lack of correlation between the blood and peritoneal TNF levels and the pathogenicity of EBOV infection in experimental animals. The guinea pigs infected with wild-type Mayinga or lethal adapted 8mc EBOV demonstrated similar, rather low, levels of TNF activity in blood and no TNF activity in peritoneal exudates (Table 3). Contrarily, when rabbits, which are completely resistant to EBOV infection, were inoculated with a wild-type EBOV, a rather high serum TNF activity was detected early (day 3 p/i) and was progressively increasing to extraordinary high values later on (days 5 and 9 p/i). In rabbits, TNF activity was also detected in peritoneal exudates (Table 3) [23]. The previously published data report the elevated proinflammatory cytokine levels in the lethal wild-type EBOV infections in humans and nonhuman primates [24, 25] and in baboons infected with guinea pig-adapted EBOV. High levels of TNF-α production by peripheral blood macrophages infected in vitro by another filovirus, Marburg virus, were proposed to be the major pathogenetic factor of Marburg virus infection due to its ability to induce hemorrhagic shock [26]. Thus, our data on TNF activity in the rodent models of EBOV infection (guinea pigs and rabbits) are contradictory to the proposed causative role of TNF-induced hemorrhages in primate infections.

Since coagulopathies, such as disseminated vascular coagulation (DIC) or massive hemorrhages, are the hallmark of EBOV disease in primates [27] and considering the tight and clinically relevant cross talk between the coagulation and complement systems [28, 29], it seems important to discuss

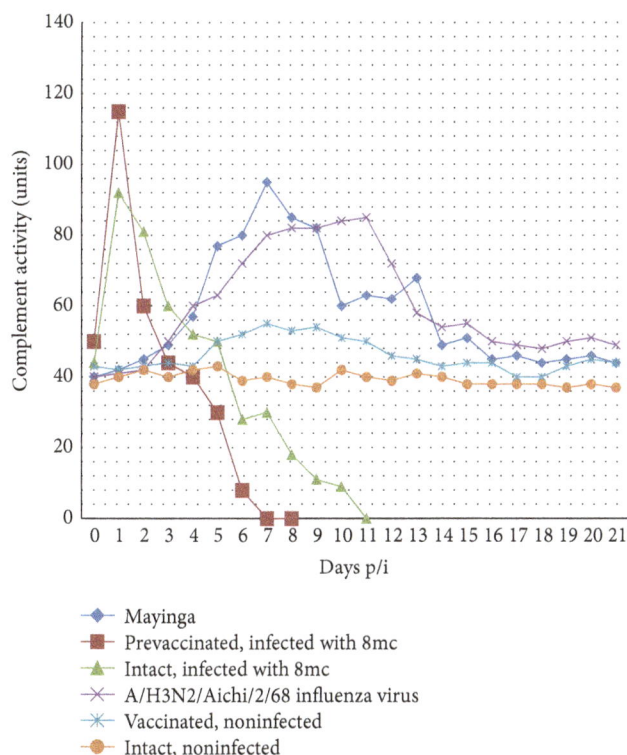

FIGURE 4: Complement activity in the intact and prevaccinated guinea pigs infected with lethal GPA-EBOV-8mc strain or nonlethal wild-type EBOV Mayinga strain. Animals infected with nonlethal influenza virus A/Aichi/2/68 (H3N2) strain, intact animals, and guinea pigs vaccinated with inactivated nonlethal Mayinga strain EBOV while not infected were used as different controls of complement activity. Slow lagging dynamics of complement activity in guinea pigs infected with nonlethal Mayinga strain EBOV is contrasting to the rapid onset/drop peak of complement activity in the intact and prevaccinated animals infected with a lethal 8mc strain GPA-EBOV.

The rate of complement activity growth in the lethally infected guinea pigs suggests the involvement of an alternative pathway of complement activation. In preimmunized animals, the classic activation can additionally occur, due to the presence of anti-Ebola immunoglobulins, which may be the possible cause of higher complement activities than in nonimmunized animals. Alternatively, slower kinetics of complement activation in guinea pigs infected with nonlethal strain indicates classic activation with the two peaks corresponding to IgM (before day 7) and IgG production (days 7–14). Rapid complement activation by alternative pathway appears to be a unique ability of the 8mc lethal EBOV strain to immediately hyperactivate complement production with subsequent fast and complete exhaustion of its synthesis [30]. Importantly, the retrospective study of the sera from days 1 and 5 and later of a single fatal case of a laboratory staff EBOV infection accident reveals the similar pattern of a sharp increase and an immediate drop of complement activity, suggesting the relevance of this data for humans [12].

Interestingly, the pattern of serum concentrations of circulating immune complexes (CICs) is closely resembling the kinetics of complement activity both in intact and in preimmunized lethally infected animals, with a typical rapid rise in the first day and an immediate decline to near-zero values by days 8-9 or 5-6 in intact or preimmunized animals, respectively, followed by the animal death. Slow CIC and complement kinetics are also very similar in the nonlethal EBOV infections of guinea pigs. The significance of circulating immune complexes (CICs) in the pathogenesis of Ebola disease still remains to be studied [30].

Since no coagulation abnormalities are occurring in the mouse-adapted EBOV model, which is a general feature of mouse models for acute viral infections [19], the guinea pig-adapted EBOV remains a unique nonprimate model for the study of EBOV-induced coagulopathies.

the role of complement involvement in the experimental EBOV infection in guinea pigs.

The dynamics of complement activity in wild-type EBOV-infected guinea pigs and in the intact or EBOV-preimmunized animals infected with a lethal adapted EBOV strain demonstrates striking differences, which can be important for the understanding of EBOV-induced coagulopathies. In wild-type EBOV-infected animals, the complement activity shows a double-peak profile with a 2-day lag, the first, higher peak at days 4–7 and second, lower peak at days 9-10. Contrarily, in animals infected with the adapted lethal 8mc strain, the complement activity demonstrates a rapid peak at 24 h p/i followed by an abrupt decline on day 2, return to the baseline by days 4-5, and further drop to the background levels by days 9–11, followed by the animal death. Finally, the guinea pigs preimmunized with formalin-inactivated EBOV and infected by a lethal 8mc strain showed even a more steep rise of complement activity on day 1 and a more abrupt fall on day 2 p/i with a further decline to near-zero values by day 6, also followed by the animal death by day 8 (Figure 4).

6. Conclusion

Since the first isolation of wild-type EBOV strains, the problems with the animal model for the study of biology and therapy/prevention of this infection became evident. Resistance of the most convenient rodent model animals (mice, guinea pigs, hamsters, and rabbits) to EBOV infection prompted the researchers to use adaptation of wild-type EBOV strains to the small animal models. Practically, the EBOV adaptation to guinea pigs was the easier and the first to be achieved. The lethality of the guinea pig-adapted EBOV variant to the nonhuman primates remained unchanged [31]. In the adaptation passage series of EBOV stocks differing in their passage histories described here and previously, the emergence of the fully lethal GPA-EBOV variants was readily achieved in 7 passages or less. EBOV adaptation to mice required much more efforts (M. Bray, personal communication). In our own attempt of EBOV adaptation to mice, a paradoxical nonlethal strain was obtained, which demonstrated high-level replication and persistence of virus in the animal's liver, while lacking any clinical symptoms of the disease. The historically first GPA-EBOV strain designated 8mc was originally established for the vaccine development and heterologic immunoglobulin production [32]. However, it was soon realized that this variant not only represents a convenient small animal model, but also offers the opportunity to compare the genetic differences between the wild-type and adapted EBOV strains and establish the correlation between the genetic determinants and the emerging and evolving virulence and lethality in a new host [16]. Also, the comparison of pathomorphologic, immunologic, hematologic, and coagulation features of EBOV infection by the wild-type and adapted virus allows one to establish the most important physiologic parameters, which influence the course of EBOV disease [9, 11, 12, 23].

We and others were able to demonstrate the mutations in EBOV VP24 protein to be the most important determinants of the virus virulence and lethality [8, 9, 16, 18].

The need to reproduce the consistency of processes occurring in the course of adaptation and establish the details of adaptation process required the repeated adaptation series starting from the virus stocks with different passage histories including the cloned EBOV stocks.

The differences in the dynamics of hemolytic complement activity found in the infections of guinea pigs by the wild-type and adapted EBOV strains allowed us to be able to predict the outcome of EBOV infection in the first hours p/i [30].

Also, our studies indicate strong suppression of neutrophilic phagocytosis in the infections of guinea pigs with GPA-EBOV strain, while only its mild activation on day 5 of wild-type EBOV infection was observed. This suggested that the reproduction of EBOV in macrophages, on the one side, with concomitant suppression of neutrophils, on the other, results in the disturbance of neutrophil/macrophage interaction as a driving force of a lethal EBOV disease.

Another interesting discovery was the presence of young thrombocytes in GPA-EBOV-infected animals. The phenomenon, which was lacking in the wild-type EBOV-infected animals, together with the increase of megakaryocyte counts in the bone marrow, can be the evidence of the activation of megakaryocytic hematopoiesis and the exit of nonmature platelets into the circulation.

Previously, the elevated levels of proinflammatory cytokines have been reported to occur in the course of EBOV disease and contribute to the infection lethality in humans and NHPs, due to their role in the development of EBOV coagulopathies. However, in guinea pigs we, paradoxically, found higher (while comparable) TNF-α levels in the animals infected with a nonlethal wild-type than in those infected with lethal adapted EBOV, thus, demonstrating lack of TNF involvement in GPA-EBOV pathogenesis.

Acknowledgment

The authors are grateful to Professor L. V. Shestopalova for her incredible help in the preparation of electron microscopy images used in the preparation of this paper.

References

[1] D. Bente, J. Gren, J. E. Strong, and H. Feldmann, "Disease modeling for Ebola and Marburg viruses," *Disease Models & Mechanisms*, vol. 2, no. 1-2, pp. 12–17, 2009.

[2] V. Wahl-Jensen, L. Bollinger, D. Safronetz, F. de Kok-Mercado, D. P. Scott, and H. Ebihara, "Use of the Syrian hamster as a new model of Ebola virus disease and other viral hemorrhagic fevers," *Viruses*, vol. 4, no. 12, pp. 3754–3784, 2012.

[3] H. Feldmann, S. Jones, H.-D. Klenk, and H.-J. Schnittler, "Ebola virus: from discovery to vaccine," *Nature Reviews Immunology*, vol. 3, no. 8, pp. 677–685, 2003.

[4] E. T. W. Bowen, G. S. Platt, G. Lloyd, R. T. Raymond, and D. I. Simpson, "A comparative study of strains of Ebola virus isolated from southern Sudan and northern Zaire in 1976," *Journal of Medical Virology*, vol. 6, no. 2, pp. 129–138, 1980.

[5] A. A. Chepurnov, I. V. Chernukhin, V. A. Ternovoi et al., "Attempts of creating a vaccine against Ebola fever," *Voprosy Virusologii*, vol. 40, no. 6, pp. 257–260, 1995.

[6] E. Ryabchikova, L. Kolesnikova, M. Smolina et al., "Ebola virus infection in Guinea pigs: presumable role of granulomatous inflammation in pathogenesis," *Archives of Virology*, vol. 141, no. 5, pp. 909–921, 1996.

[7] B. M. Connolly, K. E. Steele, K. J. Davis et al., "Pathogenesis of experimental Ebola virus infection in guinea pigs," *The Journal of Infectious Diseases*, vol. 179, supplement 1, pp. S203–S217, 1999.

[8] E. Subbotina, A. Dadaeva, A. Kachko, and A. Chepurnov, "Genetic factors of Ebola virus virulence in guinea pigs," *Virus Research*, vol. 153, no. 1, pp. 121–133, 2010.

[9] A. A. Chepurnov, N. M. Zubavichene, and A. A. Dadaeva, "Elaboration of laboratory strains of Ebola virus and study of pathophysiological reactions of animals inoculated with these strains," *Acta Tropica*, vol. 87, no. 3, pp. 321–329, 2003.

[10] M. Bray, K. Davis, T. Geisbert, C. Schmaljohn, and J. Huggins, "A mouse model for evaluation of prophylaxis and therapy of Ebola hemorrhagic fever," *Journal of Infectious Diseases*, vol. 179, supplement 1, pp. S248–S258, 1999.

[11] A. A. Dadayeva, L. P. Sizikova, Y. L. Subottina, and A. A. Chepurnov, "Hematological and immunological parameters during Ebola virus passages in guinea-pigs," *Voprosy Virusologii*, vol. 51, no. 4, pp. 32–37, 2006.

[12] A. A. Chepurnov and L. V. Shestopalova, *Genetic and Pathophysiological Factors of Ebola Virus Virulence*, Nauka, Novosibirsk, Russia, 2010 (Russian).

[13] L. V. Gubareva, J. M. Wood, W. J. Meyer et al., "Codominant mixtures of viruses in reference strains of influenza virus due to host cell variation," *Virology*, vol. 199, no. 1, pp. 89–97, 1994.

[14] B. Kissi, H. Badrane, L. Audry et al., "Dynamics of rabies virus quasispecies during serial passages in heterologous hosts," *Journal of General Virology*, vol. 80, no. 8, pp. 2041–2050, 1999.

[15] E. T. W. Bowen, G. Lloyd, W. J. Harris, G. S. Platt, A. Baskerville, and E. E. Vella, "Viral haemorrhagic fever in southern Sudan and northern Zaire. Preliminary studies on the aetiological agent," *The Lancet*, vol. 309, no. 8011, pp. 571–573, 1977.

[16] V. E. Volchkov, A. A. Chepurnov, V. A. Volchkova, V. A. Ternovoj, and H.-D. Klenk, "Molecular characterization of guinea pig-adapted variants of Ebola virus," *Virology*, vol. 277, no. 1, pp. 147–155, 2000.

[17] V. A. Volchkova, A. A. Chepurnov, H. Feldmann, V. Ternovoj, H.-D. Klenk, and V. E. Volchkov, "Genetic variability of Ebola virus during host adaptation," in *Proceedings of the 10th International Conference on Negative Strand Viruses*, p. 207, Dublin, Ireland, September 1997.

[18] M. Mateo, C. Carbonnelle, O. Reynard et al., "VP24 Is a molecular determinant of Ebola virus virulence in guinea pigs," *The Journal of Infectious Diseases*, vol. 204, supplement 3, pp. S1011–S1020, 2011.

[19] H. Ebihara, A. Takada, D. Kobasa et al., "Molecular determinants of Ebola virus virulence in mice," *PLoS Pathogens*, vol. 2, no. 7, article e73, 2006.

[20] A. Baskerville, S. P. Fisher-Hoch, G. H. Neild, and A. B. Dowsett, "Ultrastructural pathology of experimental Ebola haemorrhagic fever virus infection," *The Journal of Pathology*, vol. 147, no. 3, pp. 199–209, 1985.

[21] E. I. Ryabchikova, S. G. Baranova, V. K. Tkachev, and A. A. Grazhdantseva, "The morphological changes in Ebola infection in guinea pigs," *Voprosy Virusologii*, vol. 38, no. 4, pp. 176–179, 1993 (Russian).

[22] J. S. Owen, D. J. Brown, D. S. Harry et al., "Erythrocyte echinocytosis in liver disease. Role of abnormal plasma high density lipoproteins," *The Journal of Clinical Investigation*, vol. 76, no. 6, pp. 2275–2285, 1985.

[23] A. A. Dadaeva, L. P. Sizikova, and A. A. Chepurnov, "Functional activity of peritoneal macrophages in experimental Ebola fever," *Vestnik Rossiiskoi Akademii Meditsinskikh Nauk*, no. 8, pp. 7–11, 2004 (Russian).

[24] F. Villinger, P. Rollin, S. Brar et al., "Markedly elevated levels of interferon (INF)-γ, INF-α, interleukin (IL)-2, IL-10, and tumor necrosis factor-α associated with fatal Ebola virus infection," *The Journal of Infectious Diseases*, vol. 179, pp. 188–191, 1999.

[25] L. E. Hensley, H. A. Young, P. B. Jahrling, and T. W. Geisbert, "Proinflammatory response during Ebola virus infection of primate models: possible involvement of the tumor necrosis factor receptor superfamily," *Immunology Letters*, vol. 80, no. 3, pp. 169–179, 2002.

[26] H. Feldmann, H. Bugany, F. Mahner, H.-D. Klenk, D. Drenckhahn, and H.-J. Schnittler, "Filovirus-induced endothelial leakage triggered by infected monocytes/macrophages," *Journal of Virology*, vol. 70, no. 4, pp. 2208–2214, 1996.

[27] M. Bray and S. Mahanty, "Ebola hemorrhagic fever and septic shock," *Journal of Infectious Diseases*, vol. 188, no. 11, pp. 1613–1617, 2003.

[28] U. Amara, D. Rittirsch, M. Flierl et al., "Interaction between the coagulation and complement system," *Advances in Experimental Medicine and Biology*, vol. 632, pp. 71–79, 2008.

[29] S. Kurosawa and D. J. Stearns-Kurosawa, "Complement, thrombotic microangiopathy and disseminated intravascular coagulation," *Journal of Intensive Care*, vol. 2, article 61, 2014.

[30] N. M. Zubavichene and A. A. Chepurnov, "The complement dynamics in experimental Ebola virus infections," *Voprosy Virusologii*, vol. 2, pp. 21–25, 2004.

[31] G. M. Ignatiev, A. A. Dadaeva, S. V. Luchko, and A. A. Chepurnov, "Immune and pathophysiological processes in baboons experimentally infected with Ebola virus adapted to guinea pigs," *Immunology Letters*, vol. 71, no. 2, pp. 131–140, 2000.

[32] N. M. Kudoyarova-Zubavichene, N. N. Sergeyev, A. A. Chepurnov, and S. V. Netesov, "Preparation and use of hyperimmune serum for prophylaxis and therapy of Ebola virus infections," *Journal of Infectious Diseases*, vol. 179, supplement 1, pp. S218–S223, 1999.

10

Molecular and Phylogenetic Analysis of Bovine Papillomavirus Type 1

Mohammed A. Hamad,[1] Ahmed M. Al-Shammari,[2] Shoni M. Odisho,[3] and Nahi Y. Yaseen[2]

[1]*College of Veterinary Medicine, Al-Fallujah University, Al-Anbar 31002, Iraq*
[2]*Iraqi Center for Cancer and Medical Genetic Research, Al-Mustansiriya University, Al-Qadisiyah, Baghdad 1001, Iraq*
[3]*College of Veterinary Medicine, Baghdad University, Baghdad 1001, Iraq*

Correspondence should be addressed to Ahmed M. Al-Shammari; ahmed.alshammari@iccmgr.org

Academic Editor: Subhash C. Verma

This study aimed to provide the first molecular characterization of bovine papillomavirus type 1 (BPV-1) in Iraq. BPV is a widely spread oncogenic virus in Iraqi cattle and is associated with the formation of both benign and malignant lesions, resulting in notable economic losses in dairy and beef cattle. In the current study, 140 cutaneous papilloma specimens were collected from cattle in central Iraq. These samples were submitted to histopathological examination, PCR, and sequencing analysis. The histopathology revealed that the main lesion type among the specimens was fibropapilloma. BPV-1 DNA was detected in 121 of the samples (86.42%) in Iraqi cattle as the main causative agent for the disease. A partial sequence for the E2, L2 genes, and complete sequence for the E5 gene were deposited in GenBank. Phylogenetic analysis confirmed the presence of BPV-1 and showed that the origin of infection may be imported European cattle. Obtaining a complete E5 gene sequence enabled us to perform structural predictions. This study presents the first report of BPV-1 infection in the Iraqi cattle and contributes to extending the knowledge of the origin of the spread of this disease. The results of this study will aid in the development of appropriate control measures and therapeutic strategies.

1. Introduction

Bovine papillomavirus (BPV) contains a double-stranded, circular, 8 kb DNA genome. BPVs display tropism for mucosal tissues and squamous epithelium as well as mesenchymal tissue [1] and are associated with the development of both benign and malignant lesions [2, 3]. Although BPVs are species-specific viruses, BPV-1, BPV-2, and BPV-13 may infect equids as well as cattle and can cause the development of tumors in these species [4–6]. Fourteen BPV types have been defined, and they are classified into four genera: *Xipapillomavirus*, *Deltapapillomavirus*, *Epsilonpapillomavirus*, and *Dyoxipapillomavirus* [7–9]. E5, a small membrane-associated protein, is the main transforming protein of BPV and possesses a strong biological effect [10]. The E5 protein induces cellular transformation through its stimulation of platelet-derived growth factor receptor beta (PDGFβ-R) [11]. Furthermore, reductions in the expression of major histocompatibility complex class I (MHCI) molecules on the cell surface

enable the virus to evade immunosurveillance, leading to the inhibition of intracellular transport by means of abnormal connexin expression [5]. Reference [12] documented a tri-component complex composed of E5/PDGFβR/subunit D in vivo. E5 oncoprotein was previously shown to bind to the proteolipidic D component of V1-ATPase proton pump. Reference [12] suggests that the E5/PDGFβR/subunit D complex may perturb proteostasis, organelle, and cytosol homeostasis, which can result in altered protein degradation and in autophagic responses. Reference [13] proposed that E2 has a role in the initiation of BPV DNA replication by support E1 binding to the BPV origin via DNA-protein and protein-protein interactions. E2 is a multifunctional protein that serves main roles in transcriptional activation and genome maintenance and cooperates with the viral E1 helicase to initiate viral DNA replication. The BPV genome contains seventeen E2 binding sites, mainly concentrated within the long control region, and a single E1 binding site at the origin of viral replication [14]. Another study by [15] suggests the important participation of L2 protein in the packaging of BPV genome within PV virions, which involves interaction of L2 protein with specific DNA sequences.

In Iraq, our group previously investigated methods for growing BPV in cell cultures derived from skin warts collected from cattle to establish a cell culture technique to enable further studies. Cells from abdominal skin, neck, and udders were cultured, and the cultured cells show both epithelial and mesenchymal morphology. Successful long-term culture was achieved, and the cultured cells were used to prepare vaccines for the treatment of papillomas in BPV-infected cattle [16]. The Holstein and crossbred Holstein Friesian breeds are the main types of cattle in Iraq and are an important source of dairy and beef products [17, 18]. Bovine papillomatosis, caused by BPV genotypes, is responsible for significant economic losses due to the associated growth retardation, weight loss, and decreased milk production in BPV-infected animals [19]. For these reasons, gaining knowledge about this disease is of importance to cattle breeders in Iraq. The natural carrier and primary source of BPV is cattle. The virus enters the body through scratches or other injuries, and infection occurs via both direct and indirect contact. The infection appears to be spread through contact with contaminated materials, milking machines, and semen. Other factors, including malnutrition, hormonal imbalances, mutations, and long-term exposure to sunlight, can increase the risk of infection in cases of immunodeficiency [20]. Moreover, peripheral blood mononuclear cells were shown to be a reservoir of BPV-1 and BPV-2 DNA in affected animals [21].

This study aimed to identify and characterize BPV-1 that is circulating in central Iraq. The results of this study will aid in the development of appropriate control measures and therapeutic strategies.

2. Materials and Methods

2.1. Animals and Sample Collection. In this study, 140 cutaneous papilloma samples were collected from 140 farm cattle in different areas in central Iraq by registered veterinarians (Anbar, Baghdad, and Diwaniyah cities). The study sample included cows suffering from bovine papillomatosis that were brought to private clinics by their owners from December 2013 to May 2015. Specimens were collected for the study during routine treatment and care as well as through site visits to selected farms. The collected samples had varying diameters (from 1 to 10 cm) and came from different parts of the body (e.g., udder, teat, abdomen, and back). Each sample was immediately divided into 2 parts, which were either frozen in a deep freezer for subsequent molecular biology analysis or fixed in 10% neutral buffered formalin for histological analysis.

2.2. Histopathology. Tissue samples were fixed in formalin and processed by standard techniques. The samples were cut into 5 μm thick sections, placed on slides, and stained using hematoxylin and eosin (H&E). The slides were evaluated under a microscope at different magnification.

TABLE 1: PCR amplification protocol.

Step	Temperature	Duration	Cycles
Initial denaturation	95°C	3 min	1
Denaturation	95°C	15 sec	
Annealing	53.5°C	15 sec	35
Extension	72°C	15 sec	
Final extension	72°C	1 min/kb	1

2.3. PCR. A Bosphore® Tissue Genomic Manual DNA Extraction Spin Kit (Anatolia Geneworks, Turkey) and a Magnesia® Genomic DNA Tissue Kit (automated Magnesia DNA Extraction machine) (Anatolia Geneworks, Turkey) were used for this study. The kits were used to extract DNA from 140 frozen tissue samples according to the manufacturer's instructions. To accomplish this, a specifically designed primer set for BPV-1 was used (forward 5′-AGGAGG-GTCATGCTTTGCTC-3′; reverse 5′-GCTGTTCGGAGT-GGTGTGTA-3′) to obtain DNA fragments of 847 bp. These primers were designed to target conserved regions (identical nucleic acid sequence) for alignment of the following BPV type 1 complete genomes (X02346, NC_001522, AB626705, and JX678969). This newly designed primer was validated including testing for inclusivity and exclusivity. Amplification was performed using a SureCycler 8800 Thermal Cycler (Agilent Technologies, USA) in a final volume of 25 μL, containing 100–300 ng DNA, 2 mM MgCl$_2$, 1.25 μL primers (0.5 μM), and 12.5 μL 1X KAPA2G Robust HotStart ReadyMix (Kapa Biosystems, Cape Town, South Africa). The amplification protocol used for this work is shown in Table 1. The PCR products of the viral DNA were detected by electrophoresis on a 1.5% agarose gel containing ethidium bromide, which was placed in TBE buffer and run at a constant voltage (100 V) for approximately 35 min. DNA was visualized using a VISION Gel Documentation System (Scie-Plas, UK). As a negative control, DNA was extracted from skin tissues collected from clinically healthy slaughtered cattle that had previously shown negative results by both histological and PCR analysis.

2.4. Sequencing. A total of 121 BPV-1-positive specimens (as determined by PCR), which were selected as representative of BPV's geographical distribution, were sequenced to confirm viral genome type. For sequencing analysis, PCR products which contain E2, E5, and L2 genes were purified using a StrataPrep DNA Gel Extraction Kit (Agilent Technologies, USA); sequencing was performed at the National Instrumentation Center for Environmental Management (NICEM), College of Agriculture and Life Sciences, Seoul National University (South Korea). Sequencing reactions were performed using both forward and reverse primers in a 10 μL total reaction volume (ABI BigDYE V3.1 Ready-Reaction Kit; Applied Biosystems, USA) according to the manufacturer's recommendations. The samples were analyzed on a 3730XL DNA Analyzer (Applied Biosystems, USA). Forward and reverse complementary sequences were aligned using ApE (A plasmid Editor) software (v2.0.49, 2015), and the obtained results were submitted to GenBank and analyzed via BLAST search (http://blast.ncbi.nlm.nih.gov/) on the GenBank database. ApE software was used to detect corresponding amino acid sequences.

2.5. Phylogenetic Analysis. The sequences obtained in this study were submitted to phylogenetic analysis. As described above, the sequences were generated using a BPV-1-specific primer set, and the products were deposited in GenBank under accession number KT203919, along with the following reference strains for all 13 BPV genotypes: BPV-1 (accession number X02346), BPV-2 (accession number M20219), BPV-3 (accession number NC_004197), BPV-4 (accession number X05817), BPV-5 (accession number AJ620206), BPV-6 (accession number AJ620208), BPV-7 (accession number DQ217793), BPV-8 (accession number DQ098913), BPV-9 (accession number AB331650), BPV-10 (accession number AB331651), BPV-11 (accession number AB543507), BPV-12 (accession number JF834523), and BPV-13 (accession number JQ798171). Sequences were aligned using ApE software. To identify evolutionary relationships among the analyzed sequences, phylogenetic analysis was performed via the neighbor-joining method using MEGA software version 6 [22].

2.6. Protein Structure. To study the protein structures corresponding to the sequenced genes, we used the I-TASSER server, which is an Internet-based software product that enables protein structure and function predictions. I-TASSER allows automated generation of high-quality predictions of the 3D structures and biological functions of protein molecules based on their amino acid sequences [23, 24].

3. Results

3.1. Histopathology. All 140 of the collected samples could be clinically described by the presence of multiple exophytic warts (Figure 1(a)). Most of them located on the head and neck (46.6%), udder and teats (19%), legs (16%), and back and abdomen (18.4%). Histopathological examination indicated that the samples were fibropapilloma. In Figures 1(b) and 1(c), the epidermal and dermal interdigitations (papillary projections) of representative samples are shown. Fibroblast proliferation, collagen deposition, and lymphocyte infiltration were observed (Figure 1(d)). Furthermore, koilocytes that are keratinocytes with perinuclear halos or with swollen, clear cytoplasm and pyknotic nuclei were present (Figures 1(e) and 1(f)).

3.2. PCR. BPV-1 DNA was detected in 121 of the 140 collected papilloma samples. These BPV-1-positive samples produced DNA fragments of 847 bp in length for E2, E5, and L2 genes, which were amplified using BPV-1-specific primers (Figure 2). PCR analysis showed that 86.42% of the analyzed bovine papillomatoses were induced by BPV-1 in the assessed Iraqi cattle populations, which included both imported breeds and crossbreeds being raised in central Iraq.

3.3. Sequencing. Sequencing analysis was conducted on the PCR products for E2, E5, and L2 genes amplified from the collected samples that showed identical sequence. The results confirmed the presence of BPV-1, with 97% identity for the majority of the NCBI BLAST-searched BPV-1 sequences. As we used BPV-1-specific primers to amplify the extracted DNA samples, BPV-1 was the predominant genotype detected in all 121 BPV-positive (100%) cattle wart tissue samples. This finding is the first genotyped confirmation of the presence of BPV-1 as a primary causative agent for bovine papillomatosis in Iraqi cattle in the central Iraqi region.

3.4. Phylogenetic Analysis. A phylogenetic tree was generated using retrieved genome sequences that were deposited under accession number KT203919 and analyzed against 13 BPV genotype reference sequences (Figure 3). BPV-1 was the main BPV genotype identified (121 samples). The aligned sample sequences were classified as BPV-1 (genus *Deltapapillomavirus*). The aligned sequences showed high similarity both to the nucleotide sequence of BPV-1 (accession number X02346) and to a sequence of a BPV isolate from Japan (accession number AB626705).

We were able to obtain a complete E5 gene sequence, which we translated into an amino acid sequence that we deposited into GenBank under accession number ALB72915. The amino acid sequence was mpnlwfllfl glvaamqlll llfmllfflv ywdhfecscs nlpf. A BLAST search of the NCBI database using the identified Iraqi BPV-1 transforming protein E5 sequence showed a 100% identity match with a BPV-1 E5 sequence obtained from a South African sarcoid-affected zebra (accession number ACR09659) and a 98% identity match with a BPV-1 E5 sequence obtained from an equine sarcoid in the United Kingdom (accession number AAP69967). A distance tree was created using the NCBI database, and it confirmed these results (Figure 4).

3.5. Protein Structure. The protein structure of the complete amino acid sequence of transforming transmembrane protein E5 from the isolated Iraqi BPV-1 was analyzed using the I-TASSER server, an Internet-based software program that can be used to generate protein structure and function predictions. I-TASSER generates high-quality predictions of the 3D structures and biological functions of protein molecules based on their amino acid sequences (Figure 5(a)). Based on this analysis, a ligand-binding site was predicted on E5 that facilitates its binding to PDGFβ-R (Figure 5(b)).

4. Discussion

In the current work, clinically and histologically diagnosed cases of bovine papillomatosis were studied to identify and characterize the BPV-1 genotype which was the most prevalent in the central Iraq region, which is a major location for large cattle breeding farms. The identification and characterization of the BPV-1 genotype present in this region are important for effective disease control. We used genotype-specific primers to identify and characterize BPV-1 confirmed

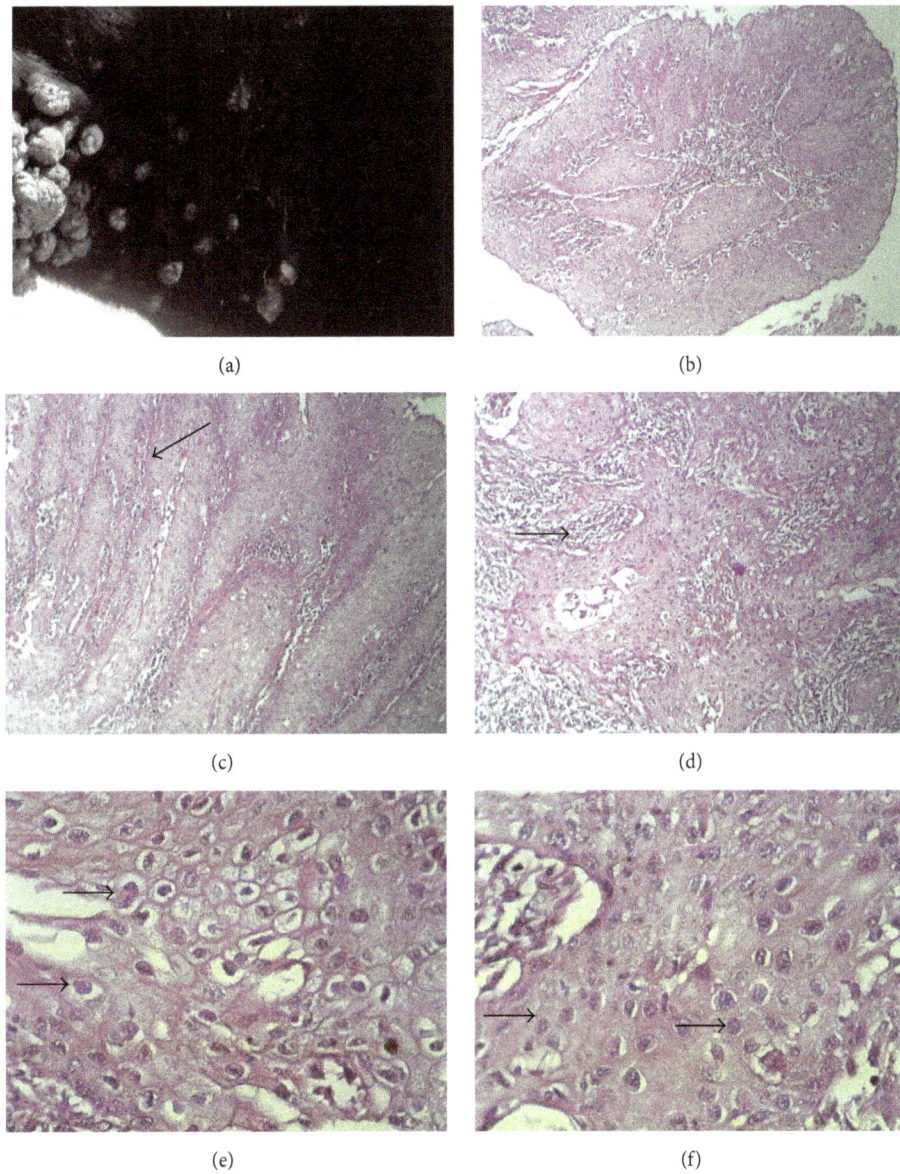

FIGURE 1: Cutaneous papillomas of the skin. (a) Neck, cow. Multiple exophytic, irregular verrucous papilloma masses arising in the skin. (b) Histopathological section showing papillary projections composed of a hyperkeratotic epidermis with a central collagenous core (10x). (c) Interdigitated epidermal and dermal papillary projections (shown by arrows, 10x). (d) Fibroblast proliferation, collagen deposition, and lymphocyte infiltration (shown by arrows, 10x). (e) Koilocytes (arrows) and keratinocytes with swollen perinuclear halos (40x). (f) Koilocytes with clear cytoplasm and pyknotic nuclei (shown by arrows, 40x, stained with H&E).

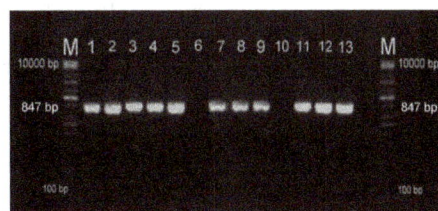

FIGURE 2: Skin wart samples. PCR products for E2, E5, and L2 genes visualized in an ethidium bromide-stained 1.5% agarose gel following electrophoresis in TBE buffer. M: 100–10,000 bp marker; lanes: 1–5, 7–9, and 11–13: BPV-1-positive samples with bands at 847 bp; lane 6: no sample; lane 10: negative control.

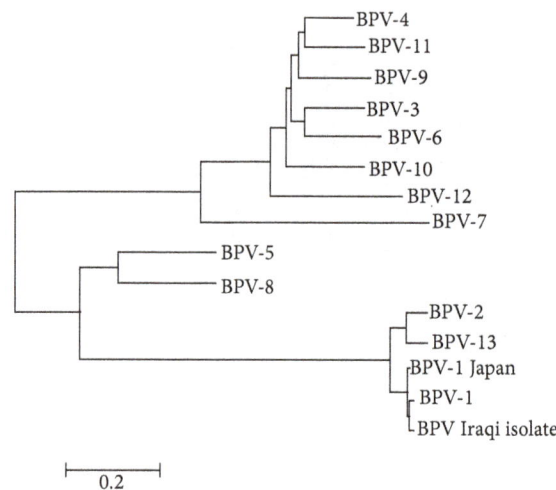

FIGURE 3: Phylogenetic tree showing the identified Iraqi BPV sequence. This is the first report of a BPV-1 sequence in Iraq (KT203919); the sequence was found to belong to the genus *Deltapapillomavirus*. The sequence was constructed via the neighbor-joining method using MEGA 6 software.

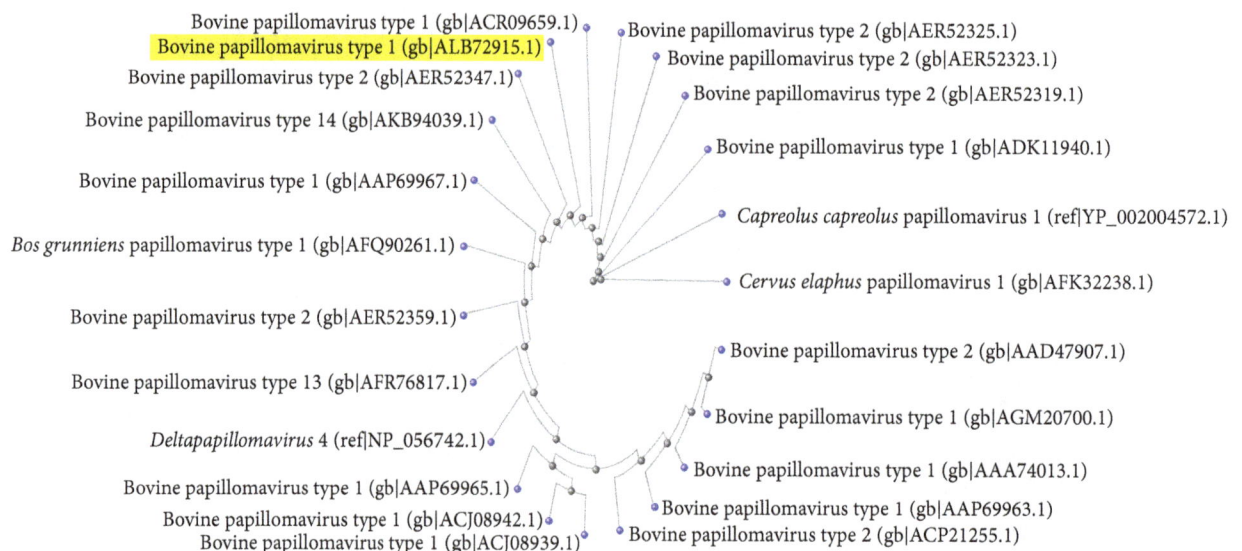

FIGURE 4: Distance tree created using the NCBI database after searching for Iraqi BPV-1 transforming protein E5. A 100% identity match was found with a BPV-1 E5 protein sequence isolated from a South African sarcoid-affected zebra (accession number ACR09659) and a 98% identity match was found with a BPV-1 E5 protein sequence isolated from an equine sarcoid in the United Kingdom (accession number AAP69967). The tree was created using the neighbor-joining method.

by sequencing and phylogenetic analysis, which are considered to be the best methods for these purposes according to the literature [25, 26].

Histological findings showed that the wart specimens evaluated in this study were cutaneous fibropapillomas, which showed characteristic features of papillomatosis as described by Zachary and McGavin [27]. In our molecular analysis, BPV-1 DNA was detected in 121 samples. Amplicons obtained by PCR reactions were submitted for sequencing and found to be identical, confirming the presence of BPV-1, which belongs to the genus *Deltapapillomavirus*. The current study revealed that highly pathogenic BPV-1 is widespread in Iraq; this genotype is associated with the development of

cutaneous papillomatosis (fibropapilloma) [28]. To the best of our knowledge, this is the first study to report the presence of BPV-1 in Iraq.

In the present investigation, we were able to obtain a complete E5 gene sequence. Interestingly, based on distance analysis, this sequence was found to exhibit high similarity to E5 amino acid sequences isolated from a South African zebra and from equine sarcoids in the United Kingdom. These results suggest the possibility of disease transmission via British army horses during the 1920s while they were present in Iraq. Another possibility is that BPV-1 in Iraq originated from the importation of livestock from other countries because Holstein Friesian cattle [17, 18] are heavily

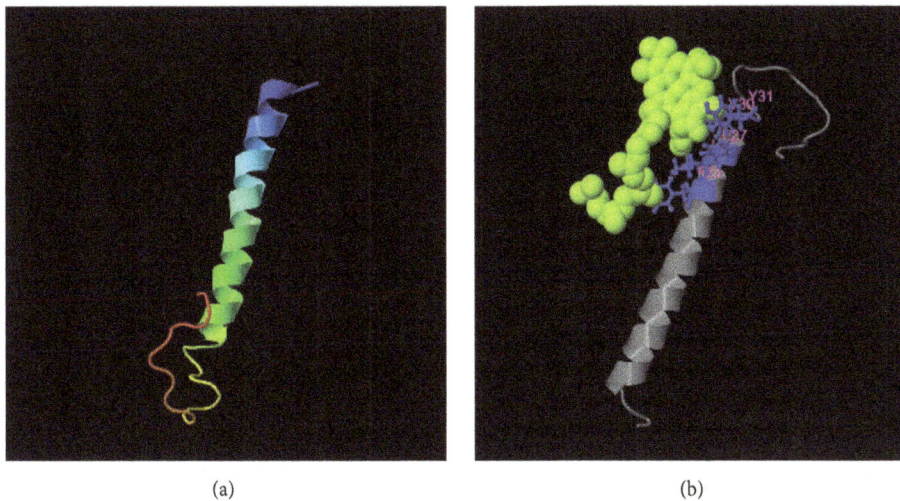

(a)   (b)

FIGURE 5: Predicted protein structure for the complete transforming transmembrane protein E5 generated using the I-TASSER server. (a) The predicted E5 protein structure created by the program. (b) A predicted ligand-binding site on E5, this site is a possible location for E5/PDGFβ-R interactions.

imported into Iraq. Fibropapilloma viruses encode the most highly conserved E5 proteins [29]. To characterize BPV-1, the structure of the E5 protein and its ligand-binding site were predicted using a special program. E5 is the smallest known oncoprotein that regulates cell transformation. This regulation is achieved via the activation of PDGFR-β [30]. The E5 protein forms a dimer in transformed infected cells. The dimer contains a membrane-spanning segment that directly binds to the transmembrane domain of PDGFβ-R. This binding then induces receptor dimerization, autophosphorylation, and sustained mitogenic signaling [3, 31]. The BPV-1 E5 protein has been shown to be localized to transformed basal keratinocytes within fibropapilloma tissues [32]. Targeting E5 as a possible therapeutic agent has also been described [10]. Thus, studies of this protein are important as well as other virus proteins to better understand the carcinogenesis molecular pathway such as Calpain 3 that is expressed in papillomavirus-associated urothelial cancers of the urinary bladder in cattle [33].

The current study is the first aimed at the detection and characterization of BPV-1 genotype in central Iraq. The results of this study are important for aiding in the development of prophylactic and therapeutic measures to reduce the economic losses associated with bovine papillomatosis in Iraq.

Ethical Approval

The animals used in this study were defined as "farm animals," and no experimental work was performed on them; therefore, approval was not required from IACUC or an ethics committee. The owner of the animals provided permission for these studies. The ethics committee at the Iraqi Center for Cancer and Medical Genetic Research reviewed the work and approved the waiver.

Disclosure

This study was conducted in the Experimental Therapy Department, Iraqi Center for Cancer and Medical Genetic Research, Al-Mustansiriya University, Baghdad, Iraq.

References

[1] S. Shafti-Keramat, C. Schellenbacher, A. Handisurya et al., "Bovine papillomavirus type 1 (BPV1) and BPV2 are closely related serotypes," *Virology*, vol. 393, no. 1, pp. 1–6, 2009.

[2] S. Roperto, R. Brun, F. Paolini et al., "Detection of bovine papillomavirus type 2 in the peripheral blood of cattle with urinary bladder tumours: possible biological role," *Journal of General Virology*, vol. 89, no. 12, pp. 3027–3033, 2008.

[3] K. Talbert-Slagle and D. DiMaio, "The bovine papillomavirus E5 protein and the PDGF β receptor: it takes two to tango," *Virology*, vol. 384, no. 2, pp. 345–351, 2009.

[4] F. Bocaneti, G. Altamura, A. Corteggio, E. Velescu, F. Roperto, and G. Borzacchiello, "Bovine papillomavirus: new insights into an old disease," *Transboundary and Emerging Diseases*, vol. 63, no. 1, pp. 14–23, 2016.

[5] A. Corteggio, G. Altamura, F. Roperto, and G. Borzacchiello, "Bovine papillomavirus E5 and E7 oncoproteins in naturally occurring tumors: are two better than one?" *Infectious Agents and Cancer*, vol. 8, article 1, 2013.

[6] M. Lunardi, B. K. de Alcântara, R. A. A. Otonel, W. B. Rodrigues, A. F. Alfieri, and A. A. Alfieri, "Bovine papillomavirus type 13 DNA in equine sarcoids," *Journal of Clinical Microbiology*, vol. 51, no. 7, pp. 2167–2171, 2013.

[7] G. Borzacchiello and F. Roperto, "Bovine papillomaviruses, papillomas and cancer in cattle," *Veterinary Research*, vol. 39, no. 5, p. 19, 2008.

[8] M. Lunardi, A. A. Alfieri, R. A. A. Otonel et al., "Genetic characterization of a novel bovine papillomavirus member of the *Deltapapillomavirus* genus," *Veterinary Microbiology*, vol. 162, no. 1, pp. 207–213, 2013.

[9] J. S. Munday, N. Thomson, M. Dunowska, C. G. Knight, R. E. Laurie, and S. Hills, "Genomic characterisation of the feline sarcoid-associated papillomavirus and proposed classification as Bos taurus papillomavirus type 14," *Veterinary Microbiology*, vol. 177, no. 3-4, pp. 289–295, 2015.

[10] A. Venuti, F. Paolini, L. Nasir et al., "Papillomavirus E5: the smallest oncoprotein with many functions," *Molecular Cancer*, vol. 10, article 140, 2011.

[11] S. Roperto, G. Borzacchiello, I. Esposito et al., "Productive infection of bovine papillomavirus type 2 in the placenta of pregnant cows affected with urinary bladder tumors," *PLoS ONE*, vol. 7, no. 3, Article ID e33569, 2012.

[12] S. Roperto, V. Russo, G. Borzacchiello et al., "Bovine papillomavirus type 2 (BPV-2) E5 oncoprotein binds to the subunit D of the V1-ATPase proton pump in naturally occurring urothelial tumors of the urinary bladder of cattle," *PLoS ONE*, vol. 9, no. 2, Article ID e88860, 2014.

[13] Y.-S. Seo, F. Müller, M. Lusky et al., "Bovine Papilloma Virus (BPV)-encoded E2 protein enhances binding of E1 protein to the BPV replication origin," *Proceedings of the National Academy of Sciences of the United States of America*, vol. 90, no. 7, pp. 2865–2869, 1993.

[14] S. M. Melanson and E. J. Androphy, "Topography of bovine papillomavirus E2 protein on the viral genome during the cell cycle," *Virology*, vol. 393, no. 2, pp. 258–264, 2009.

[15] K.-N. Zhao, X.-Y. Sun, I. H. Frazer, and J. Zhou, "DNA packaging by L1 and L2 capsid proteins of bovine papillomavirus type 1," *Virology*, vol. 243, no. 2, pp. 482–491, 1998.

[16] M. A. Hamad, A. S. Al-Banna, and N. Y. Yaseen, "Cell culture established from warts of bovine papilloma," *Al-Anbar Journal of Veterinary Sciences*, vol. 4, pp. 77–81, 2011.

[17] F. R. Al-Samarai, N. N. Al-Anbari, and Y. K. Al-tmimi, "Genetics aspects of reproductive performance for Holstein," *The Iraqi Journal of Veterinary Medicine*, vol. 30, pp. 95–107, 2006.

[18] M. Al-Kinani, A. A. Al-Zahir, and M. Al-Baiti, "The study of relationship between effect of some environmental condition in some physiological haematological in cross bread Holstein Friesian Dairy cattle," *The Iraqi Journal of Veterinary Medicine*, vol. 34, pp. 15–21, 2010.

[19] E. U. D. Santos, M. A. R. Silva, N. E. Pontes et al., "Detection of different bovine papillomavirus types and co-infection in bloodstream of cattle," *Transboundary and Emerging Diseases*, vol. 63, no. 1, pp. e103–e108, 2016.

[20] C. J. Lindsey, M. E. Almeida, C. F. Vicari et al., "Bovine papillomavirus DNA in milk, blood, urine, semen, and spermatozoa of bovine papillomavirus-infected animals," *Genetics and Molecular Research*, vol. 8, no. 1, pp. 310–318, 2009.

[21] S. Brandt, R. Haralambus, A. Schoster, R. Kirnbauer, and C. Stanek, "Peripheral blood mononuclear cells represent a reservoir of bovine papillomavirus DNA in sarcoid-affected equines," *Journal of General Virology*, vol. 89, no. 6, pp. 1390–1395, 2008.

[22] K. Tamura, G. Stecher, D. Peterson, A. Filipski, and S. Kumar, "MEGA6: molecular evolutionary genetics analysis version 6.0," *Molecular Biology and Evolution*, vol. 30, no. 12, pp. 2725–2729, 2013.

[23] J. Yang, R. Yan, A. Roy, D. Xu, J. Poisson, and Y. Zhang, "The I-TASSER suite: protein structure and function prediction," *Nature Methods*, vol. 12, no. 1, pp. 7–8, 2015.

[24] Y. Zhang, "I-TASSER server for protein 3D structure prediction," *BMC Bioinformatics*, vol. 9, article 40, 2008.

[25] R. P. Araldi, R. F. Carvalho, T. C. Melo et al., "Bovine papillomavirus in beef cattle: first description of BPV-12 and putative type BAPV8 in Brazil," *Genetics and Molecular Research*, vol. 13, no. 3, pp. 5644–5653, 2014.

[26] A. Grindatto, G. Ferraro, K. Varello et al., "Molecular and histological characterization of bovine papillomavirus in North West Italy," *Veterinary Microbiology*, vol. 180, no. 1-2, pp. 113–117, 2015.

[27] J. F. Zachary and M. D. McGavin, *Pathologic Basis of Veterinary Disease*, Elsevier Health Sciences, Philadelphia, Pa, USA, 2013.

[28] F. Jelínek and R. Tachezy, "Cutaneous papillomatosis in cattle," *Journal of Comparative Pathology*, vol. 132, no. 1, pp. 70–81, 2005.

[29] K. Van Doorslaer, "Evolution of the papillomaviridae," *Virology*, vol. 445, no. 1-2, pp. 11–20, 2013.

[30] A. L. Halpern and D. J. McCance, "Papillomavirus E5 proteins," *Transformation*, vol. 9, article 52, 1996.

[31] D. DiMaio and L. M. Petti, "The E5 proteins," *Virology*, vol. 445, no. 1-2, pp. 99–114, 2013.

[32] S. Burnett, N. Jareborg, and D. DiMaio, "Localization of bovine papillomavirus type 1 E5 protein to transformed basal keratinocytes and permissive differentiated cells in fibropapilloma tissue," *Proceedings of the National Academy of Sciences of the United States of America*, vol. 89, no. 12, pp. 5665–5669, 1992.

[33] S. Roperto, R. de Tullio, C. Raso et al., "Calpain3 is expressed in a proteolytically active form in papillomavirus-associated urothelial tumors of the urinary bladder in cattle," *PLoS ONE*, vol. 5, no. 4, article e10299, 2010.

11

Novel Gyroviruses, including Chicken Anaemia Virus, in Clinical and Chicken Samples from South Africa

Heidi E. M. Smuts

Division Medical Virology/National Health Laboratory Service, Department of Clinical Sciences, Faculty of Health Sciences, University of Cape Town, Observatory 7925, South Africa

Correspondence should be addressed to Heidi E. M. Smuts; heidi.smuts@uct.ac.za

Academic Editor: Finn S. Pedersen

Introduction. Chicken anaemia virus, CAV, was until recently the only member of the *Gyrovirus* genus. 6 novel gyroviruses, AGV2, HGyV1, and GyV3-6, have since been discovered in human and chicken samples. *Methods.* PCR amplification of the VP2 gene was used to detect AGV2/HGyV1, GyV3, and CAV in a range of clinical samples including stool, respiratory, CSF, and HIV-positive plasma. Screening of fresh local chicken meat was also performed. *Results.* AGV2/HGyV1 or GyV3 was detected in stools from healthy children (17/49, 34.7%) and patients with diarrhoea (22/149, 14.8%). 1.2% (3/246) nasopharyngeal respiratory samples were positive. No AGV2/HGyV1 or GyV3 was detected in nasal swabs from wheezing patients, in CSF from patients with meningitis, and in HIVpositive plasma. CAV was found in 51% (25/49) of stools from healthy children and 16% (24/149) in diarrhoea samples. Screening of 28 chicken samples showed a higher prevalence of gyrovirus (20/28, 71%) compared to CAV (1/28, 3.6%). Phylogenetic analysis of the CAV VP1 gene showed South African sequences clustering with Brazilian isolates from genotypes D2 and A2. *Conclusion.* Novel gyroviruses, including CAV, are present in the South African population with diarrhoea and respiratory illness as well as in healthy children. Their presence suggests an origin from chicken meat consumption.

1. Introduction

Until recently chicken anaemia virus (CAV) was the only member of the genus *Gyrovirus* in the Circoviridae family. This genus is characterized by small nonenveloped DNA viruses with a negative sense single-stranded circular DNA of about 2.3 kb [1]. Circoviruses, in contrast, have an ambisense genome. The similarity of the gyrovirus genome organization to annelloviruses, with 3 overlapping open reading frames (ORFs), has led to the recommendation that gyroviruses become a subfamily, Gyrovirinae, within the Anelloviridae-family [2].

In early 2011 Rijsewijk et al. [3] reported the discovery of a distant relative to CAV, avian gyrovirus 2 (AGV2), in diseased chicken from Brazil, with only 40% homology to CAV. Later that year, Sauvage et al. [4] identified a very closely related gyrovirus on human skin (HGyV1). Subsequently 4 other novel gyroviruses have been described. Gyrovirus 3 (GyV3) was identified by viral metagenomics in faeces from Chilean children with acute gastroenteritis and also in chicken meat [5]. A phylogenetically distinct gyrovirus (GyV4) was also discovered in both human stool samples and chicken meat by 454 pyrosequencing [6]. Further 2 divergent gyroviruses, GyV5 and GyV6, were found in the stools of Tunisian children with diarrhoea [7].

CAV is an economically important pathogen in the poultry industry causing severe anaemia and immunosuppression in young 2-3-week-old chicken that lack protective maternal antibodies [8]. In adult chickens CAV infection is subclinical, but financial losses may be incurred by poultry farmers due to lack of weight gain and susceptibility to secondary infections.

The role of CAV in the African poultry context has been addressed by a number of researchers [9–16]. Seroprevalence in Nigeria, Egypt, Central African Republic, and Cameroon ranged from 37% to 89% depending on age of chicken. Further, CAV DNA could be detected in the majority (77%) of seropositive chickens, indicating persistent virus shedding in the presence of antibodies. To date there has only been one brief report on CAV in South African chickens [17], where 3 broiler chickens were seropositive.

The aim of this study was to determine if some of the novel gyroviruses and CAV are present in the South African population and in chickens from this region.

2. Materials and Methods

2.1. Clinical Samples. Anonymized stool samples from 49 healthy children, aged 6–36 months, were obtained with parental/guardian consent from a crèche over 2 periods: summer (February/March 2006) and winter (July/August 2006). Stool samples from patients with diarrhoea submitted to the virology and microbiology diagnostic laboratory over the same time periods in 2006 were also examined ($n = 149$).

246 nasopharyngeal respiratory samples from children aged 1–60 months previously screened for the 7 common respiratory viruses (adenovirus, human respiratory syncytial virus, human metapneumovirus, influenza A and B, parainfluenza virus 1–3, and human rhinovirus A) were tested, of which 152 were negative and the remainder ($n = 94$) were positive for one of the above viruses.

Nasal swabs ($n = 48$) collected in May 2004 from children aged 6–25 months with acute wheezing were also screened. Informed consent from a parent or guardian had been obtained.

The presence of gyrovirus in plasma from HIV-infected patients ($n = 48$) was evaluated as Maggi et al. [18] had identified HGyV1 in one Italian patient. The CD4/μL count ranged from 13 to 1065 with a mean of 397.

94 cerebrospinal fluid (CSF) samples from patients with suspected meningitis were also screened.

2.2. Chicken Meat. Fresh chicken meat for human consumption was purchased in August 2012 from 4 retail stores in Cape Town, South Africa. These included 4 thighs and 4 drum sticks from 3 of 4 stores and 4 thighs from the remaining store.

A sterile scalpel was used to remove a small piece of the skin and underlying meat from each sample. This was placed in a sterile 1.5 mL Eppendorf tube and stored at −20°C until extracted.

2.3. DNA Extraction. Total nucleic acid was extracted from nasopharyngeal respiratory samples using the MagNA Pure LC automated extraction method as per manufacturer's instructions (Roche Diagnostics GmbH, Penzberg, Germany). Nucleic acid was extracted from stool, nasal swab, CSF, plasma, and chicken meat samples using the QIAamp DNA stool mini kit and QIAamp DNA mini kit, with protocols appropriate for body fluid or tissue as per manufacturer's instructions (Qiagen, Hilden, Germany).

2.4. PCR for Detection of Gyrovirus or CAV. Consensus primers targeting the conserved VP2 region of the gyroviruses, CAV, AGV2/HGyV1, GyV3, and GyV6, were used as outer primers as described by Phan et al. [5]. Nested primers specific for either CAV (CAV F1n 5′ GGCAGTGAATCG-GCGCTTAGCCG and CAV R1n 5′ AGTCGCTTGAGGTG-GTGCCACCG) or AGV2/HGyV1 and GyV3 (ConGy F1n 5′ GGCAGTGAATTGCCGCTTAGGC and ConGy R1n 5′

CGCAGTCTGTGTCTCCAGTGC) were used to improve sensitivity. The inner PCR product was ~550 bp in size. The PCR conditions for the first round were as follows: denaturation at 95°C for 3 minutes, 40 cycles of 95°C for 15 sec, 45°C for 25 sec, and 72°C for 35 sec followed by a final 72°C elongation step for 7 min. The second round of amplification was the same as above with an increase in the annealing temperature to 55°C. PCR products were visualised by electrophoresis through a 2% agarose gel, ethidium bromide staining, and UV illumination. GyV4, GyV5, and GyV6 are not amplified with the nested primers and therefore this study did not measure their prevalence.

2.5. Sanger Sequencing. The VP2 amplicons were sequenced directly in both directions using either CAV or GyV nested PCR primers. The BigDye terminator cycle sequencing kit was used (Applied Biosystems, Foster City CA, USA). The VP2 genes were aligned with reference sequences from Gen-Bank using ClustalW [19] and phylogenetic trees constructed using MEGA 5.05 [20] with 1000 bootstrap resamplings. BLAST analysis was also undertaken.

Improved phylogenetic resolution of CAV positive samples was investigated by amplification of the 1349 bp of the VP1 and overlapping VP2 and VP3 genes using primers previously described by Natesan et al. [21] and Eltahir et al. [22]. Increased sensitivity was achieved by the design of a nested VP1 forward primer (5′CCGCAAGAAGTATAAGAC).

3. Results

3.1. Gyrovirus in Clinical Samples. AGV2/HGyV1 or GyV3 was detected in stools from both healthy children (17/49, 34.7%) and patients with diarrhoea (22/149, 14.8%) (Table 1). The detection rate in respiratory samples was considerably lower at 1.3% (2/152) in samples negative for the common respiratory viruses and 1.1% (1/94) in positive samples (Table 1). In the latter sample, parainfluenza 1–3 was previously detected using the Seeplex RV7 assay (Seegene, Seoul, South Korea). No AGV2/HGyV1 or GyV3 was detected in the nasal swabs from children with acute wheezing, in plasma from HIV-infected individuals, or in the CSF from patients with suspected meningitis.

3.2. CAV in Stool Samples. CAV was detected in 51% (25/49) stool samples from healthy children and 16.1% (24/149) in diarrhoea samples (Table 1). Nasopharyngeal respiratory samples, nasal swabs, HIV-positive plasma, and CSF were not screened for the presence of CAV.

Dual infection with both CAV and AGV2/HGyV1/GyV3 was found in 10/49 (20.4%) and 8/149 (5.4%) stools from healthy children and patients with diarrhoea, respectively. Codetection of CAV and AGV2/HGyV1/GyV3 was not statistically linked ($P = 0.85$).

3.3. CAV/Gyrovirus in Chicken Meat. Screening of 28 chicken samples for the presence of CAV DNA or AGV2/HGyV1/GyV3 DNA showed a considerably higher prevalence of gyrovirus (20/28, 71.4%) compared to CAV (1/28, 3.6%).

TABLE 1: PCR screening of clinical and chicken samples for the presence of AGV2/HGyV1 and CAV.

Samples	AGV2/HGyV1 Number (%)	CAV Number (%)
Control stool	17/49 (34.7%)	25/49 (51%)
Diarrhoea stool	22/149 (14.8%)	24/149 (16.1%)
Negative respiratory virus NPA	2/152 (1.3%)	N/D
Positive respiratory virus NPA	1/94 (1.1%)	N/D
HIV-positive plasma	0/48	N/D
Acute wheezing nasal swabs	0/48	N/D
Meningitis CSF	0/94	N/D
Chicken meat store P	7/8 (87.5%)	0/8
Chicken meat store W	8/8 (100%)	0/8
Chicken meat store C	1/8 (12.5%)	0/8
Chicken meat store S	4/4 (100%)	1/4 (25%)

NPA: nasopharyngeal aspirates; N/D: not done.

From one store, C, 7/8 samples were negative for both gyrovirus and CAV, while chicken meat obtained from the remaining 3 stores was positive for AGV2/HGyV1, with only one sample coinfected with CAV (Table 1).

3.4. Phylogenetic and Amino Acid Analysis. Phylogenetic analysis of the VP2 region of samples successfully sequenced showed the presence of only AGV2/HGyV1, with 56.3% (18/32) grouping with AGV2 sequences and 43.5% (14/32) with HGyV1 sequences (Figure 1(a)). No GyV3 was detected. All 3 respiratory samples clustered with AGV2 sequences. Of the chicken samples successfully sequenced, 6/9 had sequence homology to HGyV1 and the remaining 3 samples homology with AGV2 sequences.

The VP1 region of CAV provided phylogenetic information for the classification of isolates into different genotypes (Figure 1(b)). Analysis of the 1349 bp region showed that 6/7 CAV-positive samples grouped together with genotype D, particularly D2 isolates from USA, Japan, Malaysia, and Australia. The remaining sample clustered within genotype A, but formed a separate lineage with a high bootstrap value (data not shown). Phylogenetic analysis of a truncated VP1 region (481 bp) to allow inclusion of VP1 sequences from Brazil (AY855079-88) retained the phylogeny as determined using the larger VP1 region, but now showed that all South Africa isolates clustered with the Brazilian sequences of either genotype A or D (Figure 1(b)).

Analysis of the deduced 410 amino acids of CAV VP1 protein revealed that no amino acids were characteristic of the South African isolates, although a proline (P) at position 286 was found in all sequences and in common with 2 isolates from Japan and 1 each from Australia and Malaysia. The region responsible for virulence [23] showed a glutamine (Q) at position 394 instead of histidine, indicative of a highly virulent strain (data not shown).

4. Discussion

The recent identification of novel gyroviruses in the human population led to the screening of a range of clinical samples from patients and healthy children from South Africa. The present study confirms the presence of AGV2/HGyV1 and CAV in this region. GyV3 was not detected and this study did not test for GyV4, GyV5, and GyV6. As limited studies on gyroviruses in healthy and sick individuals are available, the pathogenesis and clinical importance are not well understood. HGyV1 may be a member of the skin virome [4], although Chu et al. [6] were unable to detect gyroviruses in skin swabs from healthy individuals. Novel gyroviruses have been detected in stools from patients with diarrhoea with a prevalence of 1–9.3%, while no gyrovirus was detected in stools from healthy individuals [5, 6]. The present study showed a higher prevalence of gyroviruses (AGV2/HGyV1) in stools from patients with diarrhoea (15%), while 35% of healthy children also had evidence of AGV2/HGyV1 DNA. Chu et al. [6] demonstrated that gyroviruses were more commonly detected in patients younger than 20 years of age.

Viruses found in the stool samples may also play a role in respiratory and systemic diseases. This was investigated by screening respiratory samples from young patients hospitalized with respiratory illness and children attending an outpatient hospital clinic with acute wheezing. AGV2 was detected in 3 hospitalized patients, with one patient coinfected with parainfluenza virus 1–3. Further studies are required to determine if gyroviruses can cause respiratory infections requiring hospitalization.

Gyrovirus was not detected in blood from HIV-infected individuals, although other studies have reported a low prevalence in both blood healthy donors [24] and immuno-compromised HIV-positive and kidney transplant patients [18]. Our results may reflect the small number of samples screened.

Circoviruses are able to cross the blood-brain barrier and cause infections of the central nervous system. Porcine circovirus type 2 infection in piglets results in cerebellar vasculitis [25], while in humans TTV and novel cycloviruses were found in the CSF of patients with subacute dementia, unexplained paraplegia, and acute CNS infections of unknown aetiology [26–28]. Screening of CSF samples from patients with possible meningitis showed no evidence of gyrovirus infection.

CAV was detected more frequently in stools from healthy children (>50%) compared to those with diarrhoea (16%). Prior studies by Phan et al. [5] and Chu et al. [6] also reported a high CAV prevalence in faecal samples from healthy donors of 25% and 53%, respectively. This high detection rate suggests that consumption of infected chicken meat may possibly play a role. However, in this report screening of fresh chicken meat purchased from a number of different stores in the study area does not support this assumption, as only one positive CAV sample was found. In contrast, a significant proportion of chicken meat was positive for AGV2/HGyV1. This discrepancy may be explained by the fact that only fresh chicken meat purchased in 2012 was screened, while the clinical samples were collected from 2004–2006

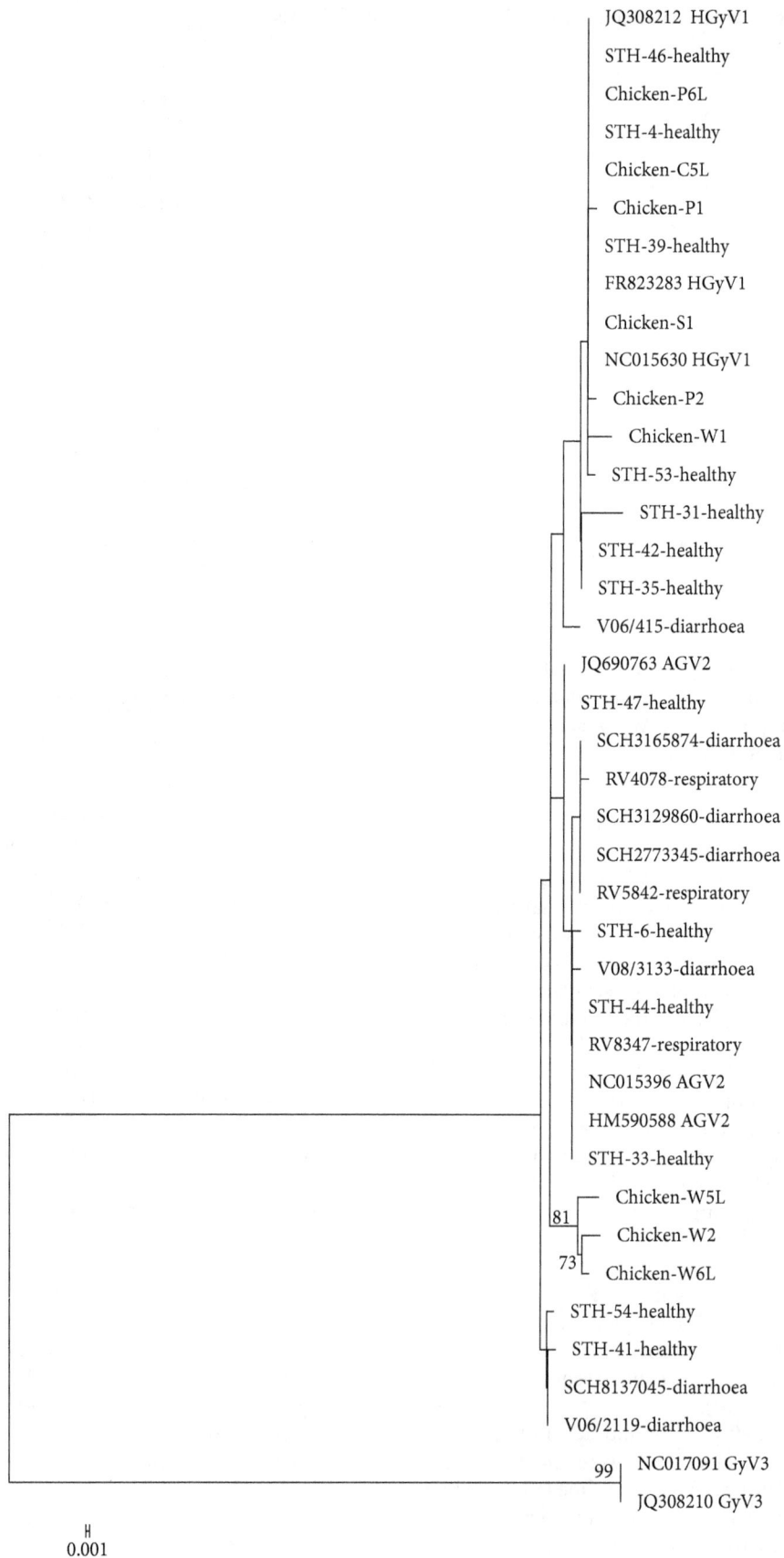

(a)

FIGURE 1: Continued.

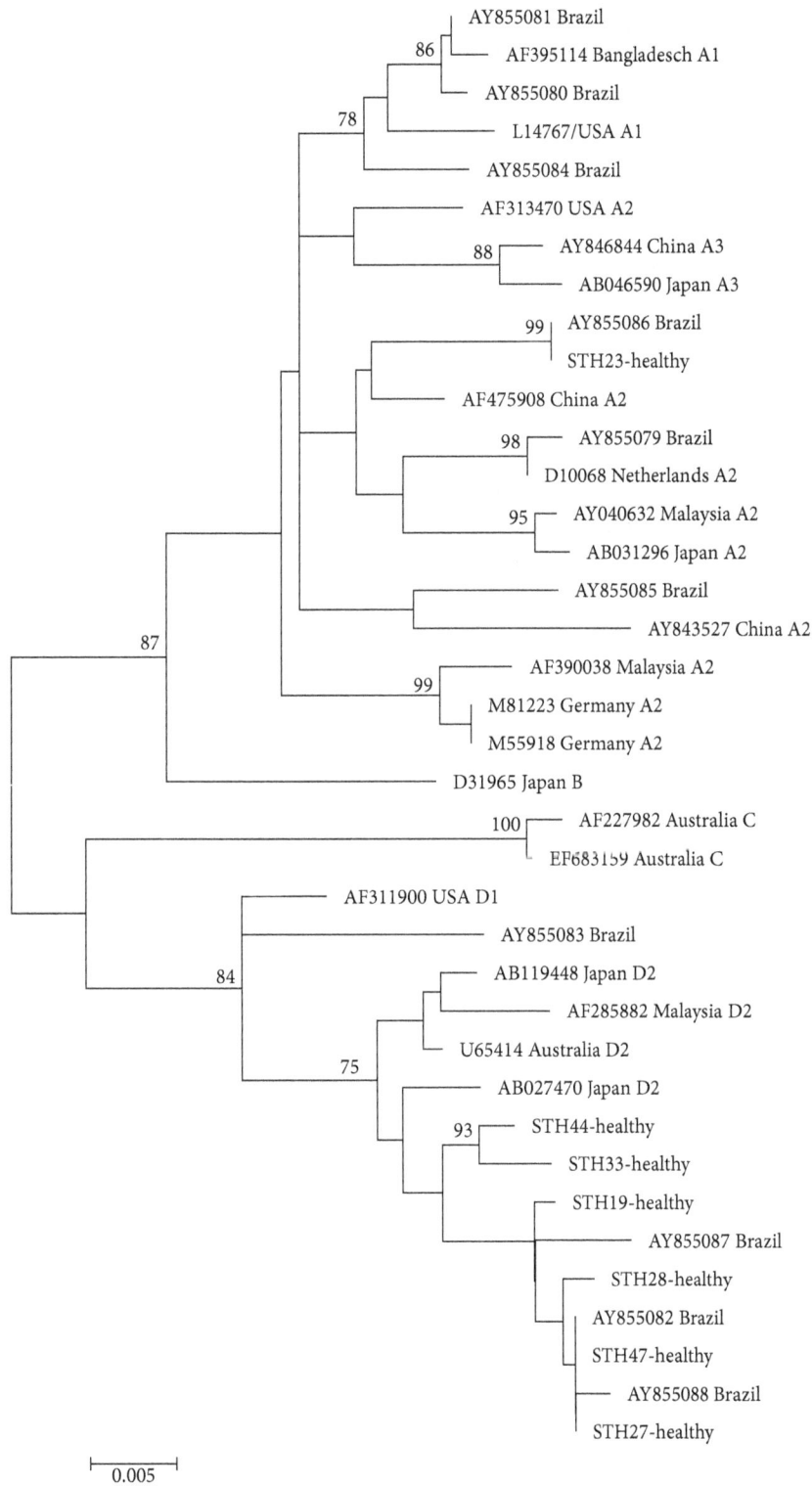

(b)

FIGURE 1: Phylogenetic trees generated by neighbour-joining analysis of the VP2 region of AGV2, HGyV1, and GyV3 (a) and CAV VP1 (b) of South African isolates of human and chicken origin. Reference sequences of AGV2, HGyV1, GyV3, and CAV were retrieved from the NCBI GenBank database and are indicated by accession numbers and country of origin. Bootstrap values greater than 75% are indicated at the nodes of the tree. The branch lengths are proportional to the evolutionary distances as shown on the scale.

when imported frozen chicken products were more readily available for consumption.

A number of live attenuated CAV vaccines are available and used in the poultry industry. However, evidence of this practice occurring in the South African poultry industry is not readily available. If undertaken, breeder hens are vaccinated to obtain high levels of circulating antibodies which can be passed onto progeny preventing early infections and disease caused by CAV (personal communication, Dr. Nkuna, South African Poultry Association).

From 2001 a significant amount of in-bone frozen chickens were imported from Brazil, which in 2010 accounted for over 70% of the South African import market of chickens [29]. This dropped substantially since 2012 with the introduction of stricter antidumping legislation. These imported products were significantly cheaper than the locally sourced chickens and may have been preferentially purchased and consumed by a large proportion of the South African population. Simionatto et al. [30] reported that CAV was detected in 90% of field samples collected from commercial breeders, broilers, and free-range chickens from different regions of Brazil. Whether these chickens are infected with CAV either naturally or through vaccination programs is not known.

Phylogenetic analysis of the VP1 region provides further evidence that CAV detected in this study may originate from Brazil. All the South African isolates, of either genotype D or A, clustered together with Brazilian isolates. Sourcing of imported chicken products from the earlier time of human sample collection to confirm this association was not possible in 2013.

5. Conclusion

The role and clinical relevance of gyroviruses in human disease require further investigation. Larger studies on patients with a variety of medical conditions are needed to elucidate the pathogenesis of gyrovirus infection.

Conflict of Interests

The author declares that there is no conflict of interests regarding the publication of this paper.

References

[1] P. Biagini, M. Bendinelli, S. Hino et al., Eds., Virus Taxonomy: Ninth Report of the International Committee on Taxonomy of Viruses, Elsevier Academic press, New York, NY, USA, 2011.

[2] P. Biagini, "Restructuring and expansion of the family Anelloviradae. Anellviradae-Circoviradae study group," International Committee on Taxonomy of Viruses, ICTV files and discussion, http://talk.ictvonline.org/files/proposals/taxonomy-proposals.vertebrat1/m/vert01/3911.aspx.

[3] F. A. M. Rijsewijk, H. F. dos Santos, T. F. Teixeira et al., "Discovery of a genome of a distant relative of chicken anemia virus reveals a new member of the genus Gyrovirus," Archives of Virology, vol. 156, no. 6, pp. 1097–1100, 2011.

[4] V. Sauvage, J. Cheval, V. Foulongne et al., "Identification of the first human Gyrovirus, a virus related to chicken anemia virus," Journal of Virology, vol. 85, no. 15, pp. 7948–7950, 2011.

[5] T. G. Phan, L. Li, M. G. O'Ryan et al., "A third gyrovirus species in human faeces," Journal of General Virology, vol. 93, no. 6, pp. 1356–1361, 2012.

[6] D. K. W. Chu, L. L. M. Poon, S. S. S. Chiu et al., "Characterization of a novel gyrovirus in human stool and chicken meat," Journal of Clinical Virology, vol. 55, no. 3, pp. 209–213, 2012.

[7] T. G. Phan, N. P. Vo, K. Sdiri-Loulizi et al., "Divergent gyroviruses in the feces of Tunisian children," Journal of Virology, vol. 446, no. 1-2, pp. 346–348, 2013.

[8] K. A. Schat, "Chicken anemia virus," Current Topics in Microbiology and Immunology, vol. 331, pp. 151–183, 2009.

[9] C. J. Snoeck, G. F. Komoyo, B. P. Mbee et al., "Epidemiology of chicken anaemia virus in Central Africa Republic and Cameroon," Journal of Virology, vol. 9, pp. 189–197, 2012.

[10] A. M. Hegazy, F. M. Abdallah, L. K. Abd-El Samie, and A. A. Nazim, "Chicken infectious anemia virus (CIAV) in broilers and laying hens in Sharkia Province, Egypt," Journal of American Science, vol. 6, pp. 752–758, 2010.

[11] D. O. Oluwayelu, D. Todd, and O. D. Olaleye, "Sequence and phylogenetic analysis of chicken anaemia virus obtained from backyard and commercial chickens in Nigeria," Onderstepoort Journal of Veterinary Research, vol. 75, no. 4, pp. 353–357, 2008.

[12] M. F. Ducatez, A. A. Owoade, J. O. Abiola, and C. P. Muller, "Molecular epidemiology of chicken anemia virus in Nigeria," Archives of Virology, vol. 151, no. 1, pp. 97–111, 2006.

[13] B. O. Emikpe, D. O. Oluwayelu, O. G. Ohore, O. A. Oladele, and A. T. Oladokun, "Serological evidence of chicken anaemia virus infection in Nigerian indigenous chickens," Onderstepoort Journal of Veterinary Research, vol. 72, no. 1, pp. 101–103, 2005.

[14] D. O. Oluwayelu, D. Todd, N. W. Ball et al., "Isolation and preliminary characterization of chicken anemia virus from chickens in Nigeria," Avian Diseases, vol. 49, no. 3, pp. 446–450, 2005.

[15] A. A. Owoade, D. O. Oluwayelu, O. A. Fagbohun, W. Ammerlaan, M. N. Mulders, and C. P. Muller, "Serologic evidence of chicken infectious anemia in commercial chicken flocks in southwest Nigeria," Avian Diseases, vol. 48, no. 1, pp. 202–205, 2004.

[16] H. A. Hussein, M. Z. Sabry, E. A. El-Ibiary, M. El-Safty, and A. I. Abd El-Hady, "Chicken infectious anaemia virus in Egypt: molecular diagnosis by PCR and isolation of the virus from infected flocks," Arab Journal of Biotechnology, vol. 5, no. 2, pp. 263–274, 2002.

[17] J. D. Wicht and S. B. Maharaj, "Chicken anaemia agent in South Africa," Veterinary Record, vol. 133, no. 6, pp. 147–148, 1993.

[18] F. Maggi, L. Macera, D. Focosi et al., "Human gyrovirus DNA in human blood, Italy," Emerging Infectious Diseases, vol. 18, no. 6, pp. 956–959, 2012.

[19] J. D. Thompson, D. G. Higgins, and T. J. Gibson, "CLUSTAL W: improving the sensitivity of progressive multiple sequence alignment through sequence weighting, position-specific gap penalties and weight matrix choice," Nucleic Acids Research, vol. 22, no. 22, pp. 4673–4680, 1994.

[20] K. Tamura, D. Peterson, N. Peterson, G. Stecher, M. Nei, and S. Kumar, "MEGA5: molecular evolutionary genetics analysis using maximum likelihood, evolutionary distance, and maximum parsimony methods," Molecular Biology and Evolution, vol. 28, no. 10, pp. 2731–2739, 2011.

[21] S. Natesan, J. M. Kataria, K. Dhama, S. Rahul, and N. Baradhwaj, "Biological and molecular characterization of chicken anaemia virus isolates of Indian origin," Virus Research, vol. 118, no. 1-2, pp. 78–86, 2006.

[22] Y. M. Eltahir, K. Qian, W. Jin, P. Wang, and A. Qin, "Molecular epidemiology of chicken anemia virus in commercial farms in China," *Journal of Virology*, vol. 8, pp. 145–152, 2011.

[23] S. Yamaguchi, T. Imada, N. Kaji et al., "Identification of a genetic determinant of pathogenicity in chicken anaemia virus," *Journal of General Virology*, vol. 82, no. 5, pp. 1233–1238, 2001.

[24] P. Biagini, S. Bedarida, M. Touinssi, V. Galicher, and P. de Micco, "Human gyrovirus in healthy blood donors, France," *Emerging Infectious Diseases*, vol. 19, no. 6, pp. 1014–1015, 2013.

[25] F. A. Seeliger, M. L. Brügmann, L. Krüger et al., "Porcine circovirus type 2-associated cerebellar vasculitis in postweaning multisystemic wasting syndrome (PMWS)-affected pigs," *Veterinary Pathology*, vol. 44, no. 5, pp. 621–634, 2007.

[26] S. Honma, S. Nakata, Y. Sakai, M. Tatsumi, K. Numata-Kinoshita, and S. Chiba, "Low prevalence of TT virus in the cerebrospinal fluid of viremic patients with central nervous system disorders," *Journal of Medical Virology*, vol. 65, no. 2, pp. 418–422, 2001.

[27] S. L. Smits, E. E. Zijlstra, J. J. van Hellemond et al., "Novel cyclovirus in human cerebrospinal fluid, Malawi, 2010-2011," *Emerging Infectious Diseases*, vol. 19, no. 9, pp. 1511–1513, 2013.

[28] L. V. Tan, H. R. van Doorn, H. D. Nghia et al., "Identification of a new cyclovirus in cerebrospinal fluid of patients with acute central nervous system infections," *MBio*, vol. 4, no. 3, pp. e00231–e00213, 2013.

[29] D. Esterhuizen, "South African poultry update: the supply and demand for broiler meat in South Africa," http://www.thepoultrysite.com/reports/?id=1795.

[30] S. Simionatto, C. A. da Veiga Lima-Rosa, E. Binneck, A. P. Ravazzolo, and C. W. Canal, "Characterization and phylogenetic analysis of Brazilian chicken anaemia virus," *Virus Genes*, vol. 33, no. 1, pp. 5–10, 2006.

12

Adaptation and Molecular Characterization of Two Malaysian Very Virulent Infectious Bursal Disease Virus Isolates Adapted in BGM-70 Cell Line

Nafi'u Lawal,[1,2] **Mohd Hair-Bejo,**[1,3] **Siti Suri Arshad,**[1]
Abdul Rahman Omar,[1,3] **and Aini Ideris**[3,4]

[1]*Department of Veterinary Pathology and Microbiology, Faculty of Veterinary Medicine, Universiti Putra Malaysia (UPM), 43400 Serdang, Selangor, Malaysia*
[2]*Department of Veterinary Microbiology, Faculty of Veterinary Medicine, Usmanu Danfodiyo University, Sokoto (UDUS), 2346 Sokoto, Nigeria*
[3]*Laboratory of Vaccine and Immunotherapeutics, Institute of Bioscience, Universiti Putra Malaysia (UPM), 43400 Serdang, Selangor, Malaysia*
[4]*Department of Veterinary Clinical Studies, Faculty of Veterinary Medicine, Universiti Putra Malaysia (UPM), 43400 Serdang, Selangor, Malaysia*

Correspondence should be addressed to Mohd Hair-Bejo; mdhair@upm.edu.my

Academic Editor: Subhash C. Verma

Two Malaysian very virulent infectious bursal disease virus (vvIBDV) strains UPM0081 and UPM190 (also known as UPMB00/81 and UPM04/190, respectively) isolated from local IBD outbreaks were serially passaged 12 times (EP12) in specific pathogen free (SPF) chicken embryonated eggs (CEE) by chorioallantoic membrane (CAM) route. The EP12 isolate was further adapted and serially propagated in BGM-70 cell line up to 20 passages (P20). Characteristic cytopathic effects (CPEs) were subtly observed at P1 in both isolates 72 hours postinoculation (pi). The CPE became prominent at P5 with cell rounding, cytoplasmic vacuoles, granulation, and detachment from flask starting from day 3 pi, up to 7 days pi with titers of $10^{9.50}$ TCID$_{50}$/mL and log$10^{9.80}$ TCID$_{50}$/mL for UPM0081 and UPM190, respectively. The CPE became subtle at P17 and disappeared by P18 and P19 for UPM0081 and UPM190, respectively. However, the presence of IBDV was confirmed by immunoperoxidase, immunofluorescence, and RT-PCR techniques. Phylogenetic analysis showed that these two isolates were of the vvIBDV. It appears that a single mutation of UPM190 and UPM0081 IBDV isolates at D279N could facilitate vvIBDV strain adaptability in CEE and BGM-70 cultures.

1. Introduction

Infectious bursal disease (IBD) is a disease of high economic importance that is highly contagious and immunosuppressive affecting young chickens especially between 3 and 6 weeks of age. The etiologic agent, IBD virus (IBDV), is a naked icosahedral virus having segmented double stranded RNA genome belonging to the genus *Avibirnavirus*, family Birnaviridae [1]. The genome segment A encoding the viral polyprotein has been extensively studied using molecular techniques with the viral outer capsid protein (VP2) identified as the basis for antigenic and pathotypic variation among IBDV strains [2, 3].

It was also reported that specific amino acid changes in the hypervariable region of the VP2 protein determine the cell culture adaptation and attenuation of IBD virus [3]. The wild type IBD virus was reported to be extremely difficult to adapt to cell culture especially the very virulent IBDV (vvIBDV) unless passaged few times in chicken embryonated eggs (CEE) [4]. Traditional isolation of IBDV by CAM inoculation of 9- to 11-day-old SPF chicken embryos is expensive coupled with high risk of contamination especially for vaccine development and production [5]. Successful adaptation of IBDV isolates in chicken embryo fibroblast (CEF), chicken embryo kidneys, and chicken embryo bursas was reported [6, 7], but the cells being of primary avian origin have limited lifespan, produce low virus titer, and may contain extraneous avian viruses that may contaminate vaccines developed using them [8, 9]. Many continuous cell lines of mammalian origin were reported to support the growth of IBDV isolates including MA-104 [10], OK [11], BGM-70 [10, 12], Vero cells [10, 13–15], and RK-13 [14, 16]. These cell lines are easier to maintain and free from avian viral contaminants [9]. Various levels of viral titers were obtained using these cell lines making them better choices for IBDV propagation especially when higher viral titers are required as is the case in vaccine production. The objective of this study was to determine the adaptation and molecular characteristics of Malaysian vvIBDV isolates in BGM-70 cell line.

2. Materials and Methods

2.1. Viruses and Cell Line. The two local vvIBDV isolates were separately obtained from severe outbreaks of infectious bursal disease (IBD) in Malaysia in the years 2000 and 2004 and were designated UPM0081 (AY520910) [22] and UPM04/190 (AY791998) [23] also named as UPM190, respectively. These isolates were isolated from infected bursae that were ground, centrifuged, and filtered through a $0.2\,\mu m$ filter (Millipore, Merck). The filtrates were serially passaged via chorioallantoic membrane (CAM) inoculation of specific pathogen-free chicken eggs (SPF CEE) (MVP, Malaysia). After 7 days of incubation, the CAM were harvested, homogenized, and filtered and the CAM homogenate was stored at -80°C until required.

The cell line BGM-70 (ECACC cat number 90092601) is an epithelial-like cell derived from baby grivet monkey kidney (ECACC, Porton Down, Salisbury, SP4 0JG, UK) that was maintained in minimum essential medium (MEM) with 5% CO_2 at 37°C.

2.2. Virus Adaptation in Specific Pathogen-Free Chicken Embryonated Eggs. To activate the vvIBDV isolates, 11-day-old SPF CEE were inoculated with the CAM homogenates of the two viruses via CAM route using an established method [24] and incubated at 37°C in an incubator. The CEE were observed daily for seven days for mortality discarding any dead embryo 48 hours postinoculation (pi). At 7 days pi, dead and surviving embryos were chilled at 4°C overnight and the CAM and embryos were aseptically harvested, homogenized with phosphate buffered saline (PBS, NaCl$_2$-8 g/L, KH$_2$PO$_4$-0.2 g/L, NaH$_2$PO$_4$-1.15 g/L, KCl$_2$-0.2 g, pH 7.2), and clarified at 1500 ×g for 20 minutes at 4°C. The supernatants for each isolate were pooled and 1% antibiotic and antifungal agents (penicillin 10,000 IU/mL, streptomycin 10,000 μg/mL, and amphotericin B-25 μg/mL) were added and filtered using $0.2\,\mu$m filter and the filtrates were serially used for eleven more passages to give EP12 of both UPM0081 and UPM190 which were used for BGM-70 cell inoculation.

2.3. Adaptation of Viruses to BGM-70 Cell Line. Confluent monolayers of BGM-70 cells were infected with 500 μL of EP12 vvIBDV at multiplicity of infection of 1 mean tissue culture infective dose (TCID$_{50}$) of virus per cell following established method [25]. The viruses were adsorbed at 37°C for 2 hours with periodic gentle shaking of the flasks after which 5 ml of 2% MEM was added to each flask and were incubated at 37°C in 5% CO_2 and examined twice daily for 7 days for development of cytopathic effects (CPE). The propagated viruses were harvested using three freeze-thaw cycles, following previously described method [26], filtered with 0.2 μm (Millipore, Merck) aliquots, and labeled as BGMP1. This was serially repeated 19 times to obtain BGMP20. The TCID$_{50}$ at BGMP5 was determined following standard method [27].

2.4. Detection of IBDV in BGM-70 Cell. The presence of vvIBDV in the cell culture supernatant was evaluated by apoptosis assay, immunofluorescence, immunoperoxidase [28], and reverse transcriptase-polymerase chain reaction (RT-PCR) [29].

2.5. Acridine Orange/Propidium Iodide Apoptosis Assay. The BGM-70 adapted viruses were evaluated for their ability to induce apoptosis in infected cells by double staining with acridine orange (AO) and propidium iodide (PI) DNA binding dyes [30]. Briefly, confluent monolayer of BGM-70 cells was infected with the adapted viruses as described before while another flask was kept as uninoculated control. The medium from infected flasks and control were separately collected 24 hrs pi and the monolayer was washed with warm PBS and trypsinized and the detached cells were aspirated into appropriately labeled tubes and centrifuged at 4°C at 1000 ×g. The supernatant was discarded while the pellets were resuspended with PBS and centrifuged again at 4°C at 1000 ×g and the supernatant was discarded, leaving only a small quantity of PBS to resuspend the cells. In a dark room, 5 μL of AO dye stock solution (10 mg/mL, A3568, ThermoFisher Scientific) diluted in PBS (0.5 μL of AO stock solution in 49.5 μL of PBS) was mixed with 5 μL of PI dye stock solution (1.0 mg/mL, P3566, ThermoFisher Scientific) diluted in PBS (5 μL of PI stock solution in 45 μL of PBS) and the mixture was added to 10 μL of the infected cells or uninfected control, gently mixed on a glass slide, and immediately covered with cover slip. The slides were then viewed within 30 minutes with an immunofluorescence microscope (Leica Microsystems Limited, Heerbrugg, Switzerland).

2.6. Indirect Immunoperoxidase Assay. Four 6-well plates (Corning®, Sigma-Aldrich, Germany) containing confluent BGM-70 cells monolayer were taken out of the incubator and the medium was discarded and rinsed twice with prewarmed PBS, and the individual wells were inoculated with 200 μL of the harvested cell culture supernatant of passages 5, 10, 15, 16, 17, 18, and 19 of both the UPM0081 and UPM190 and incubated for 120 minutes for adsorption at 37°C and 5% CO_2. A volume of 1.8 mL of maintenance medium (MEM + 2% FBS) was added to each well, while the uninfected control wells were filled with 2 ml of the medium. The plates were then incubated at 37°C and 5% CO_2 and observed daily for 4 days. The plates were fixed with 4% paraformaldehyde (P6148, Sigma-Aldrich, Germany) for 30 minutes at room temperature and washed twice using ice cold PBST (PBS containing

0.5% Tween 20) for 5 minutes and quenched with 3% hydrogen peroxide (H_2O_2) for 30 minutes at room temperature. The plates were washed twice with PBST for 5 minutes each and the VP2 IBDV antigen was retrieved with citrate buffer in a microwave (50 power level) for 10 minutes. The plates were rinsed with PBST twice for 5 minutes and blocked with 5% BSA in PBST for 1 hour at room temperature. The cells were rinsed twice as before and 40 μl of monoclonal chicken anti-VP2-IBDV specific primary antibody (Charles River Laboratories, USA) diluted with distilled water at 1 : 200 was dispensed on the cells and then incubated at 4°C in humidified chamber overnight. The plates were rinsed two times with PBST for 5 minutes and 40 μl of rabbit anti-chicken-IgY-Fc-HRP-conjugated secondary antibody (ThermoFisher Scientific) diluted with distilled water at 1 : 1000 was dispensed to each well and incubated at room temperature for 1 hour in a dark room. The plates were rinsed with PBST and 100 μL/well of 3,3$'$ diaminobenzidine (Sigma-Aldrich, Germany) was added for 5 minutes of incubation, before the plates were briefly rinsed with PBST and stained with haematoxylin for 15 seconds followed by rinsing in slow running tap water for 5 minutes. The cover slips were dried and transferred to label clean glass slides using a mountant DPX (Sigma-Aldrich, Germany) and finally observed under the microscope (Leica Microsystems Limited, Heerbrugg, Switzerland) for positive reaction seen as brownish or golden coloration within the cytoplasm of the cells [28].

2.7. Indirect Immunofluorescence Assays. Clean coverslips were placed in four 6-well tissue culture plates and allowed to stand overnight under UV light exposure. The plates were seeded with BGM-70 cells following standard established protocols [26]. Following confluence, the plates were washed twice with prewarmed PBS, and the individual wells were inoculated with 200 μl of the cell culture harvested supernatant of passages 5, 10, 15, 16, 17, 18, and 19 of both the UPM0081 and UPM190 viruses and incubated for 120 minutes for adsorption at 37°C, 5% CO_2 condition, and then 1.8 mL of maintenance medium was added to each well, while the uninfected control wells were filled with 2 ml of the medium. The plates were then incubated at 37°C and 5% CO_2 and observed daily for 3 days. The plates were fixed with 4% paraformaldehyde for 30 minutes at room temperature and washed three times for 5 minutes using ice cold PBST (PBS containing 0.5% Tween 20). After this, the plates were incubated in a 0.5% Triton X-100 in PBST (PBS 1 L pH 7.2 + 0.5 mL Tween 20) for 15 minutes to permeabilize the cells followed by rinsing with PBST three times for 5 minutes. Unspecific binding was blocked using blocking buffer (5% BSA in PBST) for 1 hour at room temperature. The plates were rinsed three times with PBST for 5 minutes and then 40 μl of chicken monoclonal anti-VP2-IBDV specific primary antibody (Charles River Laboratories, USA) diluted at 1 : 200 with sterile distilled water was dropped on the cells followed by incubation at 4°C in a dark humidified chamber overnight. The plates were washed thrice for 5 minutes with PBST and 40 μL of polyclonal rabbit anti-chicken-FITC conjugated secondary antibody raised against chicken IgY-Fc (Sigma-Aldrich, Germany) and diluted at 1 : 200 with sterile

distilled water was dropped on each slide containing wells and incubated at room temperature for 1 hour in the dark. The plates were rinsed with PBST for 5 minutes three times and 20 μl of 4$'$,6-diamidino-2-phenylindole dihydrochloride (DAPI) (Sigma-Aldrich, Germany) was added to the plates and incubated for 10 minutes at room temperature and the plates were briefly rinsed with PBST. The cover slips were dried and placed on a labeled clean glass slides using a mountant (DPX) for fluorescence microscopic examination (Leica Microsystems Limited, Heerbrugg, Switzerland) of VP2 antigen positive cells [28].

2.8. Reverse Transcriptase-Polymerase Chain Reaction (RT-PCR). The CAM homogenate from CEE passage 12 and BGM-70 cell culture supernatants at passages 1, 5, 10, 15, 16, 17, 18, 19, and 20 were used for RNA extraction, cDNA synthesis, and PCR analysis. Briefly, 250 μL of the CAM homogenate or cell culture supernatant was dispensed in 1.5 mL sterile Eppendorf tubes and 750 μl of Trizol® LS was added in 1 : 3 ratio. The mixture was resuspended by several up- and downpipetting and allowed to stand for 15 minutes at room temperature. Chloroform (200 μL) was added to the mixture, shaken vigorously for 15 seconds, and then allowed to stand at room temperature for 5 minutes before centrifugation at 12000 ×g for 15 minutes at 4°C. The upper clear aqueous phase containing RNA was gently removed from the two organic and DNA phases into new labeled 1.5 mL tube and was used for RNA precipitation. Five hundred microlitres of 100% isopropanol was added to each tube and allowed to stand at room temperature for 10 minutes before centrifugation at 12000 ×g for 10 minutes and the isopropanol was discarded while the RNA was washed with 1000 μL of 75% alcohol and centrifuged for 5 minutes at 7500 ×g. The alcohol was discarded and RNA pellet partially dried inside level 2 biosafety cabinets for 5 to 10 minutes at the end of which 35 μL of sterile RNAse free water was added to resuspend the RNA for determination of concentration, purity, and subsequent use for downstream application. The extracted RNA was used to amplify the VP2 hypervariable region of the segment A genomic RNA sequences.

2.9. cDNA Synthesis. The extracted RNA was used to synthesize cDNA using MMLV cDNA synthesis kit with the following reagent mixtures and conditions: RNA template (10 μL), RNAase free water (1.5 μL), and random oligomers (1.0 μL). The mixture was briefly centrifuged and incubated at 65°C for 2 minutes and rapidly chilled on ice for 5 minutes after which 2.0 μl of MMLV buffer, 2.0 μL of DTT, 2.0 μL of dNTPs, 0.5 μL of Riboguard, and 1.0 μL of reverse transcriptase were added to bring the total reaction volume to 20 μL. The mixture was gently mixed, briefly centrifuged, and incubated at 37°C for 60 minutes after which the temperature was raised to 85°C for 5 minutes using the cyclical conditions shown in Table 1.

2.10. PCR Amplification. The synthesized cDNA was used as template for PCR amplification using KAPA HIFI PCR kit (Kapa Biosystems, Boston, Massachusetts, USA) using

TABLE 1: cDNA synthesis using IBDV RNA templates.

Condition	Temperature (°C)	Time	Cycle
First denaturation	98	2 min	1
Second denaturation	98	30 sec	35
Annealing	56	30 sec	35
Extension	72	1 min	35
Final extension	72	10 min	1

TABLE 2: PCR cycling conditions used to amplify the synthesized cDNA templates.

Condition	Temperature	Time	Cycle
Initial denaturation	95°C	3 min	1
Denaturation	98°C	20 sec	35
Annealing	60°C	15 sec	35
Extension	72°C	15–60 sec/kb	35
Final extension	72°C	1 min/kb	1

the following reagents volume and concentrations as recommended by the manufacturers: 5x KAPA HiFi Buffer 10.0 μL (1x), 10 mM KAPA dNTP Mix 1.5 μL (0.3 mM each), 10 μM Forward Primer 1.5 μL (0.3 μM), 10 μM Reverse Primer 1.5 μL (0.3 μM), Template DNA 5 μL, 1 U/μL KAPA HiFi DNA Polymerase 1.0 μL (1 U), and 4.5 μL PCR-grade water to top up to 25 μL total reaction volume. The following primers described previously (Liu et al., 1994) were used to amplify a 643-bp region of the hvVP2 sequence: 643-1 (5'-TCACCGTCCTCAGCTTAC-3') and 643-2 (5'-TCAGGATTTGGGATCAGC-3'). The mixture was briefly centrifuged and incubated in a PCR cycling conditions as shown in Table 2.

2.11. Nucleotide Sequence Analysis. To confirm the pathotypic identity of both the CEE and BGM-70 adapted viruses, all the amplified 643 bp PCR products from all the different passages were sequenced directly by Sanger method (First BASE Laboratories, Seri Kembangan, Selangor, Malaysia) and the nucleotide sequences were analyzed using BioEdit Sequence Alignment Editor v7.2.5 (Tom Hall, Ibis Biosciences, Carlsbad, CA). Phylogenetic analysis was conducted using the *MEGA* version 7 [19]. Alignment of nucleotide sequences was done using Clustal W, and Phylogenetic Trees were designed with the neighbor-joining (NJ) methods and up to 1000 bootstrap replicates. The portion of the sequence analyzed was from nucleotide positions 637 to 879 corresponding to the amino acid positions 213 to 293 with numbering according to [31]. The sequences used for comparisons comprised very virulent, variant, and classical serotype 1 as well as serotype 2 IBDV as shown in Table 3.

3. Results

3.1. Specific Pathogen-Free Embryonated Egg Passage. Both virus strains showed typical IBD lesions including intracranial hemorrhage, marbling of the liver, oedema of the head, hyperemia, and abdominal distention from EP2 to EP12. The

mean embryo mortality was 5 days pi. The UPM0081 isolate presented lesions such as hyperemia, ecchymotic hemorrhages on the thigh, breast muscle, mottled liver (sometimes pale or yellowish), oedema of the head, intracranial hemorrhages, and dwarfing. The isolate UPM190 induced occasionally hyperemia or paleness, ecchymotic hemorrhages on the thigh and breast muscles, intracranial hemorrhages, distended abdomen, subcutaneous edema, and mottled liver (Figures 1(a)–1(d)) at EP12 of the two isolates.

3.2. Adaptation of Viruses to BGM-70 Cell Line. Normal confluent monolayer of BGM-70 cells was obtained within 72 hours with fibroblast morphology (Figure 2(a)). During the first passage, the virus induced little CPE with the monolayer remaining 100% intact up to 4 days pi. Evidence of CPE manifested from day 5 pi as the virus began adapting to the cell line. At BGMP2, CPE developed 4 days pi and reached 20% by day 7 pi and by P5; clear CPE developed within 48 hours pi. The CPE was characterized by small refractile and round cells, cytoplasmic granulation, cell detachment, and slow destruction of monolayer by day 6 pi (Figure 2(b)). The CPE became subtle at P18 onwards appearing only after 9 days pi suggesting reduction in virulence of the propagated viruses (Figures 2(c) and 2(d)). The infectious titer of the adapted viruses at BGMP5 was found to be $10^{9.98}$ TCID$_{50}$/mL and $10^{9.50}$ TCID$_{50}$/mL at 3 days pi for UPM190 and UPM0081, respectively.

3.3. Acridine Orange/Propidium Iodide Apoptosis Assay. The apoptosis assay using AO/PI dyes showed that, at 24 hours pi, the IBDV triggered few infected cells to undergo apoptosis as a means of virus dissemination (Figure 5). The AO dye stains the nucleus of both normal and apoptotic cells green as it became bound to DNA because it can easily penetrate intact membrane of living cells, whereas PI dye can only permeate cells that have damage membrane such as apoptotic and necrotic cells which it stains orange-red to red. Apoptotic cells were demonstrated by the presence of orange coloration (Figures 3(c) and 3(f)) due to the combined effects of the AO/PI dyes and membrane blebbing (Figure 3(f)) at 24 and 48 hours pi compared to the uninfected control (Figure 3(i)).

3.4. Indirect Immunoperoxidase Assay. To verify the presence of IBD viruses in infected BGM-70 cells, indirect immunoperoxidase assay was performed on infected cells grown on glass slides. The assay resulted in the presence of intracytoplasmic brown coloration that indicates the presence of the IBDV VP2 antigen in the cytoplasm of BGM-70 infected cells (Figure 4(a)) compared to the uninfected control (Figure 4(b)).

3.5. Indirect Immunofluorescence Assay. To further confirm the presence of the VP2 viral antigen within the cytoplasm of BGM-70 cells, indirect immunofluorescence assay was performed. The assay revealed positive green fluorescence for IBDV VP2 protein in the cytoplasm and on the nuclear membrane of infected cells (green) compared to the uninoculated negative control that showed only excitation for the nuclear stain DAPI (blue). The presence of the green signal for VP2

TABLE 3: The names, accession number, countries of origin, and references of the sequences used for nucleotide, amino acid, and phylogenetic analyses with the UPM0081 and UPM190 isolates.

S/number	Sequence	Strain	Accession number	Country	References
(1)	UPM94/230	vvIBDV	AY52091l.1	Malaysia	Tan et al., 2004
(2)	UPM94/273	vvIBDV	AF527039.1	Malaysia	Kong et al., 2004
(3)	UPM B0081	vvIBDV	FJ824699.1	Malaysia	Mohammed et al., 2009
(4)	UPM92-04	vvIBDV	AF262030.1	Malaysia	
(5)	Strain Harbin	vvIBDV	AF092171.1	China	Hu & Zhang, 1998
(6)	Strain SA-KZN95	vvIBDV	KF241548.1	South Africa	Vukea et al., 2014
(7)	IBDV77/Georgia Vac	Vaccine	JX424076.1	Nigeria	Adamu, 2012
(8)	Strain Edgar	cell culture adapted	AY462026.1	USA	Petkov et al., 2007
(9)	South Korea (Strain KSH)	vvIBDV	AF165151.1	South Korea	Kwon et al., 2000
(10)	UK661	vvIBDV	X92760.1	UK	Brown and Skinner, 1996
(11)	GA97	vIBDV	AY963132.1	USA	Mickael and Jackwood, 2005
(12)	IRAQI2.I27-743	IBDV	KC352669.1	Kurdistan and Iraq	Gergis and Jackwood, 2013
(13)	ISRl3	vvIBDV	AY907012.1	USA	Jackwood and Sommer, 2005
(14)	UPM0081EP12	vvIBDV	KY411641	Malaysia	Lawal, Hair-Bejo, Arshad, et al., 2016
(15)	UPM190EP12	vvIBDV		Malaysia	Lawal, Hair-Bejo, et al., 2016

S/number	Name	Strain	Accession number	Country	References
(16)	IBDV/Turkey/PA/00924/14	Serotype 2	KP642112.1	USA	Lu, Tang, Yeh, et al., 2015
(17)	OKYM	vvIBDV	D49706.1	Japan	Yamaguchi, Ogawa, Inoshima, et al., 1995
(18)	Thai4 classic	caIBDV	AY907014	Thailand	Jackwood and Sommer, 2005
(19)	JNeto-BR	IBDV	AY780423	Brazil	Hayashi, Brentano and Ferreira, 2004
(20)	Strain E	vIBDV	AY819703	USA	Khatri and Sharma, 2004
(21)	Strain IM	vIBDV	AY819702	USA	Khatri and Sharma, 2004
(22)	Strain STC	caIBDV	AY819701	USA	Khatri and Sharma, 2004
(23)	Spain 1	vvIBDV	AY907007	Spain	Jackwood and Sommer, 2005
(24)	D78	vvIBDV	EU162087.1	USA	Jackwood, D. J., Sreedevi, LeFever et al., 2008
(25)	Strain B00/81 (Pre-adaptation)	vvIBDV	AY520910.1	Malaysia	Tan et al., 2004
(26)	HK46	vvIBDV	AF092943	Hong Kong	Lim, Cao, Yu et al., 1999
(27)	Cevac-Gumbo-L	Vaccine	EU544158	Brazil	Gomes, Abreu, Resende et al., 2008
(28)	Singapore97S181	IBDV	DQ916216	Singapore	Jackwood and Sommer-Wagner, 2006
(29)	OH strain	Serotype 2	U30818.1	Canada	Kibenge, McKenna and Dybing, 1995
(30)	UPM190BGMP15	vvIBDV	KY418010	Malaysia	Lawal, Hair-Bejo, Arshad, et al., 2016
(31)	UPM190BGMP20	vvIBDV	KY418009	Malaysia	Lawal, Hair-Bejo, Arshad, et al., 2016
(32)	UPM0081BGMP20	vvIBDV	KY418011	Malaysia	Lawal, Hair-Bejo, Arshad, et al., 2016

TABLE 3: Continued.

S/number	Name	Strain	Accession number	Country	References
(33)	UPM04/190 (Pre-adaptation)	vvIBDV	KU958716.1	Malaysia	Liew, Hair-Bejo, Omar et al., 2016
(34)	UPM190EP1	vvIBDV		Malaysia	Lawal, Hair-Bejo, Arshad, et al., 2016
(35)	UPMBGMP008IP15	vvIBDV	KY418012	Malaysia	Lawal, Hair-Bejo, Arshad, et al., 2016
(36)	UPMBGMP008IP16	vvIBDV		Malaysia	Lawal, Hair-Bejo, Arshad, et al., 2016
(37)	UPMBGMP008IP17	vvIBDV		Malaysia	Lawal, Hair-Bejo, Arshad, et al., 2016
(38)	UPMBGMP008IP18	vvIBDV		Malaysia	Lawal, Hair-Bejo, Arshad, et al., 2016
(39)	UPMBGMP008IP19	vvIBDV		Malaysia	Lawal, Hair-Bejo, Arshad, et al., 2016
(40)	UPMBGMP008IP10	vvIBDV		Malaysia	Lawal, Hair-Bejo, Arshad, et al., 2016
(41)	UPMBGMP008IP5	vvIBDV		Malaysia	Lawal, Hair-Bejo, Arshad, et al., 2016
(42)	UPMBGMP008IP1	vvIBDV		Malaysia	Lawal, Hair-Bejo, Arshad, et al., 2016
(43)	UPMBGMP190P16	vvIBDV		Malaysia	Lawal, Hair-Bejo, Arshad, et al., 2016
(44)	UPMBGMP190P17	vvIBDV		Malaysia	Lawal, Hair-Bejo, Arshad, et al., 2016
(45)	UPMBGMP190P18	vvIBDV		Malaysia	Lawal, Hair-Bejo, Arshad, et al., 2016
(46)	UPMBGMP190P19	vvIBDV		Malaysia	Lawal, Hair-Bejo, Arshad, et al., 2016
(47)	UPMBGMP190P10	vvIBDV		Malaysia	Lawal, Hair-Bejo, Arshad, et al., 2016
(48)	UPMBGPM190P5	vvIBDV		Malaysia	Lawal, Hair-Bejo, Arshad, et al., 2016
(49)	UPMBGMP190P1	vvIBDV		Malaysia	Lawal, Hair-Bejo, Arshad, et al., 2016
(50)	UPM190EP1	vvIBDV		Malaysia	Lawal, Hair-Bejo, Arshad, et al., 2016
(51)	South Korean IBDV	vvIBDV	AF508177.1	South Korea	Kim and Yeo, 2002

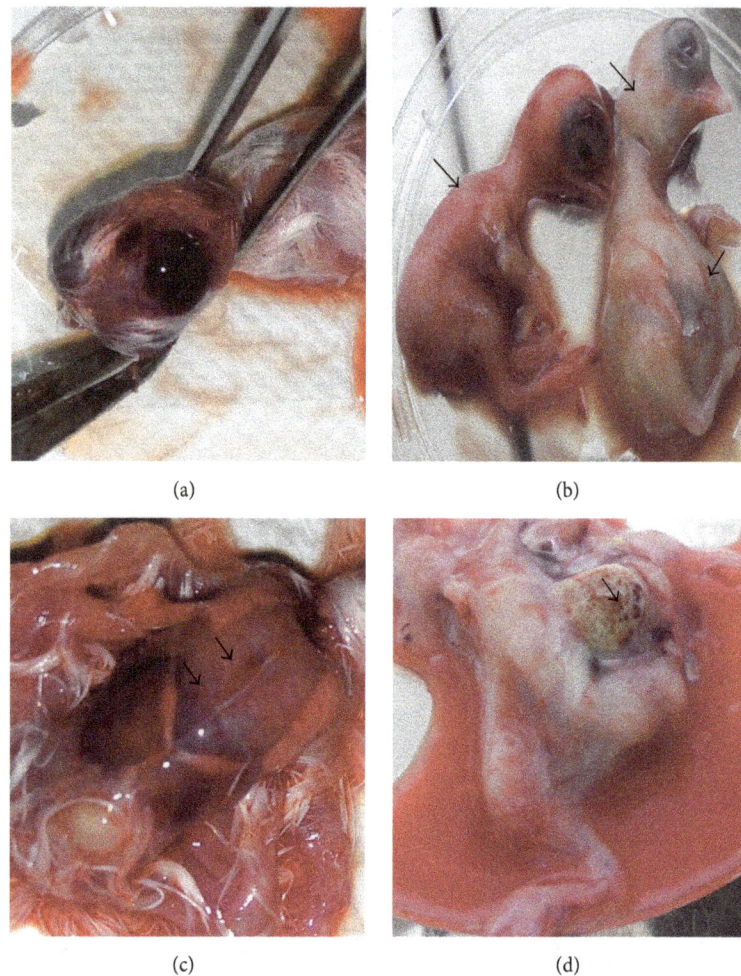

(a)

(b)

(c)

(d)

FIGURE 1: vvIBDV infected SPF embryos with (a) intracranial hemorrhage (UPM0081), (b) hyperemia, abdominal distention, and subcutaneous edema (UPM190), (c) petechial hemorrhages on the breast muscle (UPM0081), and (d) mottled liver (UPM0081) at EP12.

antigen therefore indicates the presence of IBD virus in the cytoplasm and on the nuclear membrane of infected BGM-70 cells.

3.6. Reverse Transcriptase-Polymerase Chain Reaction (RT-PCR). The identification of CEE and BGM-70 adapted viruses through embryonic lesions and CPE was confirmed by the appearance of a distinct 643 bp band when an RT-PCR of the CAM homogenate and BGM-70 cell culture supernatant and the products were analyzed by gel electrophoresis and ethidium bromide staining (Figure 6).

3.7. Nucleotide Sequence Analysis. To confirm the identity of the RT-PCR products as IBDV genome, the RT-PCR products were directly sequenced and analyzed using BioEdit *v7* and MEGA *v7*. The nucleotide sequences of the two isolates were aligned by ClustalW together with other reference sequences (Figure 7). The aligned sequences revealed that, at nucleotide positions 642 and 645, there were changes from C and A to T and G nucleotides in the sequences of preadaptation UPM04/190 parent virus, UPM190EP1, UPM190EP12, UPM190BGMP5, and UPM190BGMP10. From positions 648

to 650, UPM04/190 had TAG compared to the CTC possessed by the rest of the isolates including the reference sequences. At nucleotide positions 652 to 654, there were nucleotide mutations from TCA to AGC in UPM04/190. Other nucleotide mutations observed were C660T, A663G, A666G, T669C, A675G, A693C, T696C, T699C, C702T, C708G, C711T, A714C, C720G, C726T, G729C, A732C, A752C, C759G, T758G, T777C, and C780G. Others include C786T, C789T, T792G, G807C, T810C, A816G, C819T, A823C, and A825T. Further changes were detected at T828G, C834G, A837G, C840T, T843C, G846C, A849G, G852C, C855G, T861C, C864T, T870G, A876G, and C879T. Moreover, the isolates UPM190EP1, UPM190EP12, UPMBGMP5, and UPM-BGMP10 nucleotide changes were observed in some reference sequences.

When the nucleotide sequences of the preadaptation, CEE, BGM-70 adapted, and reference isolates were translated to amino acids, the putative motifs identifying vvIBDV pathotypes were seen revealing isoleucine (I) at positions 242, 256, and 294 and serine (S) at position 299 (Figure 8). The IDA motifs at amino acid positions 234 to 236 were present in both the preadaptation and CEE and BGM-70 adapted

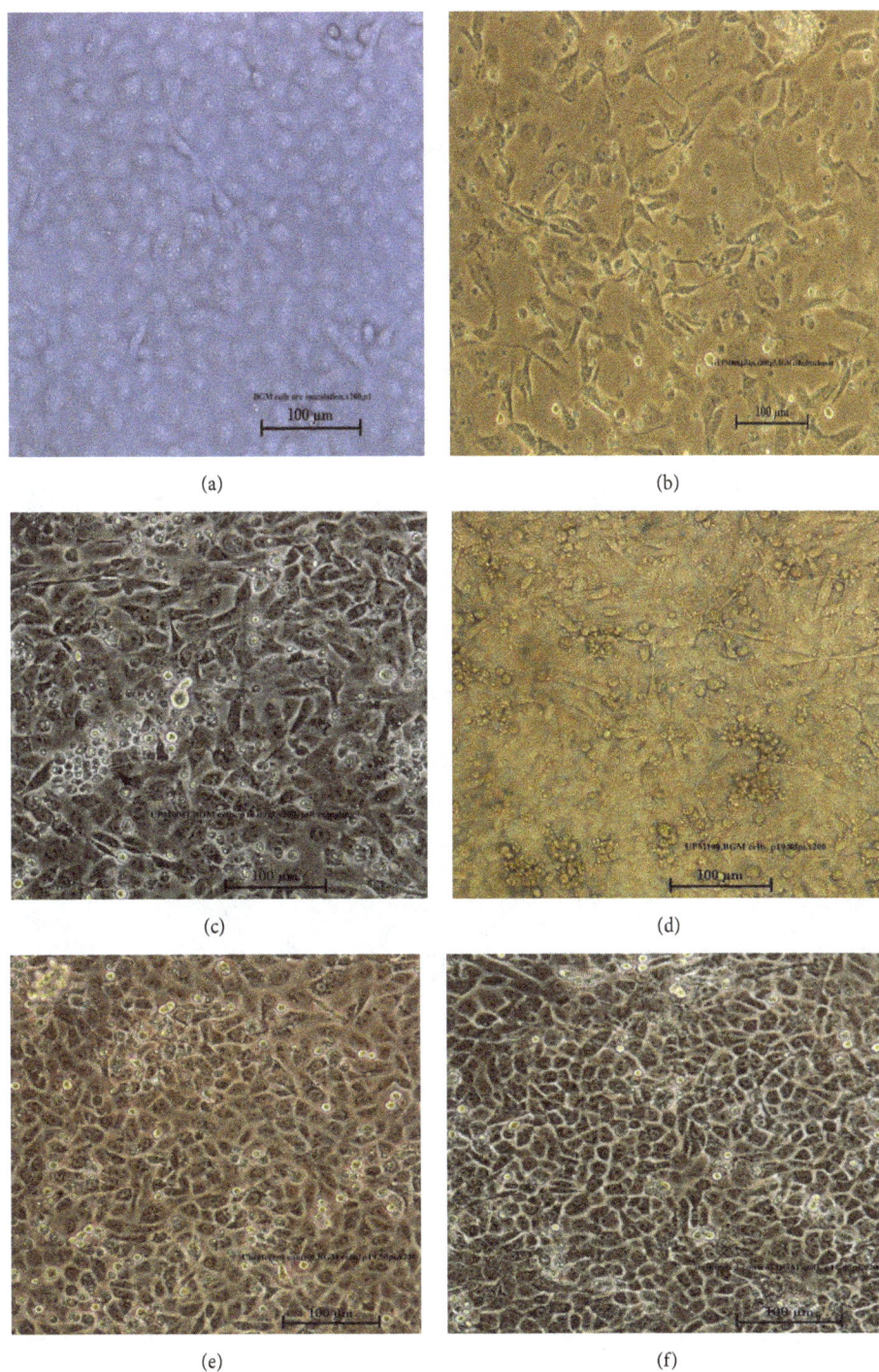

FIGURE 2: (a) A normal confluent monolayer of BGM-70 cells compared with (b) UPM0081, BGMP5 induced CPE on BGM-70 infected cells including small refractive cells, cytoplasmic granulation, cell rounding, and detachment at 6 days pi. (c) BGM-70 cells infected with UPM0081 at BGMP18 and (d) UPM190 BGMP19 at days 9 and 8, respectively, showing little CPE compared with (e) uninfected controls at day 5 and (f) at day 7. Bar = 100 μm.

viruses (Figure 8). At position 249, UPM04/190, UPM190EP1, UPM190EP12, UPM190BGMP1, and UPM190BGMP5 possessed amino acid E249 in place of Q249 possessed by the rest of the CEE and BGM-70 adapted strains. Similarly, all the reference sequences possessed Q249 except for

KF241548.1 that possessed H249. Similarly, at position 270, UPM B0081 preadaptation virus, UPM04/190, UPM190EP1 and UPM190EP12, UPM190BGMP5 and UPM190BGMP10, and other reference sequences possessed Alanine at that position while the other CEE and BGM-70 adapted viruses had

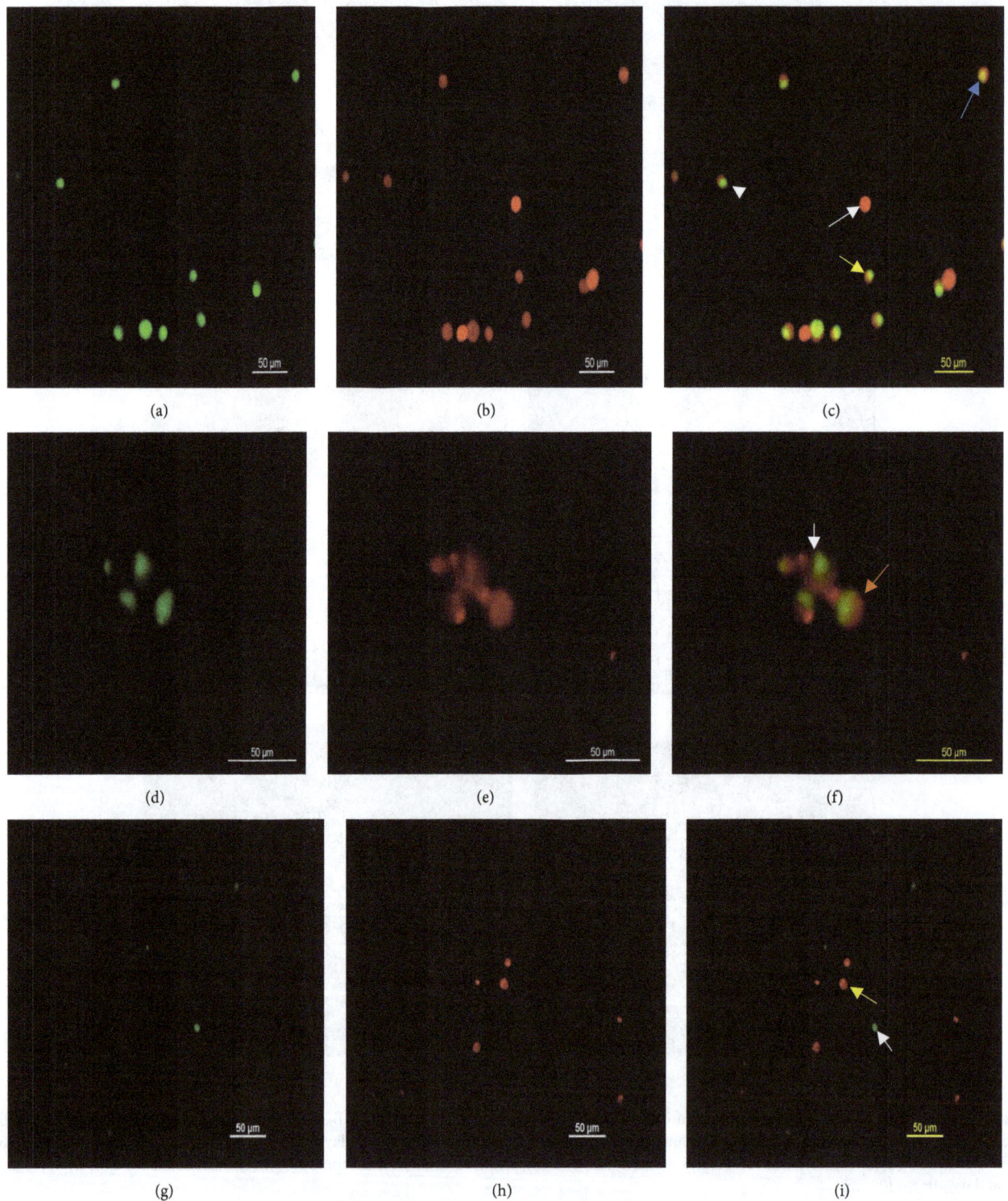

FIGURE 3: (a) AO stained, (b) PI stained, and (c) merged UPM0081 infected BGM-70 cells showing green-orange fluorescence as an indicator of early (white arrowhead), intermediate (yellow arrow), and late apoptosis (blue arrow) and necrosis (white arrow) at 24 hours pi. Bar = 50 μm. (d) AO stained, (e) PI stained, and (f) merged UPM190 infected BGM-70 cells showing membrane blebbing (white arrow) and positive orange color induced by the virus at 48 hours pi as a sign of apoptosis. Bar = 50 μm. (g) AO stained, (h) PI stained, and (i) merged uninfected control BGM-70 cells showing normal unapoptotic (white arrow) and necrotic cells (yellow arrow) at 24 hours after culture. Bar = 50 μm.

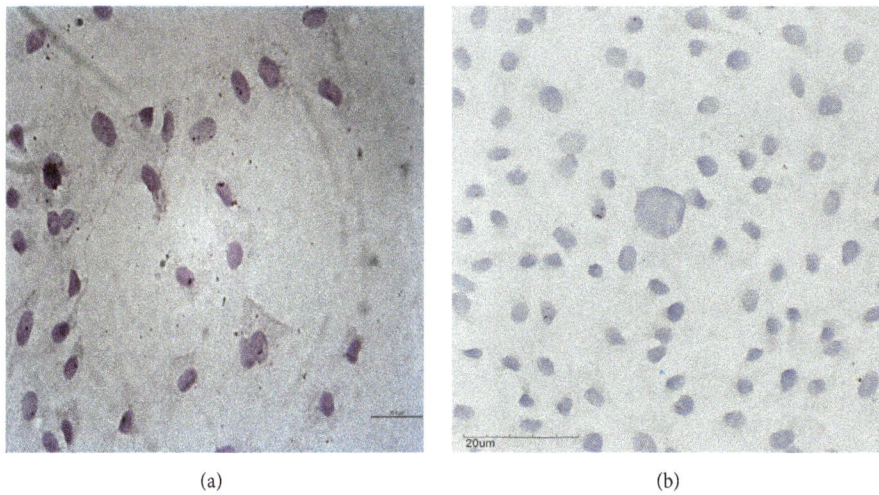

(a)   (b)

FIGURE 4: (a) Immunoperoxidase positive BGM-70 cells showing brown cytoplasmic precipitate compared to (b) the uninfected BGM-70 cells.

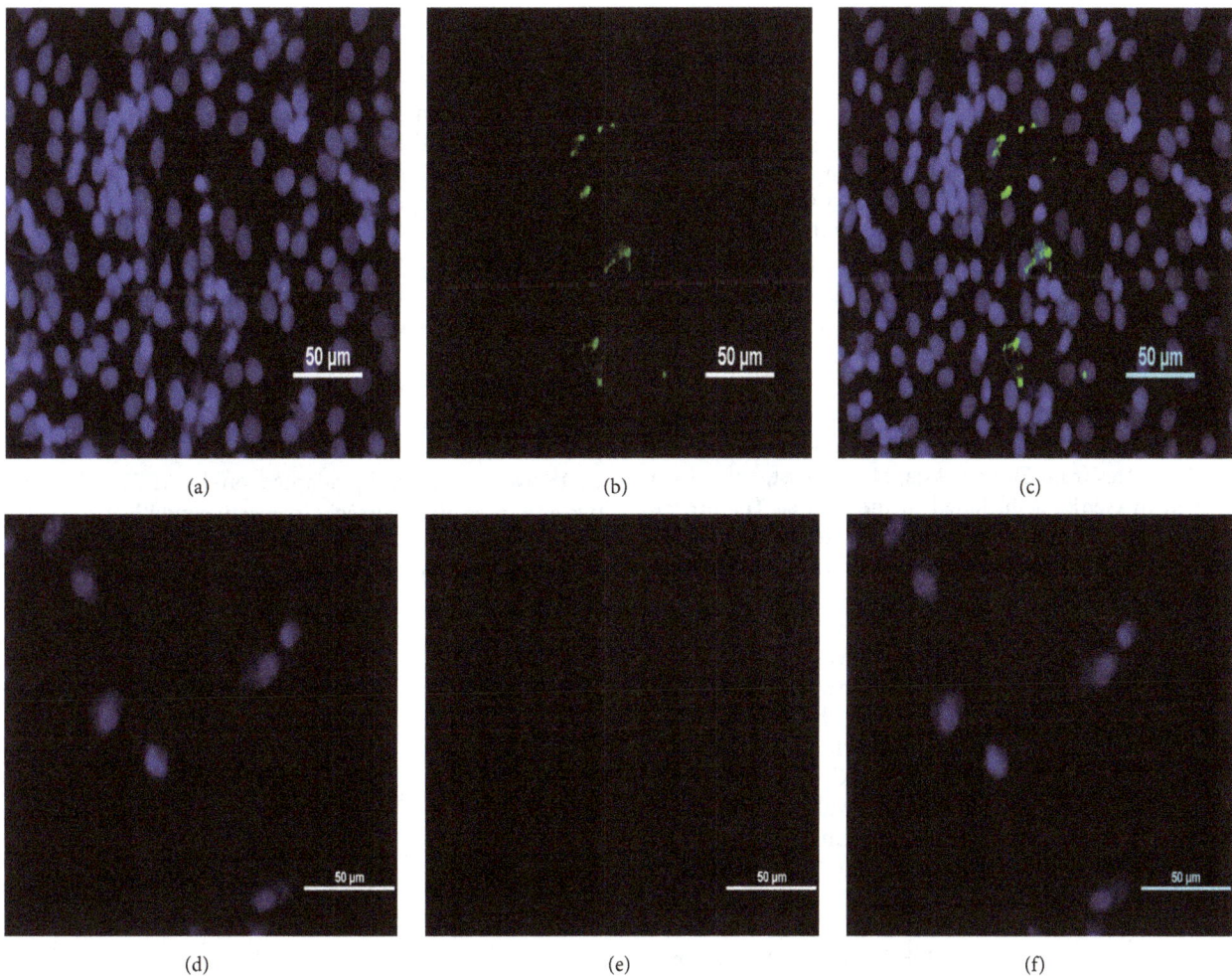

(a)   (b)   (c)

(d)   (e)   (f)

FIGURE 5: IBDV infected BGM-70 cells showing (a) blue fluorescence when stained with DAPI (b) green fluorescence when stained with FITC-labeled anti-chicken antibody indicating the presence of VP2 antigen and (c) the fluorescence when the two channels were merged (c). The uninfected BGM-70 control (d, e, and f) showing no green fluorescence due to the absence of IBDV VP2 antigen within the cells.

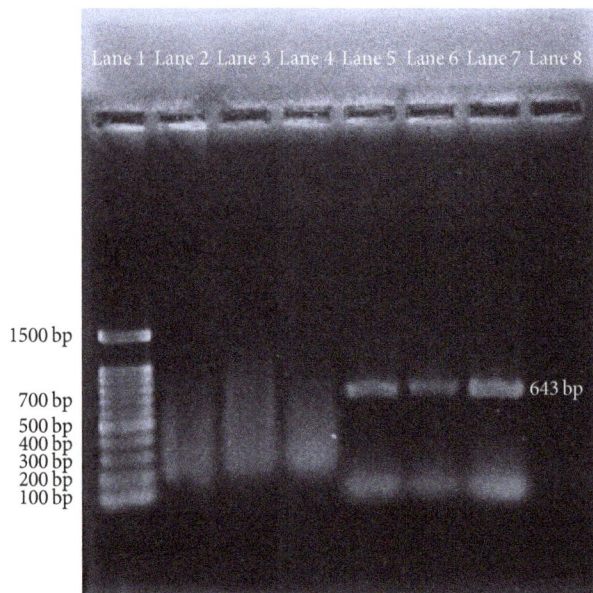

FIGURE 6: RT-PCR products of the BGM-70 cell culture supernatants showing 100 bp molecular ladder (Lane 1), nontemplate control (Lanes 2 and 3), negative control (Lane 4), positive control (Lane 5), UPM0081 (Lane 6), and UPM190 (Lane 7).

glutamic acid (E270) at that position. The reference sequences however possessed A, T, S, or V in that position except AF527039.1 and U30818.1 which possessed the E270 amino acid. At amino acid position 279, only UPM190EP12, UPM-BGM190P1, and UPMBGM190P5 possessed an Asparagine (N) while the preadaptation parent virus and other CEE and BGM-70 adapted isolates possessed D (Figure 8). The N279 mutation however reverted back as the viruses were further serially passaged in the BGM-70 cell line.

Phylogenetic analysis of the nucleotide sequences revealed that our isolates cluster with the sequences of the vvIBDV isolates from Europe, Asia, Middle East, and Africa deposited in GenBank included in the analysis (Figure 9). Distance matrix (Figure 10) revealed pairwise similarity index ranging from UPM B0081 was 0.8% different with AF508177, 10.9% different with the cell culture adapted Edgar strain, 11.5% different with AY819701, 9% different with AY963132, 8% different with JX424076.1, 43.4% different with U30818, and 45.9% different with KP642112.1. When compared with the UPM190 and UPM0081 sequences, the preadaptation UPM B0081 was 33.8% different with UPM04/190 and 0.4% to 3.4% different with the rest of the CEE and BGM-70 adapted isolates. On the other hand, UPM04/190 was 33.2% different with AF508177 and 34.5% different with all the CEE and BGM-70 except UPM190BGMP1 and UPM190BGMP5 and UPM190EP12 that differs by 32.5% and 31.8% with UPM190P1. Moreover, when UPM04/190 was compared with the serotype 2 isolates, U30818.1 was 62.9% different with it while KP642112 differs with it by 64.9%. The rest of the CEE and BGM-70 adapted isolates differed with UPM04/190 between 0.4% and 3.9%. The sequences used to construct the Phylogenetic Tree and to compute distance matrix are shown in Table 3.

4. Discussion

Outbreaks of vvIBDV in chickens as confirmed through RT-PCR and restriction fragment length polymorphism (RFLP) techniques were reported in Malaysia [22] and other parts of the world. Primary SPF CEE and several continuous avian and mammalian cell lines including BGM-70 cells were reported to support the growth and propagation of many viruses infecting vertebrates and invertebrate species including IBDV [9, 10, 12, 21]. In this study, two Malaysian vvIBDV isolates designated UPM0081 and UPM190 were adapted and serially passaged 12 times in CEE and were later adapted to grow in BGM-70, a continuous cell line of mammalian origin. The advantages of continuous mammalian cell lines over CEE include among other things such as absence of contamination with avian viruses, ease of handling, low cost, infinite lifespan, and ease of maintenance [9]. Most of the commercially available vaccines for the control of IBDV infection especially the very virulent IBDV (vvIBDV) pathotype are egg based, making their production laborious, costly, and a possible source of vertical transmission for important avian viruses to the vaccinated flocks. The need for shift from egg based to cell culture based IBD vaccine development using vvIBDV as the seed virus is very crucial in order to reduce the labor and high cost of production involved, but the problem is that vvIBDV has been reported to be difficult to adapt to cell culture [32, 33]. The unsuccessful attempt to adapt vvIBDV isolates from Holland, Taiwan, and Turkey on BGM-70 cell line after 10 blind passages has been previously documented [25]. In that study, the vvIBDV strains were passaged 8 times in SPF CEE before using it for serial inoculation of BGM-70 cultures up to 10 times without CPE development. In this study, two Malaysian vvIBDV isolates UPM0081 and UPM190 were successfully adapted on BGM-70 cell line with distinctive CPE development by passage 5. This is similar to the observation of Hassan and coworkers [9] and Abdel-Alim and Saif [34] where classical (STC) and variant (IN) IBDV were successfully adapted on BGM-70 cells within two and three blind passages, respectively, with characteristic CPE development. Furthermore, the reports of El-mahdy et al. [12] on the adaptation of local Egyptian vaIBDV isolates on BGM-70 cell line at passage 1 and with high virus yield ($\log_{10}7.5$ TCID$_{50}$/mL) agreed with our findings as IBDV UPM190 and UPM0081 yielded high virus titer of $10^{9.98}$ TCID$_{50}$/mL and $10^{9.50}$ TCID$_{50}$/mL, respectively, 72 hours after infection at passage 5.

Earlier investigations on the usefulness of BGM-70 cell line for the propagation of IBDV indicated that serial propagation of classic (STC) and variant (IN) IBDV as low as 4 passages resulted in loss of pathogenicity [9]; similarly, serial passaging as high as 30 passages (variant IN strain) or 40 passages (variant E strain) leads to the loss of ability of the viruses to replicate in the bursa of SPF chickens when used as live vaccines but protects chickens against experimental challenge when the viruses were used as inactivated vaccines [26]. In this study, the two viruses were passaged 20 times only in BGM-70 cells with high virus titer yield (log10 9.98 TCID$_{50}$/mL and log10 9.50 TCID$_{50}$/mL for UPM190 and

```
                              640       650       660       670       680       690       700       710       720       730
                              ...|....|....|....|....|....|....|....|....|....|....|....|....|....|....|....|....|....|....|..

AF508177.1|                   GATT ACCAATTCTC ATCACAGTAC CAAGCAGGTG GGGTAACTAT CACACTGTTC TCAGCTAATA TCGATGCCAT CACAAGCCTC AGCATTGGGG GAGAAC
FJ824699.1_UPM B0081_(Pre-adap  .... .......... .......... .......... ......A... .......... .......... .......... .......C.. .......... ......
UPM0081EP1                      .... .......... .......... .......... ......A... .......... .......... .......... .......C.. .......... ......
KY411641_(UPM0081EP12)          .... .......... .......... .......... ......A... .......... .......... .......... .......C.. .......... ......
UPM0081BGMP1                    .... .......... .......... .......... ......A... .......... .......... .......... .......C.. .......... ......
UPM0081BGMP5                    .... .......... .......... .......... ......A... .......... .......... .......... .......C.. .......... ......
UPM0081BGMP10                   .... .......... .......... .......... ......A... .......... .......... .......... .......C.. .......... ......
UPM0081BGMP15                   .... .......... .......... .......... ......A... .......... .......... .......... .......C.. .......... ......
UPM0081BGMP16                   .... .......... .......... .......... ......A... .......... .......... .......... .......C.. .......... ......
UPM0081BGMP17                   .... .......... .......... .......... ......A... .......... .......... .......... .......C.. .......... ......
UPM0081BGMP18                   .... .......... .......... .......... ......A... .......... .......... .......... .......C.. .......... ......
UPM0081BGMP19                   .... .......... .......... .......... ......A... .......... .......... .......... .......C.. .......... ......
KY418011_(UPM0081BGMP20)        .... .......... .......... .......... ......A... .......... .......... .......... .......C.. .......... ......
KY418009_(UPM190BGMP20)         .... .......... .......... .......... ......A... .......... .......... .......... .......C.. .......... ......
UPM190BGMP19                    .... .......... .......... .......... ......A... .......... .......... .......... .......C.. .......... ......
UPM190BGMP18                    .... .......... .......... .......... ......A... .......... .......... .......... .......C.. .......... ......
UPM190BGMP17                    .... .......... .......... .......... ......A... .......... .......... .......... .......C.. .......... ......
UPM190BGMP16                    .... .......... .......... .......... ......A... .......... .......... .......... .......C.. .......... ......
KY418010_(UPM190BGMP15)         .... .......... .......... .......... ......A... .......... .......... .......... .......C.. .......... ......
UPM190BGMP10                    .... .......... .......... .......... ......A... .......... .......... .......... .......C.. .......... ......
UPM190BGMP5                     .... .T..G..... .......... .......... ......A... .......... .......... .......... .......C.. .......... ......
UPM190BGMP1                     .... .T..G..... .......... .......... ......A... .......... .......... .......... .......C.. .......... ......
UPM190EP12                      .... .T..G..... .......... .......... ......A... .......... .......... .......... .......C.. .......... ......
UPM190EP1                       .... .T..G..... .......... .......... ......A... .......... .......... .......... .......C.. .......... ......
KU958716.1_UPM04/190_(pre-adap  .... .T..G..TAG CAGC.....T ..G..G..C. .C..G..C.. T..C.....T AGC..G..C. .T.....G.. T..C.....G .......C. .C....
EU162087.1                      .... .......... .......... .C...... .......A... .......... .C..C..T.. .......... .......... ...G...... ..G.
AJ878898.1                      A... .......... .......... .......... ......A... .......... .......... .......... .......C.. .......... ......
AY462026.1                      .... .......... .......... .T...... .......A... .......... .C..C..T... .T....... .......... ......G.
KF241548.1                      .... .......... .......... .......... ......A... .......... ....A..... .......... .......C.. .......... ......
AF051838.1                      .... .......... .......... .......A.. ......A... .......... .......... .......... .......C.. .......... ......
X92760.1                        .... .......... .......... .......... ......A... .......... .......... .......... .......C.. .......... ......
AY907014                        .... .......T .......... ..C...... .......A... .......... .C..C..T...T .......... .......... ...G...... ..G.
AY780423                        .... .......... .......... .......... ......A... .......... .......... .......... .......C.. .......... ......
AY819703                        A... .......... .......... ...A...... ......A... .......... .C..C..T .T...... .......... ...G...... ..G.
AY819702                        A... .......... .......... ...A...... ......A... .......... .C..C..T .T...... .......... ...G...... ..G.
AY819701                        A... .......... .......... ...A...... ......A... .......... .C..C..T .T...... .......... ...G...... ..G.
JX424076.1                      .... .......... .......... ..C...... ......A... .......... .C..C..T.. .......... .......... ...G...... ..G.
KC352669.1                      .... .......... .......... ......A... ......A... .......... .......... .G........ ....C..... .G....
AY963132.1                      A... .......... .......... ...A...... ......A... .......... .C..C..T .T...... .......... ...G...... ....
AY907012.1                      .... .......... .......... ......G. ......A... .......... .......... .......... .......C.. .......... ......
AY907007                        .... .......... .......... .......... ......A... .......... .......... .......... .......C.. .......... ......
AJ586926.1                      .... .......... .......... .......... ......A... .......... .C..C. .......... .......C.. .......... ......
AF092171.1                      .... .......... .......... .......... ......A... .......... .......... .......T.. .......C.. .......... ......
EU544158                        .... .......... .......... ..C...... ......G... .......... .C..C..T.. .......... .......... ...G...... ..G.
DQ916216                        .... .......... .......... ..T...... ......A... .......... .......... .......... .......C.. .......... ......
AF262030.1                      .... .......... .......... .......... ......A... .......... .......... .......... .......C.. .......... ......
D49706.1                        .... .......... .......... .......... ......A... .......... .......... .......... .......C.. .......... ......
AF527039.1                      .... .......... .......... .......... ......A... .......... .C....... .......... .......C.. .......... ......
KP642112.1                      ..G. .T..G..... G...AGACT. GTCC..A... .A..G.AG.C .......... A.C..C..C. .A...TC. T........G ..TG....T. .T..G.
U30818.1                        ..G. .......... G..G..ACT. ATCC..A... .A..G.AG.C T......... A.C..C..C. .......TC. T......... .TG....T. .T..G.
```

FIGURE 7: Continued.

```
              740       750       760       770       780       790       800       810       820       830
         ...|....|....|....|....|....|....|....|....|....|....|....|....|....|....|....|....|....|....|....|....|.
AF508177.1|                    TCGT GTTT  CAA ACAAGCGTCC AAGGCCTTAT ACTGGGTGCT ACCATCTACC TTATAGGCTT TGATGGGACT GCGGTAATCA CCAGAGCTGT GGCCGC
FJ824699.1_UPM B0081_(Pre-adap  .... ....  ...  .......... .......... .......... .......... .......... .......... .......... .......... ......
UPM0081EP1                      .... ....  ...  .......... .......... .......... .......... .......... .......... .A........ .......... ......
KY411641_(UPM0081EP12)          .... ....  ...  .......... .......... .......... .......... .......... .......... .A........ .......... ......
UPM0081BGMP1                    .... ....  ...  .......... .......... .......... .......... .......... .......... .A........ .......... ......
UPM0081BGMP5                    .... ....  ...  .......... .......... .......... .......... .......... .......... .A........ .......... ......
UPM0081BGMP10                   .... ....  ...  .......... .......... .......... .......... .......... .......... .A........ .......... ......
UPM0081BGMP15                   .... ....  ...  .......... .......... .......... .......... .......... .......... .A........ .......... ......
UPM0081BGMP16                   .... ....  ...  .......... .......... .......... .......... .......... .......... .A........ .......... ......
UPM0081BGMP17                   .... ....  ...  .......... .......... .......... .......... .......... .......... .A........ .......... ......
UPM0081BGMP18                   .... ....  ...  .......... .......... .......... .......... .......... .......... .A........ .......... ......
UPM0081BGMP19                   .... ....  ...  .......... .......... .......... .......... .......... .......... .A........ .......... ......
KY418011_(UPM0081BGMP20)        .... ....  ...  .......... .......... .......... .......... .......... .......... .A........ .......... ......
KY418009_(UPM190BGMP20)         .... ....  ...  .......... .......... .......... .......... .......... .......... .A........ .......... ......
UPM190BGMP19                    .... ....  ...  .......... .......... .......... .......... .......... .......... .A........ .......... ......
UPM190BGMP18                    .... ....  ...  .......... .......... .......... .......... .......... .......... .A........ .......... ......
UPM190BGMP17                    .... ....  ...  .......... .......... .......... .......... .......... .......... .A........ .......... ......
UPM190BGMP16                    .... ....  ...  .......... .......... .......... .......... .......... .......... .A........ .......... ......
KY418010_(UPM190BGMP15)         .... ....  ...  .......... .......... .......... .......... .......... .......... .A........ .......... ......
UPM190BGMP10                    .... ....  ...  .......... .......... .......... .......... .......... .......... .A........ .......... ......
UPM190BGMP5                     .T.. ....  G..  .......... .......... .......C.. .......... .......G.. .......... ...T...... .......... ......
UPM190BGMP1                     .T.. ....  G..  .......... .......... .......C.. .......... .......G.. .......... ...T...... .......... ......
UPM190EP12                      .T.. ....  G..  .......... .......... .......C.. .......... .......G.. .......... ...T...... .......... ......
UPM190EP1                       .T.. ....  G..  .......... .......... .......C.. .......... .......G.. .......... ...T...... .......... ......
KU958716.1_UPM04/190_(pre-adap  .G.. ....  G..  .C.....G. .G.....G. T.....C.G  .T..T. .G.G...... .C..C..... .G..T. ..C.T.G...  ...G..
EU162087.1                      .... ....  ...  .C.....G. ....C..C  .......... .C........ .......A A......... ...G...... ......
AJ878898.1                      .... ....  ...  .......... .......... .......... .......... .......... .......... .......... ......
AY462026.1                      .... ..C.  .T.  .C.....GC ..AC..C  .......... .......... ...A.A.... .......... ......T. ......
KF241548.1                      .... ....  ...  ..A....... ..T..A.. .......... .......... .......... .......... ...A..... ......
AF051838.1                      .... ....  ...  .......... .......... .......... .......... .......... ..T....... .......... ......
X92760.1                        .... ....  ...  .......... .......... .......... .......... .......... .......... .......... ......
AY907014                        .... ....  ...  ..T....... ..G....... .C..C.... .......... .A........ ...G...... ......
AY780423                        .... ....  ...  .......... .......... .......... .......... .......... .......... .......... ......
AY819703                        ..A. ...C  A..  .CA....GA ....C..C  .......... .......... .......... .......... .......T
AY819702                        ..A. ...C  A..  .CA....GA ....C..C  .......... .......... .......... .......... .......T
AY819701                        ..A. ...C  A..  .CA....GA ....C..C  .......... .......... .......... .......... .......T
JX424076.1                      .... ....  ...  .C.....G. ....C..C  .C........ .......... .A A...... ...G...... ......
KC352669.1                      .T.. ....  ...  .......... .......... .......... .......... .......... ...T...... .......... ......
AY963132.1                      .... ..C.  A..  ..A....G. .C..C.... .......... .......... ...C...... .......... ......
AY907012.1                      .... ..C.  ...  .......... .......... ....C..... .......... .......T.. .......... ......
AY907007                        .... ....  ...  .......... .......... .......... .......... .......... .......... .......... ......
AJ586926.1                      .T.. ....  ...  ..A....... ..T....... .......... .......... .......... .......... ...A..
AF092171.1                      .... ....  ...  .......... .......... .......... .......... .......... .......... .......... ......
EU544158                        .... ....  ...  .C.....G. ....C..C  ....C.... .C........ A......... ...A...... ...G...... ......
DQ916216                        .... ....  ...  .......... .......... .......... .......... .......... .......... .......... ......
AF262030.1                      .... ....  ...  .......... .......... .......... .......... .......... .......... .......... ......
D49706.1                        .... ....  ...  .......C. .......... .......... .......... .......... .......... .......... ......
AF527039.1                      .... ....  ...  ..A....... .......... .......... .......... ...A...... .......... .......... ......
KP642112.1                      .T.. C..CAGC. .G GT..CGA...  .A..A..GA .G...AC.T. ..T.....T  .C..T.G.. C..C..... .A .T...CAG T..AG..... T..AA.
U30818.1                        .TA. C..CAGC... GT..CGA...  CA..A..GA .G...AC.TC  .....T..T  .C..T.G.. C..C..... .A .A..C.CAG T..A... T..AA.
```

FIGURE 7: Continued.

```
                                      840           850           860           870
                                   ...|  ....|....| ....|....| ....|....| ....|....
AF508177.1|                        AGAC AATGGGCTAA CGGCCGGCAC TGACAACCTT ATGCCATTC
FJ824699.1_UPM B0081_(Pre-adap     .... .......... .......... .......... .........
UPM0081EP1                         .... .......... .......... .......... .........
KY411641_(UPM0081EP12)             .... .......... .......... .......... .........
UPM0081BGMP1                       .... .......... .......... .......... .........
UPM0081BGMP5                       .... .......... .......... .......... .........
UPM0081BGMP10                      .... .......... .......... .......... .........
UPM0081BGMP15                      .... .......... .......... .......... .........
UPM0081BGMP16                      .... .......... .......... .......... .........
UPM0081BGMP17                      .... .......... .......... .......... .........
UPM0081BGMP18                      .... .......... .......... .......... .........
UPM0081BGMP19                      .... .......... .......... .......... .........
KY418011_(UPM0081BGMP20)           .... .......... .......... .......... .........
KY418009_(UPM190BGMP20)            .... .......... .......... .......... .........
UPM190BGMP19                       .... .......... .......... .......... .........
UPM190BGMP18                       .... .......... .......... .......... .........
UPM190BGMP17                       .... .......... .......... .......... .........
UPM190BGMP16                       .... .......... .......... .......... .........
KY418010_(UPM190BGMP15)            .... .......... .......... .......... .........
UPM190BGMP10                       .... .......... .......... .......... .........
UPM190BGMP5                        .A.. .......... .......... .......... .........
UPM190BGMP1                        .A.. .......... .......... .......... .........
UPM190EP12                         .A.. .......... .......... .......... .........
UPM190EP1                          .... .......... .......... .......... .........
KU958716.1_UPM04/190_(pre-adap     G..T ..C..C..G. .C..G..... C..T.....G .....G..T
EU162087.1                         .A.. ........G. ..A....... C......... .........
AJ878898.1                         .... ........G. .......... .......... .........
AY462026.1                         .... ........G. .TA......T C.....T... .... ....
KF241548.1                         .... .......... .......... .......... .........
AF051838.1                         .... .......... .......... .......... .........
X92760.1                           .... ........G. .......... .......... .........
AY907014                           .... ........G. .......... C.....T... .........
AY780423                           .... ........G. .......... .......... .........
AY819703                           .A..T ........G. ..A......T C.....T... .........
AY819702                           .A.. ........G. ..A......T C.....T... .........
AY819701                           .A.. ........G. ..A......T C.....T... .........
JX424076.1                         .A.. ........G. ..A....... C......... .........
KC352669.1                         .... .......... .......... .......... .........
AY963132.1                         .A.. ........G. ..........T C.....T... .........
AY907012.1                         .... .......... .......... C......C.. .........
AY907007                           G... .......... .......... .......... .........
AJ586926.1                         T... .......... .......... .......... .........
AF092171.1                         .... .......... .......... .......... .........
EU544158                           .A.. ........G. ..A....... ..........T .........
DQ916216                           T... .......... .......... .......... .........
AF262030.1                         .... .......... .......... .......... .........
D49706.1                           .... .......... .......... .......... .........
AF527039.1                         .... .......... .......... .......... .........
KP642112.1                         .... TT......G. .AA.T..G.. GA........ G........
U30818.1                           .... TT......G. .AA.T..G.. GA........ G........
```

FIGURE 7: Nucleotide sequences of the isolates. Nucleotide sequences of 645 bp fragment of the hypervariable region of VP2 comparison between CEE and BGM-70 adapted Malaysian isolates and reference sequences. Dots (.) indicate consensus with the AF508177.1, a South Korean IBDV isolate, and dash (-) indicates gaps.

```
              220       230       240       250       260       270       280       290
              ..|....|  ....|....|  ....|....|  ....|....|  ....|....|  ....|....|  ....|....|  ....|....|  ...
AF508177.1|   DYQFSSQY  QAGGVTITLF  SANIDAITSL  SIGGELVF-Q  TSVQGLILGA  TIYLIGFDGT  AVITRAVAAD  NGLTAGTDNL  MPF
FJ824699.1 UPM B0081 (Pre-adap  ........  ..........  ..........  .....-..  ..........  ..........  ..........  .........  ...
UPM0081EP1    ........  ..........  ..........  .....-..  ..........  .....[E]..  ..........  .........  ...
KY411641 (UPM0081EP12)  ........  ..........  ..........  .....-..  .......  .....[E]..  ..........  .........  ...
UPM0081BGMP1  ........  ..........  ..........  .....-..  .......  .....[E]..  ..........  .........  ...
UPM0081BGMP5  ........  ..........  ..........  .....-..  .......  .....[E]..  ..........  .........  ...
UPM0081BGMP10  ........  ..........  ..........  .....-..  .......  .....[E]..  ..........  .........  ...
UPM0081BGMP15  ........  ..........  ..........  .....-..  .......  .....[E]..  ..........  .........  ...
UPM0081BGMP16  ........  ..........  ..........  .....-..  .......  .....[E]..  ..........  .........  ...
UPM0081BGMP17  ........  ..........  ..........  .....-..  .......  .....[E]..  ..........  .........  ...
UPM0081BGMP18  ........  ..........  ..........  .....-..  .......  .....[E]..  ..........  .........  ...
UPM0081BGMP19  ........  ..........  ..........  .....-..  .......  .....[E]..  ..........  .........  ...
KY418011 (UPM0081BGMP20)  ........  ..........  ..........  .....-..  .......  .....[E]..  ..........  .........  ...
KY418009 (UPM190BGMP20)  ........  ..........  ..........  .....-..  .......  .....[E]..  ..........  .........  ...
UPM190BGMP19  ........  ..........  ..........  .....-..  .......  .....[E]..  ..........  .........  ...
UPM190BGMP18  ........  ..........  ..........  .....-..  .......  .....[E]..  ..........  .........  ...
UPM190BGMP17  ........  ..........  ..........  .....-..  .......  .....[E]..  ..........  .........  ...
UPM190BGMP16  ........  ..........  ..........  .....-..  .......  .....[E]..  ..........  .........  ...
KY418010 (UPM190BGMP15)  ........  ..........  ..........  .....-..  .......  .....[E]..  ..........  .........  ...
UPM190BGMP10  ........  ..........  ..........  .....-.  .......  .....[E]..  ..........  .........  ...
UPM190BGMP5   ........  ..........  ..........  ....[E]-..  .......  ...M..  ..........  .....N...  ...
UPM190BGMP1   ........  ..........  ..........  ....[E]-..  .......  ...M..  ..........  .....N...  ...
UPM190EP12    ........  ..........  ..........  ....[E]-..  .......  ...M..  ..........  .....N...  ...
UPM190EP1     ........  ..........  ..........  ....[E]-..  .......  ...M..  ..........  .....N...  ...
KU958716.1 UPM04/190 (pre-adap  ........  ..........  ..........  ....[E]-..  .......  ...M..  ..........  .........  ...
EU162087.1    ........  .P..  ..........  .V...-..  ...H..V..  ..........  T.....  .....N...  ..T..
AJ878898.1    N.......  ..........  ..........  .....-..  .......  ..........  ..........  .........  ...
AY462026.1    ........  .S..  ..........  -H...H..A.D  .......  ..........  T.......S.  ....T.I..
KF241548.1    ........  ..........  ..........  .....-..  ...S..  ..........  ..........  .........  ...
AF051838.1    ........  ..........  ..........  .....-..  .......  ..........  ..........  .........  ...
X92760.1      ........  ..........  ..........  .....-..  .......  ..........  ..........  .........  ...
AY907014      ...L..  .P..  ..........  .V...-..  ...V..  ..........  T.......  .........  ...
AY780423      ........  ..........  ..........  .....-..  .......  ..........  ..........  .........  ...
AY819703      N.......  .T..  ..........  .V...M..-K  ..HS.E.  ..........  VN.......  ..T.I..
AY819702      N.......  .T..  ..........  .V...M..-K  ..HS.E.  ..........  VN.......  ..T.I..
AY819701      N.......  .T..  ..........  .V...M..-K  ..HS.E.  ..........  VN.......  ..T.I..
JX424076.1    ........  .P..  ..........  .V...-..  ...H..V..  ..........  T.......  .....N...  ..T..
KC352669.1    ........  ..........  ..........  .....-..  .......  ..........  ..........  .........  ...
AY963132.1    N.......  .T..  ..........  .V...-K  ..S.V..  ..........  .........N  .......I..
AY907012.1    ........  ..........  ..........  .....-..  ...S..  ..........  S.......  .........  ...
AY907007      ........  ..........  ..........  .....-..  .......  ..........  ..........  .........  ...
AJ586926.1|   ........  ..........  ..........  .....-..  ...S..  ..........  ..........  .........  ...
AF092171.1    ........  ..........  ..........  .....-..  .......  ..........  ..........  .........  ...
EU544158      ........  .P..  ..........  .V...-..  ...H..V...  ..H...L..  ..........  .....N...  ..T...L.
DQ916216      ........  .S..  ..........  .....-..  .......  ..........  ..........  .........  ...
AF262030.1    ........  ..........  ..........  .....-..  .......  ..........  ..........  .........  ...
D49706.1      ........  ..........  ..........  .....-..  .......  ..........  ..........  .........  ...
AF527039.1    ........  ..........  ..........  .....-..  ...S..  ..........  E.......  .........  ...
KP642112.1    E.....RL  VPS..KT...  T.....L...  .V......S.  VTI.SIEVDV  ...F.....  V.TVK...T.  F...T..N..  V..
U30818.1      E......L  IPS..KT...  T.....L...  .V....I.S.  VTIHSIEVDV  ...F.....  E.TVK...T.  F...T..N..  V..
```

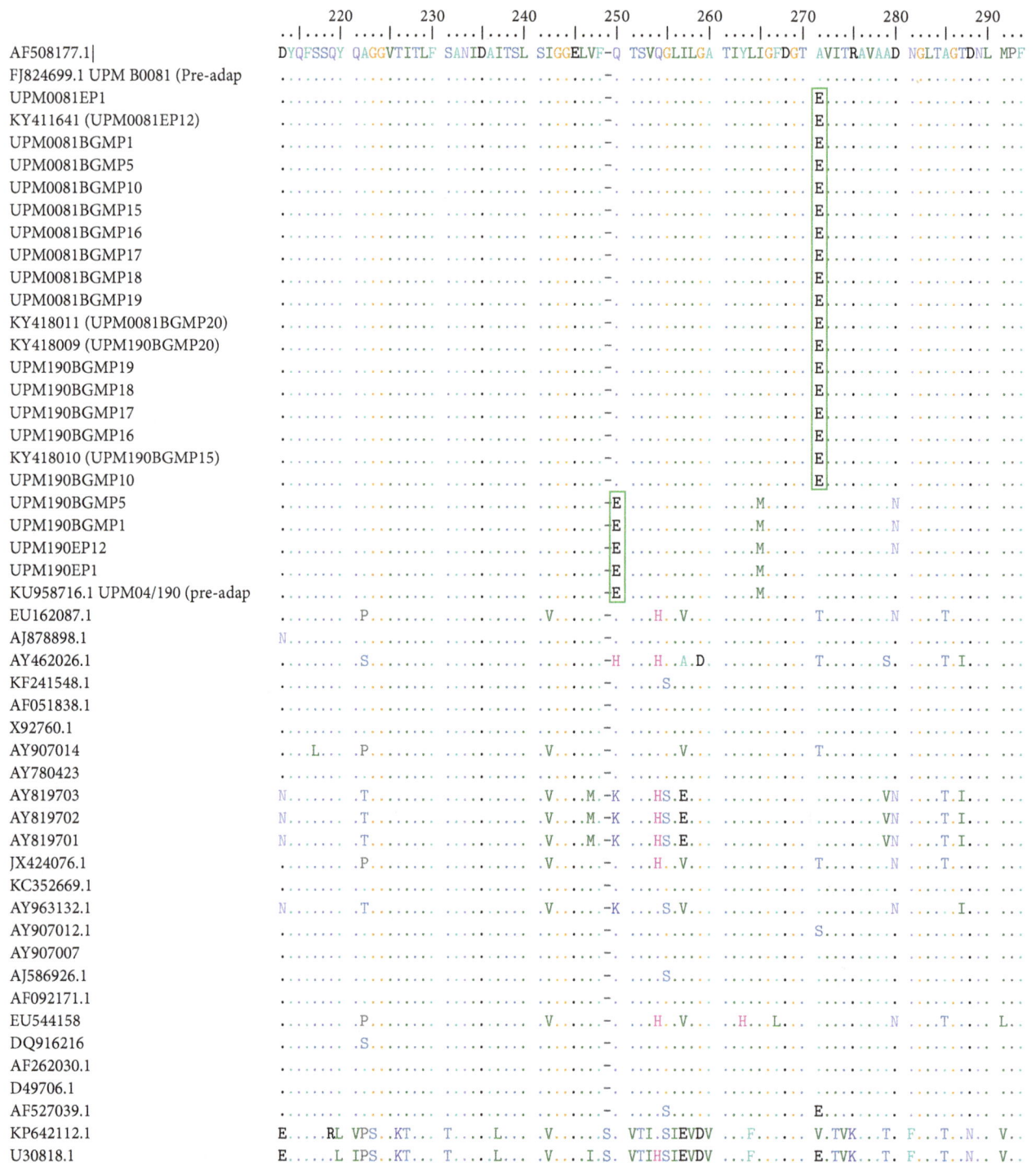

FIGURE 8: Deduced amino acid sequences of the isolates. Figure 8 shows the deduced amino acid sequences from positions 213 to 293 where both CEE and BGM-70 adapted UPM190 and UPM0081 isolates showed high similarity with the reference vvIBDV from different parts of the world such as UK661, HK46, JNeto-BR, SA-KZN95, Oyo.NIE 96-09, IRAQ12.127-743 but striking differences with the classical, variant, and serotype 2 reference isolates. Note the E249 and E270 (boxed) amino acids present in some of adapted viruses not seen in other vvIBDV except UPM94/273, a Malaysian isolate with unusual pathogenicity and serotype 2 OH strain.

UPM0081, respectively); there is the need to evaluate their pathogenicity, immunogenicity, and efficacy in experimental challenge studies to establish their usefulness as potential live attenuated or inactivated vaccine candidates.

Apoptosis is a programmed cell death that is highly regulated by cellular factors characterized by distinct morphological cytologic changes such as chromatin condensation, nuclear fragmentation, and membrane blebbing [35]. Certain

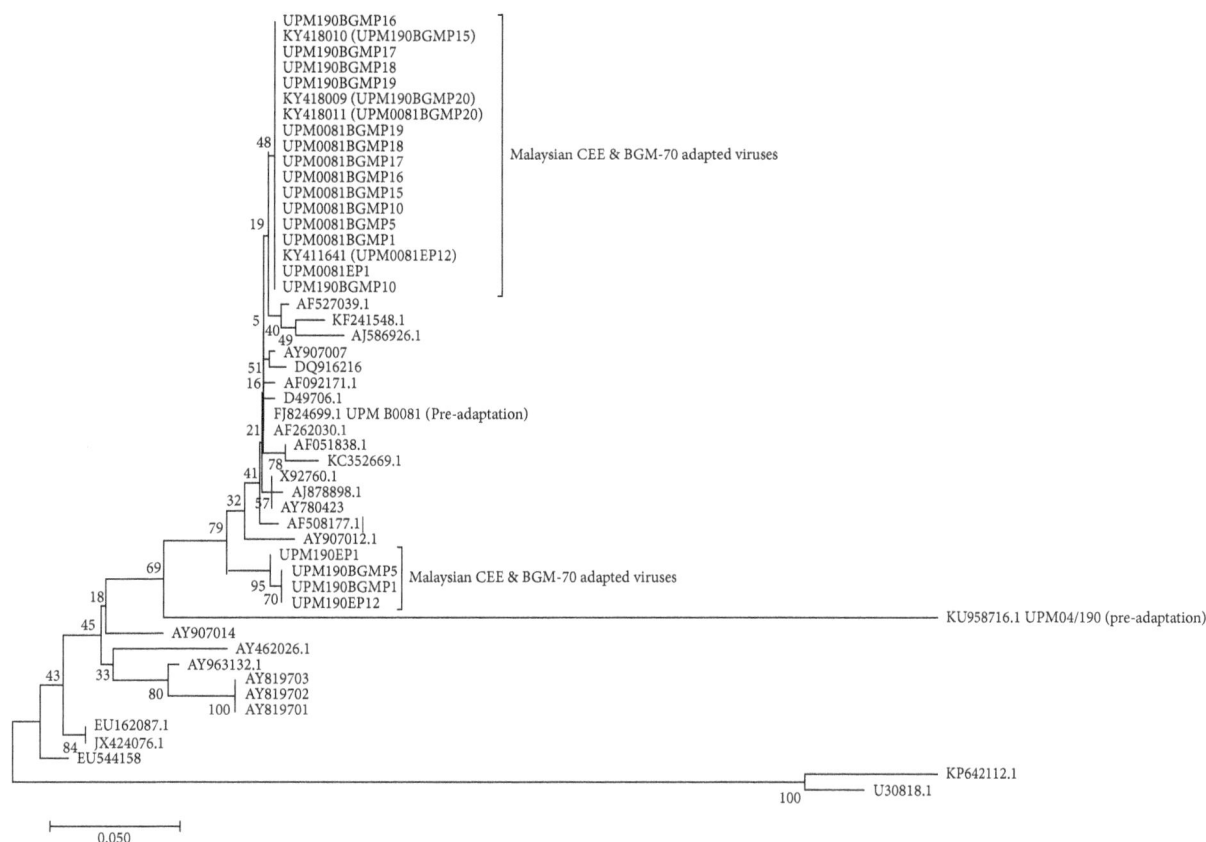

FIGURE 9: Nucleotide Phylogenetic Tree Analysis. Phylogenetic analysis of the hypervariable region of the VP2 gene of the IBDV segment A genome from nucleotide positions 637 to 876. The preadaptation, CEE, and BGM-70 adapted viruses are located on the red branch. The vvIBDV pathotypes included in the analysis were AJ878898, AF051838, KF241548, AF508177, D49706.1, X92760, AY780423, AF262030.1, AY520910.1, AF092171.1, AY907007, KC352669.1, AY907012.1, AJ586926.1, and DQ916216. JX424079.1, AY462026, EU162087, AY819703, EU544158, AY907014, AY819702, AY819701, and AY963132.1 represent the classical strains, whereas U30818.1 and KP642112.1 represent the serotype 2 sequences. The evolutionary history and distances were inferred using the neighbor-joining method [17] and the Kimura 2-parameter method [18], respectively. Evolutionary analyses were conducted in MEGA7 [19].

staining methods were developed that aid in the recognition and differentiation of apoptotic from necrotic cells which include Annexin V stain, 4′,6-diamidino-2-phenylindole (DAPI) stain, acridine orange/ethidium bromide/propidium iodide stain, and Hoechst stain. These fluorochromes emit fluorescence when they bind to DNA and are viewed at certain excitation spectra with fluorescence microscopy [36]. The productive infection of cell lines with IBDV has been associated with induction of apoptosis [30, 37, 38], a process that was linked to the nonstructural IBDV VP5 protein, seen only in IBDV infected cells [37, 39–41]. The use of AO/PI dyes to stain infected cultures was used to differentiate apoptotic from necrotic cells [30, 36]. The presence of an orange coloration after dual staining with AO/PI was considered as one of the indicators of apoptosis beside nuclear fragmentation, condensation, and membrane blebbing [42]. In this study, AO/PI dyes were used to demonstrate apoptosis induced by the VP5 nonstructural protein of IBDV that is seen only in a productive infection [30, 37–41, 43, 44]. The dual staining of IBDV infected BGM-70 cells with AO/PI dyes allowed the detection of cells undergoing apoptosis evidenced by the presence of orange coloration of the nucleus of stained cells

when viewed under fluorescence microscopy. Presence of propidium iodide in a cell indicates loss of cell membrane integrity; therefore this dye can only permeate damaged cells where it stains the nucleus red. Acridine orange on the other hand readily crosses the membrane of healthy and early apoptotic cells and stains the nucleus green. The presence of these two dyes together in a cell staining the nucleus orange to red is an evidence of the loss of membrane selective permeability that is only seen in dying cells. Staining of the nucleus red by the PI in combination of AO indicates necrotic cells whereas orange coloration is an indication of cells undergoing late apoptosis [42]. This technique is simple but elegant in its ability to differentiate dead cells from those undergoing apoptosis in response to obnoxious stimuli such as IBD virus.

To further confirm the presence of IBDV within infected BGM-70 cells, immunohistochemistry and immunofluorescence techniques were performed to identify antigen positive cells [44–48]. The presence of VP2 antigen as demonstrated by immunoperoxidase and immunofluorescence within the cytoplasm of infected cells 48 hours pi indicated the ability of BGM-70 cell line to support the growth and replication of

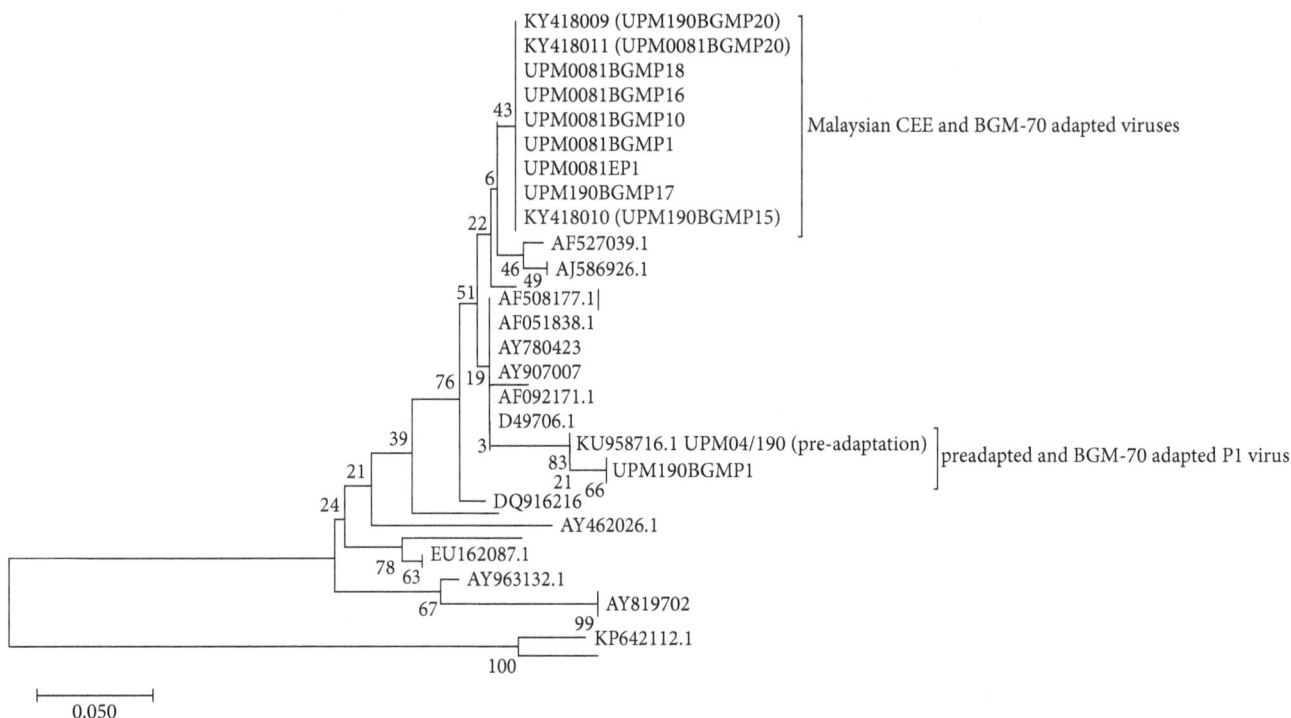

FIGURE 10: Phylogenetic Tree of the deduced amino acids. Fifty amino acid sequences were used to infer evolutionary history using the neighbor-joining method [17] and 1000 bootstrap test [20]. The Poisson correction method was used to compute the evolutionary distances [21]. Analyses were conducted in MEGA7 [19].

these two vvIBDV isolates, because the virus was reported to replicate within the cytoplasm of infected cells with generation of viral capsid proteins (VP2 and VP3) within 48 hours pi [30, 49, 50]. These two techniques are sensitive and specific and useful diagnostic tools for the detection and localization of IBDV in infected cells and tissues.

The molecular analyses using RT-PCR, sequence, and sequence analysis revealed that the two isolates are phylogenetically related to the vvIBDV found in Asia, Europe, Middle East, and Africa due to the presence of A222 [51, 52] and I242, I256, I294, and S299 [51] in their VP2 hypervariable amino acid composition compared to the caIBDV or vaIBDV that possessed V222, VA, or E256 or the serotype 2 viruses that possessed P222, V242, I or S256, N or F294 and T or P299 [51] in the same region. The presence of the 233–236 IDA motif in our strains just like other IBDV indicates that these viruses could adapt to cell culture because these amino acids were reported to be important for cell culture adaptation [51, 53] via the integrin receptors. Furthermore, during the CEE passaging, UPM190 isolate acquired a mutation at D279N at EP12, a mutation that was reported to be part of the two changes observed in attenuated and/or cell culture adapted IBD viruses [7, 54–56]. However, when the virus was passaged in BGM-70 cell, the N279 reverted back to D279 as seen in the amino acid sequences of the BGM-70 adapted viruses. The ability of this isolate with only a single mutation at D279N to replicate in BGM-70 cell culture indicated that perhaps the D279N mutation alone could facilitate cell culture adaptability to a very virulent strain of IBDV. This may

be the reason why UPM190 replicated more efficiently and with more pronounced CPE compared to UPM0081 whose amino acids remained unchanged during the CEE passages. Moreover, BGM-70 adaptation resulted in other mutations in UPM190 amino acid sequences at positions E249Q and A270E within the VP2 hypervariable region. The A270E mutation was previously reported only in UPM94/273, a vvIBDV with unusual pathogenicity, and in nonpathogenic serotype 2 OH strain [57]. It was previously reported that two amino acid changes at specific sites may lead to virus attenuation [58]. The appearance of this A270E mutation in the sequence of BGM-70 adapted UPM190 may be responsible for the decrease in CPE observed in BGM-70 cell culture suggesting attenuation. However, for UPM0081, the A270E mutation was acquired during CEE adaptation before the isolate was passaged and adapted in BGM-70 cell line. The importance of this mutation needs to be confirmed by further experiments involving reverse genetic technology.

Phylogenetically, all the isolates fall within the vvIBDV clades by clustering with other published vvIBDV reference sequences deposited in GeneBank, indicating that the BGM-70 passaging and the mutations observed did not lead to a change in the pathotypes of the isolates.

In summary, attenuated Malaysian vvIBDV was obtained by 12 serial passages in CEE followed by 20 serial passages in BGM-70 cell line. One amino acid change was seen in UPM190 at CEE passage 12 that reverted back when the isolate was passaged in BGM-70 cell line, and two amino acid changes were seen in UPM190 and one mutation was seen in UPM0081 during BGM-70 serial passages. To our knowledge, this is the first reported successful adaptation of local Malaysian vvIBDV isolates in BGM-70 cell line; therefore, this study highlight the merit of this cell line for the *in vitro* propagation of vvIBDV in the laboratory and the possible role the A270E mutation may play as a novel site for attenuation, further strengthening the possibility that many different sites within the VP2 hypervariable region may be involved in IBDV attenuation.

Acknowledgments

This study was sponsored under the TechnoFund project (6364002), Ministry of Science, Technology and Innovation, Malaysia, and HiCoE project (6369101), Ministry of High Education, Malaysia.

References

[1] P. Dobos, B. J. Hill, R. Hallett, D. T. Kells, H. Becht, and D. Teninges, "Biophysical and biochemical characterization of five animal viruses with bisegmented double-stranded RNA genomes," *Journal of Virology*, vol. 32, no. 2, pp. 593–605, 1979.

[2] T. Berg, "Acute infectious bursal disease in poultry: a review," *Avian Pathology*, 2000, http://www.tandfonline.com/doi/abs/10.1080/03079450050045431.

[3] H. J. Boot, A. J. Hoekman, and A. L. Gielkens, "The enhanced virulence of very virulent infectious bursal disease virus is partly determined by its B-segment," *Archives of Virology*, vol. 150, no. 1, pp. 137–144, 2005.

[4] J. B. McFerran, M. S. McNulty, E. R. McKillop et al., "Isolation and serological studies with infectious bursal disease viruses from fowl, turkeys and ducks: Demonstration of a second serotype," *Avian Pathology*, vol. 9, no. 3, pp. 395–404, 1980.

[5] S. B. Hitchner, "Infectivity of infectious bursal disease virus for embryonating eggs," *Poultry Science*, vol. 49, no. 2, pp. 511–516, 1970.

[6] B. R. Cho, R. G. Raymond, and R. W. Hill, "Growth of Infectious Bursal Disease Virus with Plaque Formation in Chick Embryo Fibroblast Cell Culture," *Avian Diseases*, vol. 23, no. 1, p. 209, 1979.

[7] T. Yamaguchi, T. Kondo, Y. Inoshima et al., "In vitro attenuation of highly virulent infectious bursal disease virus: Some characteristics of attenuated strains," *Avian Diseases*, vol. 40, no. 3, pp. 501–509, 1996.

[8] P. Lukert, J. Leonard, and R. Davis, "Infectious bursal disease virus: antigen production and immunity," *American Journal of Veterinary Research*, 1975, http://www.ncbi.nlm.nih.gov/pubmed/164798.

[9] M. K. Hassan, M. Q. Al-Natour, L. A. Ward, and Y. M. Saif, "Pathogenicity, Attenuation, and Immunogenicity of Infectious Bursal Disease Virus," *Avian Diseases*, vol. 40, no. 3, p. 567, 1996.

[10] D. H. Jackwood, Y. M. Saif, and J. H. Hughes, "Replication of Infectious Bursal Disease Virus in Continuous Cell Lines," *Avian Diseases*, vol. 31, no. 2, p. 370, 1987.

[11] F. S. Kibenge and P. K. McKenna, "Isolation and propagation of infectious bursal disease virus using the ovine kidney continuous cell line," *Avian Diseases*, vol. 36, no. 2, pp. 256–261, 1992.

[12] S. El-Mahdy, F. Hayam, and A. NA, "Vaccine strains in Egypt," *Am J*, 2013, http://www.usa-journals.com/wp-content/uploads/2013/09/El-mahdy_Vol110.pdf.

[13] F. S. Kibenge, A. S. Dhillon, and R. G. Russell, "Growth of serotypes I and II and variant strains of infectious bursal disease virus in Vero cells.," *Avian Diseases*, vol. 32, no. 2, pp. 298–303, 1988.

[14] I. Simoni, M. Fernandes, and R. Custódio, "Susceptibility of cell lines to avian viruses," *Microbiology*, 1999, http://www.scielo.br/scielo.php?pid=S0001-37141999000400015&script=sci_arttext.

[15] M. Ahasan, K. Hossain, and M. Islam, "Adaptation of infectious bursal disease virus (IBDV) on vero cell line," *Journal of Biological Sciences*, 2002, http://www.medwelljournals.org/ref.php?doi=jbs.2002.633.635.

[16] M. Petek, P. N. D'Aprile, and F. Cancellotti, "Biological and physico-chemical properties of the infectious bursal disease virus (ibdv)," *Avian Pathology*, vol. 2, no. 2, pp. 135–152, 1973.

[17] P. H. A. Sneath and R. R. Sokal, *Numerical Taxonomy: The Principles and Practice of Numerical Classification*, W. H. Freeman, San Francisco, Calif, USA, 1973.

[18] M. Kimura, "A simple method for estimating evolutionary rates of base substitutions through comparative studies of nucleotide sequences," *Journal of Molecular Evolution*, vol. 16, no. 2, pp. 111–120, 1980.

[19] S. Kumar, G. Stecher, and K. Tamura, "MEGA7: Molecular Evolutionary Genetics Analysis version 7.0 for bigger datasets," *Molecular Biology and Evolution*, vol. 33, no. 7, pp. 1870–1874, 2016.

[20] J. Felsenstein, "Confidence limits on phylogenies: an approach using the bootstrap," *Evolution*, vol. 39, pp. 783–791, 1985.

[21] D. Dahling and B. Wright, "Recovery of viruses from water by a modified flocculation procedure for second-step concentration. Appl Environ Microbiol," in *Accessed*, URL http,//aem.asm.org/content/51/6/1326.short, 1986, http://aem.asm.org/content/51/6/1326.short.

[22] D. Y. Tan, M. Hair-Bejo, A. R. Omar, and I. Aini, "Pathogenicity and molecular analysis of an infectious bursal disease virus isolated from Malaysian village chickens," *Avian Diseases*, vol. 48, no. 2, pp. 410–416, 2004.

[23] I. Nurulfiza, M. Hair-Bejo, Ar. Omar, and I. Aini, "Molecular characterization of recent infectious bursal disease virus isolates from Malaysia," *Acta Virol*, vol. 50, no. 1, pp. 45–51, 2017, http://cat.inist.fr/?aModele=afficheN&cpsidt=17663179.

[24] G. A. Abdel-Alim and Y. M. Saif, "Pathogenicity of Embryo-Adapted Serotype 2 OH Strain of Infectious Bursal Disease Virus in Chickens and Turkeys," *Avian Diseases*, vol. 46, no. 4, pp. 1001–1006, 2002.

[25] G. A. Abdel-Alim and Y. M. Saif, "Immunogenicity and antigenicity of very virulent strains of infectious Bursal disease viruses," *Avian Diseases*, vol. 45, no. 1, pp. 92–101, 2001.

[26] H. J. Tsai and Y. M. Saif, "Effect of Cell-Culture Passage on the Pathogenicity and Immunogenicity of Two Variant Strains of Infectious Bursal Disease Virus," *Avian Diseases*, vol. 36, no. 2, p. 415, 1992.

[27] L. Reed and H. Muench, "A simple method of estimating fifty per cent endpoints," *American Journal of Epidemiology*, vol. 27, no. 3, pp. 493–497, 1938.

[28] E. Heyderman, "Immunoperoxidase technique in histopathology: applications, methods, and controls," *Journal of Clinical Pathology*, vol. 32, no. 10, pp. 971–978, 1979.

[29] D. J. Jackwood, B. Sreedevi, L. J. LeFever, and S. E. Sommer-Wagner, "Studies on naturally occurring infectious bursal disease viruses suggest that a single amino acid substitution at position 253 in VP2 increases pathogenicity," *Virology*, vol. 377, no. 1, pp. 110–116, 2008.

[30] A. Jungmann, H. Nieper, and H. Müller, "Apoptosis is induced by infectious bursal disease virus replication in productively infected cells as well as in antigen-negative cells in their vicinity," *Journal of General Virology*, vol. 82, no. 5, pp. 1107–1115, 2001.

[31] C. D. Bayliss, U. Spies, K. Shaw et al., "A comparison of the sequences of segment A of four infectious bursal disease virus strains and identification of a variable region in VP2," *Journal of General Virology*, vol. 71, no. 6, pp. 1303–1312, 1990.

[32] oie IBD 2008.pdf.

[33] OIE, "Infectious Bursal Disease (Gumboro disease)," in *OIE Terrestial Man*, 2016, Chapter 2.3.12.

[34] G. A. Abdel-Alim and Y. M. Saif, "Pathogenicity of cell culture-derived and bursa-derived infectious bursal disease viruses in specific-pathogen-free chickens," *Avian Diseases*, vol. 45, no. 4, pp. 844–852, 2001.

[35] N. Atale, S. Gupta, U. C. S. Yadav, and V. Rani, "Cell-death assessment by fluorescent and nonfluorescent cytosolic and nuclear staining techniques," *Journal of Microscopy*, vol. 255, no. 1, pp. 7–19, 2014.

[36] B. S. Cummings, L. P. Wills, and R. G. Schnellmann, "Measurement of Cell Death in Mammalian Cells," in *Curr Protoc Phamacol*, vol. 1 (Lemasters 1999), pp. 30-10, 1999.

[37] J. C. Rodríguez-Lecompte, R. Niño-Fong, A. Lopez, R. J. Frederick Markham, and F. S. B. Kibenge, "Infectious bursal disease virus (IBDV) induces apoptosis in chicken B cells," *Comparative Immunology, Microbiology and Infectious Diseases*, vol. 28, no. 4, pp. 321–337, 2005.

[38] K. M. Tham and C. D. Moon, "Apoptosis in cell cultures induced by infectious bursal disease virus following in vitro infection," *Avian Diseases*, vol. 40, no. 1, pp. 109–113, 1996.

[39] K. Yao and V. N. Vakharia, "Induction of apoptosis in vitro by the 17-kDa nonstructural protein of infectious bursal disease virus: Possible role in viral pathogenesis," *Virology*, vol. 285, no. 1, pp. 50–58, 2001.

[40] L. L. Kong, A. R. Omar, M. Hair-Bejo, I. Aini, and H. F. Seow, "Comparative analysis of viral RNA and apoptotic cells in bursae following infection with infectious bursal disease virus," *Comparative Immunology, Microbiology and Infectious Diseases*, vol. 27, no. 6, pp. 433–443, 2004.

[41] A. F. Tapparo, D. E. Gomes, C. Silva, H. F. Ferrari, M. C. R. Luvizotto, and T. C. Cardoso, "Apoptosis detection in embryonic chicken lymphoid tissues infected with attenuated very virulent infectious bursal disease virus (vvIBDV)," *Brazilian Journal Veterinary Pathology*, vol. 2, no. 2, pp. 75–79, 2009.

[42] S. I. Abdel Wahab, A. B. Abdul, A. S. Alzubairi, M. M. Elhassan, and S. Mohan, "In vitro ultramorphological assessment of apoptosis induced by Zerumbone on (HeLa)," *Journal of Biomedicine and Biotechnology*, vol. 2009, Article ID 769568, 10 pages, 2009.

[43] C. Riccardi and I. C. Nicoletti, "Analysis of apoptosis by propidium iodide staining and flow cytometry," *Nature Protocols*, vol. 1, no. 3, pp. 1458–1461, 2006.

[44] H. Nieper, J. P. Teifke, A. Jungmann, C. V. Löhr, and H. Müller, "Infected and apoptotic cells in the IBDV-infected bursa of Fabricius, studied by double-labelling techniques," *Avian Pathology*, vol. 28, no. 3, pp. 279–285, 1999.

[45] G. Ponte and G. Fiorito, "Immunohistochemical analysis of neuronal networks in the nervous system of octopus vulgaris," *Neuromethods*, vol. 101, pp. 63–79, 2015.

[46] J. S. Cruz-Coy, J. J. Giambrone, and F. J. Hoerr, "Immunohistochemical detection of infectious bursal disease virus in formalin-fixed, paraffin-embedded chicken tissues using monoclonal antibody." *Avian Diseases*, vol. 37, no. 2, pp. 577–581, 1993.

[47] J. Singh, H. S. Banga, R. S. Brar, N. D. Singh, S. Sodhi, and G. D. Leishangthem, "Histopathological and immunohistochemical diagnosis of infectious bursal disease in poultry birds," *Veterinary World*, vol. 8, no. 11, pp. 1331–1339, 2015.

[48] P. C. Tissues, U. Monoclonal, J. J. Giambrone, and F. J. Hoerr, "Nmmunohistochemical detection of infectious bursal disease virus in formalin-fixed," *Paraffin-Embedded Chicken Tissues Using Monoclonal Antibody*, vol. 37, no. 2, pp. 577–581, 2015.

[49] M. G. J. Tacken, P. J. M. Rottier, A. L. J. Gielkens, and B. P. H. Peeters, "Interactions in vivo between the proteins of infectious bursal disease virus: Capsid protein VP3 interacts with the RNA-dependent RNA polymerase, VP1," *Journal of General Virology*, vol. 81, no. 1, pp. 209–218, 2000.

[50] T. C. Cardoso, P. Rahal, D. Pilz, M. C. B. Teixeira, and C. W. Arns, "Replication of classical infectious bursal disease virus in the chicken embryo related cell line," *Avian Pathology*, vol. 29, no. 3, pp. 213–217, 2000.

[51] N. Eterradossi, C. Arnauld, F. Tekaia et al., "Antigenic and genetic relationships between European very virulent infectious bursal disease viruses and an early West African isolate," *Avian Pathology*, vol. 28, no. 1, pp. 36–46, 1999.

[52] D. J. Jackwood and S. E. Sommer-Wagner, "Amino acids contributing to antigenic drift in the infectious bursal disease Birnavirus (IBDV)," *Virology*, vol. 409, no. 1, pp. 33–37, 2011.

[53] L. Delgui, D. González, and J. F. Rodríguez, "Infectious bursal disease virus persistently infects bursal B-lymphoid DT40 cells," *Journal of General Virology*, vol. 90, no. 5, pp. 1148–1152, 2009.

[54] E. Mundt, "Tissue culture infectivity of different strains of infectious bursal disease virus is determined by distinct amino acids in VP2," *Journal of General Virology*, vol. 80, no. 8, pp. 2067–2076, 1999.

[55] B.-L. Lim, Y. Cao, T. Yu, and C.-W. Mo, "Adaptation of very virulent infectious bursal disease virus to chicken embryonic fibroblasts by site-directed mutagenesis of residues 279 and 284 of viral coat protein VP2," *Journal of Virology*, vol. 73, no. 4, pp. 2854–2862, 1999.

[56] D. Jackwood, B. Sreedevi, and L. LeFever, "Studies on naturally occurring infectious bursal disease viruses suggest that a single amino acid substitution at position 253 in VP2 increases pathogenicity," *Virology*, vol. 377, no. 1, pp. 110–116, 2008.

[57] M. M. Hoque, A. R. Omar, L. K. Chong, M. Hair-Bejo, and I. Aini, "Pathogenicity of SspI-positive infectious bursal disease virus and molecular characterization of the VP2 hypervariable region," *Avian Pathology*, vol. 30, no. 4, pp. 369–380, 2001.

[58] D. Lazarus, M. Pasmanik-Chor, B. Gutter et al., "Attenuation of very virulent infectious bursal disease virus and comparison of full sequences of virulent and attenuated strains," *Avian Pathology*, vol. 37, no. 2, pp. 151–159, 2008.

13

Serological Investigation of Akabane Virus Infection in Cattle and Sheep in Nigeria

Daniel Oladimeji Oluwayelu, Comfort Oluladun Aiki-Raji, Emmanuel Chibuzor Umeh, Samat Odunayo Mustapha, and Adebowale Idris Adebiyi

Department of Veterinary Microbiology and Parasitology, University of Ibadan, Ibadan 20005, Nigeria

Correspondence should be addressed to Daniel Oladimeji Oluwayelu; ogloryus@yahoo.com

Academic Editor: Jay C. Brown

Akabane virus (AKAV) is recognized as an important pathogen that causes abortions and congenital malformations in ruminants. However, it has not received adequate attention in Nigeria. Therefore, in investigating this disease, serum samples from 184 (abattoir and farm) head of cattle and 184 intensively reared sheep from two states in southwest Nigeria were screened for antibodies against AKAV using enzyme-linked immunosorbent assay. An overall seropositivity of 70.1% (129/184) was obtained with antibodies being detectable in 73.8% of abattoir (trade) cattle and 40.0% in farm cattle, while 4.3% (8/184) seropositivity was observed in sheep. All the age groups of cattle tested had seropositive animals, 0-1 year (1/7, 14.3%), 2-3 years (17/34, 50.0%), 4-5 years (92/121, 76.0%), and >5 years (19/22, 86.4%), while in sheep only the age groups of 2-3 and 4-5 years showed seropositivity of 4.1% (4/97) and 8.2% (4/49), respectively. The detection of antibody-positive animals among unvaccinated cattle and sheep provides evidence of AKAV infection in Nigeria. These findings call for continuous monitoring of the disease among ruminants in order to ascertain the actual burden and increase awareness of the disease. This will facilitate early detection and aid the development of appropriate control measures against the disease in Nigeria.

1. Introduction

The family Bunyaviridae is the largest virus family with over 350 member viruses that are classified into five genera, including the *Orthobunyavirus* genus which contains a large number of viruses that share common genetic features [1]. Based on serological relationships, viruses in this genus have been divided into serogroups with the Simbu serogroup being one of the largest. Several Simbu serogroup viruses isolated from domestic and wild animals as well as mosquito and *Culicoides* vectors have been found in Africa, Australia, Asia, and the Middle East [2–6]. This serogroup, which includes Akabane, Aino, and Shamonda viruses, plays a significant role as pathogens of ruminants with Akabane virus (AKAV) being the most recognized [7]. In particular, Akabane virus, a teratogenic, *Culicoides*-borne virus, replicates in many kinds of natural host species and in several experimental animals [8]. Based on serological evidence, cattle, horses, donkeys, sheep, goats, pigs, camels, and buffaloes appear to be infected in

natural situations [9, 10]. AKAV has been identified as a cause of seasonal epizootics of reproductive disorders (abortions, premature births, and stillbirths) and congenital arthrogryposis, hydranencephaly, or microencephaly in cattle, sheep, and goats, sometimes resulting in significant economic losses [1, 6, 11].

Although virus isolation [2], histopathology, immunohistochemistry, serology, and genetic analysis [12] have been used for laboratory confirmation of AKAV infections, serology is the most practical and commonly used technique. Specific antibodies against AKAV have been detected using virus neutralization test (VNT) and enzyme-linked immunosorbent assay (ELISA) [13, 14]. In Africa, limited information based on virus isolation and/or serology revealed the presence of AKAV in Kenya [2, 10], Sudan [15, 16], South Africa [5, 17], Zimbabwe [18], and Tanzania [19] with limited information from Nigeria and perhaps West Africa. In Nigeria, although abortions and congenital malformations associated with AKAV such as arthrogryposis, kyphosis, and scoliosis have been reported in ruminants [20–22], the virus has not received adequate attention as a possible cause of these conditions. Therefore, as part of ongoing surveillance for *Culicoides*-borne arboviruses of livestock in Nigeria, we investigated the presence of specific antibodies against AKAV in cattle and sheep from Oyo and Ogun states, southwest Nigeria.

2. Materials and Methods

2.1. Study Area. This study was based on a cross-sectional design and conducted between May and September 2015 in Ogun and Oyo states of southwest Nigeria. The study area extended from latitudes $7°00'$ to $8°00'$ north and longitudes $3°35'$ to $4°00'$ east. Sera were collected in Oyo state from 184 head of trade cattle at the central municipal abattoirs in Bodija and Ogbomoso and a privately owned farm at Ido where they were kept semi-intensively. Cattle slaughtered at the abattoirs are sourced mainly from the northern part of the country and neighbouring countries, where they were reared on free-range management system that exposes them to insect vectors. Also, 184 sera were collected from semi-intensively reared sheep from farms and backyard flocks in Akinyele, Egbeda, Ido, Ibadan North, and Ona-Ara in Oyo state as well as from Imeko and Odeda in Ogun state. The semi-intensively managed cattle and sheep were allowed to graze on pastures during the day and kept indoors at night. However, the animal houses were not insect-proof.

2.2. Sample Collection. Blood (about 5 mL) was collected at slaughter from abattoir cattle while farm cattle and sheep were bled via the jugular vein into sterile plain bottles without anticoagulant. The blood was allowed to clot at room temperature after which sera were decanted into sterile Eppendorf tubes and stored at −20°C until tested.

2.3. Detection of AKAV Antibodies by Competitive ELISA. All the collected sera were analyzed using a commercially available ID Screen® competition ELISA kit (IDvet, Montpellier, France) that detects anti-G1 antibodies directed against AKAV in ruminant serum and plasma. The test, which was reported by the manufacturer to lack cross-reactivity with other viruses in the *Bunyaviridae* family, such as Schmallenberg virus (SBV), Rift Valley fever virus (RVFV), and Aino virus, and to have a high (96.52%) correlation with the VNT, was performed according to the kit protocol. For each sample, results were expressed as sample/negative percentage (S/N%) using the optical densities (OD) from the ELISA reader: $S/N\% = OD_{sample}/OD_{negative\ control} \times 100$. Samples that presented S/N% lower than 30%, between 30% and 40%, and >40% were considered positive, doubtful, and negative, respectively.

2.4. Statistical Analysis. Results of serology were analyzed using the statistical package GraphPad Prism version 5.01 (San Diego, USA). Differences in AKAV antibody seroprevalence between cattle and sheep, abattoir and farm cattle, and male and female animals were evaluated using chi-square (χ^2) test. Furthermore, seroprevalence results based on breed,

TABLE 1: Prevalence of AKAV antibodies in sheep and cattle in the study area.

	Number sampled	Positive (%)	Doubtful (%)	Negative (%)
Sheep	184	8 (4.4)	22 (12.0)	154 (83.7)
Cattle	184	129 (70.1)*	37 (20.1)	18 (9.8)
Total	364	137 (37.6)	59 (16.2)	172 (47.3)

*$P = 0.0001$.

TABLE 2: Seroprevalence of AKAV in cattle in the study area.

Variable	Group	Number sampled	Positive (%)
Sex	Female	131	92 (70.2)
	Male	53	37 (69.8)
Age (years)	0-1	7	1 (14.3)*
	2-3	34	17 (50.0)
	4-5	121	92 (76.0)
	>5	22	19 (86.4)*
Source	Abattoir	164	121 (73.8)*
	Farm	20	8 (40.0)

*$P = 0.0001$.

age group, and location were subjected to one-way ANOVA and subsequently to Tukey's posttest for performing multiple comparisons in order to assess statistically significant differences between all possible pairs of groups. The level of statistical significance was $P < 0.05$.

3. Results

Out of 184 sheep sera tested, 8 (4.4%), 22 (12.0%), and 154 (83.7%) were positive, doubtful, and negative, respectively, for AKAV anti-G1 antibodies while, of the 184 cattle sera tested, 129 (70.1%), 37 (20.1%), and 18 (9.8%) were positive, doubtful, and negative, respectively (Table 1). The prevalence of AKAV antibodies was significantly ($P < 0.005$) higher in abattoir cattle compared to farm cattle (Table 2). For the abattoir cattle, AKAV antibody prevalence was significantly higher in Bodija central abattoir compared to the Ogbomosho abattoir. Overall, based on cattle breed, AKAV antibody prevalence was 66.4% (75/113), 77.8% (28/36), 75.0% (3/4), 83.3% (10/12), and 76.5% (13/17) for White Fulani, Sokoto Gudali, Kuri, Red Bororo, and crossbreeds, respectively. However, comparison of the AKAV seroprevalence rates in sheep based on age, sex, breed, and location of sample collection revealed no significant differences.

4. Discussion

Akabane virus has been shown to be an important pathogen causing abortions and congenital malformations in ruminants [23]. Antibodies to this *Culicoides*-borne, Simbu serogroup virus have been found in ruminants from countries of Australia, Asia, Southeast Asia, the Middle East, and Africa [6, 10, 16, 24, 25]. However, since the initial isolation of Simbu group viruses from cattle and *Culicoides* biting midges in Nigeria [26, 27], there has been no report on the presence of AKAV in Nigeria. In the present study, which is part of ongoing surveillance for *Culicoides*-borne arboviruses in Nigeria [28, 29], AKAV antibody prevalence of 70.1% and 4.3%, respectively, was obtained for cattle and sheep in two states (Ogun and Oyo) of southwest Nigeria using a competition ELISA. According to the internal validation report of the kit manufacturer on the assay, known SBV-, RVFV-, and Aino virus-positive sera produced negative results with the AKAV ELISA kit, demonstrating the absence of cross-reactions with antisera against these viruses. To our knowledge, this is the first report of AKAV antibody-positive animals in Nigeria. As AKAV vaccines are currently not administered to livestock in the country, the detection of seropositive cattle and sheep in this study suggests natural exposure of these animals to AKAV. The higher seroprevalence obtained for cattle, which is similar to the findings of a recent study in Sudan [16], is an indication that they were more likely to be infected with AKAV than sheep. This possibility is buttressed by the knowledge that cattle are allowed to graze more extensively, thus making them more exposed to the *Culicoides* vectors of AKAV than sheep. Moreover, it has previously been reported [30] that some *Culicoides* species have distinct feeding preference for cattle over sheep even when kept in the same vicinity.

Furthermore, it was observed in this study that AKAV antibodies were more prevalent in trade cattle from abattoirs than in farm cattle. This higher seroprevalence may be due to the fact that, compared to farm cattle which are domiciled in one location, trade cattle for slaughter at these abattoirs are sourced from different parts of Nigeria and neighbouring countries where they are kept mostly on free-range. This makes the abattoirs convergence points for animals from diverse geographical locations where they could have had contact with infected *Culicoides* vectors. Since there is unregulated transborder movement of ruminants from neighbouring West African countries into Nigeria, it is possible that some of the seropositive cattle could have imported the disease into the country. Also, the detection of seropositive animals among trade cattle of different breeds suggests that the disease is not breed-restricted.

Previous reports of congenital malformations in cattle and sheep in Nigeria suggested that these defects have no clearly established cause [20–22, 31]. However, the increased prevalence of AKAV antibodies observed with increasing age of cattle and sheep in this study (Table 2) suggests AKAV as a possible cause of these conditions. Since it has been reported that inapparent Akabane infection in adults can lead to abortions, stillbirth, and congenital defects in newborns [10, 32], this finding suggests that AKAV may significantly increase abortion risk among adult cattle and sheep, thus constituting a potential health risk to the animals. Therefore, the findings of this study corroborate the fact that AKAV is endemic in sub-Saharan Africa and underscore the need for large-scale surveillance of the virus in Nigeria in order to establish its role as a possible cause of economic losses in ruminants through abortions, stillbirths, and con-

genital malformations and develop effective prevention and control strategies. Additionally, virus isolation and genetic characterization of isolates will be essential for understanding the molecular epidemiology and evolution of AKAV in Nigeria.

References

[1] N. J. MacLachlan and E. J. Dubovi, "Bunyaviridae," in *Fenner's Veterinary Virology*, pp. 371–383, Academic Press, London, UK, 4th edition, 2011.

[2] D. Metselaar and Y. Robin, "Akabane virus isolated in Kenya," *Veterinary Record*, vol. 99, no. 5, p. 86, 1976.

[3] W. J. Hartley and R. A. Wanner, "Bovine congenital arthrogryposis in New South Wales," *Australian Veterinary Journal*, vol. 50, no. 5, pp. 185–188, 1974.

[4] Y. Miura, Y. Inaba, T. Tsuda et al., "A survey of antibodies to arthropod-borne viruses in Indonesian cattle," *Japanese Journal of Veterinary Science*, vol. 44, no. 6, pp. 857–863, 1982.

[5] H. Zeller and M. Bouloy, "Infections by viruses of the families *Bunyaviridae* and *Filoviridae*," *Revue Scientifique et Technique*, vol. 19, no. 1, pp. 79–91, 2000.

[6] O. Markusfield and E. Mayer, "An arthrogryposis and hydranencephaly syndrome in calves in Israel, 1969-70: epidemiological and clinical aspects," *Refuah Veterinarith*, vol. 28, pp. 51–61, 1971.

[7] T. D. St George and P. D. Kirkland, "Diseases caused by Akabane and related Simbu-group viruses," in *Infectious Diseases of Livestock*, J. A. W. Coetzer and R. C. Tustin, Eds., pp. 1029–1036, Oxford University Press, Oxford, UK, 2nd edition, 2004.

[8] C.-C. Huang, T.-S. Huang, M. C. Deng, M.-H. Jong, and S.-Y. Lin, "Natural infections of pigs with Akabane virus," *Veterinary Microbiology*, vol. 94, no. 1, pp. 1–11, 2003.

[9] S. Al-Busaidy, C. Hamblin, and W. P. Taylor, "Neutralising antibodies to Akabane virus in free-living wild animals in Africa," *Tropical Animal Health and Production*, vol. 19, no. 4, pp. 197–202, 1987.

[10] F. G. Davies and D. M. Jessett, "A study of the host range and distribution of antibody to Akabane virus (genus bunyavirus, family *Bunyaviridae*) in Kenya," *Journal of Hygiene*, vol. 95, no. 1, pp. 191–196, 1985.

[11] H. Kurogi, Y. Inaba, Y. Goto et al., "Serologic evidence for etiologic role of Akabane virus in epizootic abortion-arthrogryposis-hydranencephaly in cattle in Japan, 1972-1974," *Archives of Virology*, vol. 47, no. 1, pp. 71–83, 1975.

[12] J.-K. Oem, H.-J. Yoon, H.-R. Kim et al., "Genetic and pathogenic characterization of Akabane viruses isolated from cattle with encephalomyelitis in Korea," *Veterinary Microbiology*, vol. 158, no. 3-4, pp. 259–266, 2012.

[13] Y. Miura, S. Hayashi, T. Ishihara, Y. Inaba, T. Omori, and M. Matumoto, "Neutralizing antibody against Akabane virus in precolostral sera from calves with congenital arthrogryposis-hydranencephaly syndrome," *Archiv für die Gesamte Virusforschung*, vol. 46, no. 3-4, pp. 377–380, 1974.

[14] T. Tsuda, K. Yoshida, T. Yanase, S. Ohashi, and M. Yamakawa, "Competitive enzyme-linked immunosorbent assay for the detection of the antibodies specific to Akabane virus," *Journal of Veterinary Diagnostic Investigation*, vol. 16, no. 6, pp. 571–576, 2004.

[15] M. E. Mohamed, P. S. Mellor, and W. P. Taylor, "Akabane virus: serological survey of antibodies in livestock in the Sudan," *Revue d'Elevage et de Médecine Vétérinaire des pays Tropicaux*, vol. 49, no. 4, pp. 285–288, 1996.

[16] A. M. Elhassan, M. E. A. Mansour, A. A. A. Shamon, and A. M. El Hussein, "A serological survey of Akabane virus infection in cattle in Sudan," *ISRN Veterinary Science*, vol. 2014, Article ID 123904, 4 pages, 2014.

[17] A. Theodoridis, E. M. Nevill, H. J. Els, and S. T. Boshoff, "Viruses isolated from Culicoides midges in South Africa during unsuccessful attempts to isolate bovine ephemeral fever virus," *Onderstepoort Journal of Veterinary Research*, vol. 46, no. 4, pp. 191–198, 1979.

[18] N. K. Blackburn, I. Searle, and B. J. Phelps, "Viruses isolated from *Culicoides* (Diptera: Ceratopogonidae) caught at the veterinary research farm, Mazowe, Zimbabwe," *Journal of the Entomological Society of South Africa*, vol. 48, no. 2, pp. 331–336, 1985.

[19] C. Mathew, S. Klevar, A. R. W. Elbers et al., "Detection of serum neutralizing antibodies to Simbu sero-group viruses in cattle in Tanzania," *BMC Veterinary Research*, vol. 11, article 208, 2015.

[20] I. U. Ate and L. Allam, "Multiple congenital skeletal malformations in a lamb associated with dystocia in a Yankasa ewe," *Nigerian Veterinary Journal*, vol. 23, no. 1, pp. 61–63, 2002.

[21] M. M. Bukar, M. Waziri, and U. I. Ibrahim, "Dystocia due to arthrogryposis and associated with a mummified twin in a crossed (Yankassa/Uda) ewe: a case report," *Tropical Veterinarian*, vol. 24, no. 4, pp. 85–88, 2006.

[22] N. D. Ibrahim, S. Adamu, S. M. Useh et al., "Multiple congenital defects in a Bunaji bull," *Nigerian Veterinary Journal*, vol. 27, no. 3, pp. 80–86, 2006.

[23] O. R. Coverdale, D. H. Cybinski, and T. D. St George, "Congenital abnormalities in calves associated with Akabane virus and Aino virus," *Australian Veterinary Journal*, vol. 54, no. 3, pp. 151–152, 1978.

[24] W. J. Hartley, R. A. Wanner, A. J. Della-Porta, and W. A. Snowdon, "Serological evidence for the association of Akabane virus with epizootic bovine congenital arthrogryposis and hydranencephaly syndromes in New South Wales," *Australian Veterinary Journal*, vol. 51, no. 2, pp. 103–104, 1975.

[25] S. M. Al-Busaidy, P. S. Mellor, and W. P. Taylor, "Prevalence of neutralising antibodies to Akabane virus in the Arabian Peninsula," *Veterinary Microbiology*, vol. 17, no. 2, pp. 141–149, 1988.

[26] O. R. Causey, G. E. Kemp, C. E. Causey, and V. H. Lee, "Isolation of Simbu-group viruses in Ibadan, Nigeria 1964–69, including the new types Sango, Shamonda, Sabo and Shuni," *Annals of Tropical Medicine and Parasitology*, vol. 66, no. 3, pp. 357–362, 1972.

[27] V. H. Lee, "Isolation of viruses from field populations of *Culicoides* (Diptera: Ceratopogonidae) in Nigeria," *Journal of Medical Entomology*, vol. 16, no. 1, pp. 76–79, 1979.

[28] D. O. Oluwayelu, O. Olatoye, M. Akanbi, and B. Hoffmann, "Seroprevalence of bluetongue virus infection in Oyo state, Nigeria," *Journal of Commonwealth Veterinary Association*, vol. 27, no. 2, pp. 234–238, 2011.

[29] D. O. Oluwayelu, C. O. Meseko, and A. I. Adebiyi, "Serological screening for Schmallenberg virus in exotic and indigenous cattle in Nigeria," *Sokoto Journal of Veterinary Sciences*, vol. 13, no. 3, pp. 14–18, 2015.

[30] S. Bartsch, B. Bauer, A. Wiemann, P.-H. Clausen, and S. Steuber, "Feeding patterns of biting midges of the *Culicoides obsoletus* and *Culicoides pulicaris* groups on selected farms in Brandenburg, Germany," *Parasitology Research*, vol. 105, no. 2, pp. 373–380, 2009.

[31] A. A. Bello, I. A. Nwanena, I. Hamman, and C. T. Aba, "Foetal monster in a four-year old Yankassa ewe with dystocia: a case report," *Tropical Veterinarian*, vol. 24, no. 4, pp. 89–94, 2006.

[32] P. D. Kirkland, R. D. Barry, P. A. Harper, and R. Z. Zelski, "The development of Akabane virus-induced congenital abnormalities in cattle," *Veterinary Record*, vol. 122, no. 24, pp. 582–586, 1988.

14

Farming of Plant-Based Veterinary Vaccines and their Applications for Disease Prevention in Animals

Pit Sze Liew and Mohd Hair-Bejo

Department of Veterinary Pathology and Microbiology, Faculty of Veterinary Medicine,
Universiti Putra Malaysia, 43400 Serdang, Malaysia

Correspondence should be addressed to Mohd Hair-Bejo; mdhair@upm.edu.my

Academic Editor: Jay C. Brown

Plants have been studied for the production of pharmaceutical compounds for more than two decades now. Ever since the plant-made poultry vaccine against Newcastle disease virus made a breakthrough and went all the way to obtain regulatory approval, research to use plants for expression and delivery of vaccine proteins for animals was intensified. Indeed, in view of the high production costs of veterinary vaccines, plants represent attractive biofactories and offer many promising advantages in the production of recombinant vaccine proteins. Furthermore, the possibility of conducting immunogenicity and challenge studies in target animals has greatly exaggerated the progress. Although there are no edible plant-produced animal vaccines in the market, plant-based vaccine technology has great potentials. In this review, development, uses, and advantages of plant-based recombinant protein production in various expression platforms are discussed. In addition, examples of plant-based veterinary vaccines showing strong indication in terms of efficacy in animal disease prevention are also described.

1. Introduction

Plant molecular farming is a term used to describe the application of molecular biological techniques to the synthesis of commercial products in plants, which include a variety of carbohydrates, fats, and proteins, as well as secondary products [1]. The process of manufacturing a plant-based vaccine in the plant green factory begins with the selection of a target antigen of interest. The vaccine candidate is cloned into a plant expression cassette that is capable of promoting and terminating transgene expression. The expression cassette is then delivered into a plant for the production of a recombinant protein [2].

The delivery of an expression cassette carrying the gene of interest into the plant cells could be achieved by either stable or transient transformation. Transient gene expression represents a rapid and convenient system for verification and characterisation of the target gene product. Notwithstanding, it is now a routine practice in molecular farming for the production of foreign proteins [3]. The process circumvents the long development time and low protein accumulation

levels associated with the use of transgenic plants. Besides, as the foreign protein production is only temporary, it requires no selection method to identify transformed plant cells. Compared to transient expression systems, the major advantage of stable transgenic lines is that the candidate gene sequence is incorporated into the plant genome and thus the acquired protein production trait is inherited. This allows the transfer of the desired character to the next and over multiple generations [4]. Thus, seed stock could be established, which assures the continuing availability of the stock [5].

2. Brief History of Development of Plant-Based Recombinant Protein Production

The idea of plant molecular farming was burgeoning about 26 years ago when the proof of concept recombinant plant-derived pharmaceutical proteins was reported (Table 1; [1, 6]). Among these, biologically active human interferon alpha D was produced in turnip following inoculation with mutant cauliflower mosaic virus carrying human interferon alpha D at its ORF II [7]. In the same year, tobacco plants expressing

TABLE 1: Various applications of plant-based expression system and key events related to their development.

Product	Plant host(s)	Importance	References
Human pharmaceutical proteins			
Human interferon-α	Turnip	First recombinant plant-derived pharmaceutical proteins.	[7]
Human serum albumin	Tobacco, potato	Plant-derived proteins identical to the authentic human proteins.	[9]
Antibodies			
Mouse immunoglobulin	Tobacco	First plant-derived antibody showing the ability of plants to assemble heterologous biomolecules.	[8]
Antibody against hepatitis B	Tobacco	First commercialized plant-derived antibody used for vaccine purification in Cuba.	[10]
Antibody against *Streptococcus mutans* (CaroRx)	Tobacco	EU-approved medical device for prevention of tooth decay.	[6, 11]
Industrial and agricultural recombinant enzymes			
Avidin	Maize		[12]
β-glucuronidase	Maize	Plant-derived products on the market.	[13]
Trypsin	Maize		[14]
Vaccine antigens– human use			
Hepatitis B antigen	Tobacco	Plant-made HBsAg particles antigenically and physically similar to HBsAg particles derived from human serum and recombinant yeast.	[15]
	Lettuce, lupin	Specific antibody responses in human volunteers fed with transgenic lettuce.	[16]
	Potato	Increased specific serum immune response when given orally as a booster to vaccinated human volunteers.	[17]
Escherichia coli LT-B	Potato	First proof of concept for edible plant-derived vaccines that conferred protection to mice upon oral feeding.	[18]
	Maize	Specific serum and mucosal antibody responses in human volunteers ingested transgenic corn germ meal.	[19]
Norwalk virus	Tobacco, potato	Specific serum and mucosal antibody responses in mice fed orally with transgenic plants. Phase I clinical trials completed.	[20]
Vaccine antigens– veterinary use			
Newcastle disease virus HN proteins	Tobacco suspension cell culture	First USDA-approved plant-derived veterinary vaccine.	[21]

either gamma or kappa immunoglobulin chains of mouse were crossed to generate progeny expressing both chains of immunoglobulin, showing the ability of plants to assemble heterologous biomolecules [8]. Then, the production of human serum albumin in tobacco and potato plants which was identical to the authentic human protein was reported [9].

The idea has since expanded to the production of many industrial and agricultural recombinant enzymes. The leading examples were avidin [12], β-glucuronidase [13], and trypsin [14]. Besides, the use of plants for the production of foreign proteins especially biomedically important materials is wide and varied. Several biopharmaceuticals like growth hormones, human blood components, and cytokines have been expressed in plants [6, 11]. Furthermore, many medically related proteins including antibodies or vaccines for human and veterinary use are continually being explored and developed. The monoclonal antibody against hepatitis B surface antigen (HBsAg), expressed in tobacco, was the first commercialized plant-derived antibody. Being marketed in Cuba, it has replaced the mouse derived monoclonal antibody for the routine purification of recombinant HBsAg for hepatitis B vaccine production [10]. Plant-made antibodies currently in the pipeline for commercialization include those against *Streptococcus mutans* and non-Hodgkin's lymphoma [6, 11]. The monoclonal secretory antibody against *S. mutans* made in plant was shown to prevent colonisation of microbes in the human oral cavity [22]. It has since been approved as a medical device in 2003 by the European regulatory authority for human use and commercialized as CaroRx [6].

On the other hand, a variety of vaccine antigens have been well tested for expression in plants, be it for human or veterinary applications. Among the vaccine targets intended for human use, *S. mutans* surface protein A for dental caries and HBsAg for viral hepatitis B were the first to be explored [23]. It has been demonstrated that the plant-made 22 nm particles of HBsAg were similar to HBsAg particles derived from human serum and recombinant yeast, both antigenically and physically [15]. Subsequently, various vaccine candidates including *E. coli* heat-labile enterotoxin B subunit (LT-B), Norwalk virus particles, and cholera toxin B subunit have been expressed in plants [23, 24]. The bacterial antigen LT-B made the first proof of concept for edible plant-produced vaccines by showing that the orally delivered vaccine conferred protective efficacy to mice [18]. Moreover, the vaccine targeting antigens like viral hepatitis B, LT-B, and Norwalk virus are heading towards advanced stages of development and have completed the phase I clinical trials [6]. Notwithstanding, many vaccine antigens are making their way forward although they were in the early stage of development. These include and are not limited to vaccines for rotavirus infection [25], measles [26, 27], human immunodeficiency virus type 1 [28–30], human cytomegalovirus [31], respiratory syncytial virus [32, 33], *Staphylococcus aureus* [34], *Pseudomonas aeruginosa* [35, 36], and *Plasmodium falciparum* [37].

However, it was a plant-made poultry vaccine against Newcastle disease virus (NDV) that turned out to be the first plant-based vaccine to obtain regulatory approval from the United States Department of Agriculture, Center for Veterinary Biologics [21]. The NDV vaccine was shown to confer more than 90% protection rate in chicken upon challenge with NDV. Although the proof of concept poultry vaccine has not been commercialized and there are no other veterinary vaccines introduced into the market since then, animal pathogens have become the focus for expression in plants [38]. Indeed, the number and range of candidate antigens from animal microbes and viruses that have been expressed in plants are extensive [39]. The possibility of carrying out challenge experiments in specific animal species of interest has encouraged and resulted in enthusiastic development of plant-made veterinary vaccines.

3. Merits of Plant Production System

Since the early 1990s, plants have gained an additional role of being bioreactors in molecular farming for new drugs and vaccines [38]. Whole plants, either by stable or transient transformation, were used to produce foreign target antigens of interest [40] that have the potential of being applied in routine vaccination strategies. Plants, therefore, represent attractive alternatives for vaccine production. Different parts of plants like the leaf and stem tissues, seeds, and fruits and root vegetables have been used for production of foreign proteins. Some of the commonest species of plants used include small flowering weed *Arabidopsis thaliana* that is widely used in plant science, tobaccos, alfalfa, spinach, potatoes, rice, beans, maize, tomatoes, strawberries, carrots, and many more [3]. Initially conceptualized as a platform for production of edible vaccines [41], expression of foreign proteins in plants aims to reduce the use of needles and cold chain for vaccine delivery especially in the developing countries. Besides, should the food plants be used for foreign protein expression especially for vaccines, they could be consumed directly or with only minimal processing. Nevertheless, plants offer many other advantages over other production systems.

The production cost in plants is only a fraction of that of mammalian cell systems and between 10 and 50 times lower than microbial system like *E. coli* fermentation for producing the same protein [42, 43]. The farming of transgenic plants requires relatively basic and economical propagation materials like sunlight, water, and nutrients. Furthermore, the harvest and downstream processing of transgenic plants require an uncomplicated technology and the scale-up of production is simple and rapid as they can be done by increasing the cultivation area [41].

Production of foreign proteins in plants is generally considered safe when compared to mammalian cell systems, as they are less likely to harbour microbes or prions that are pathogenic to humans or animals [41]. The conventional live veterinary vaccines especially of viral origins, intended for use in poultry, are typically propagated in chicken embryos or cell culture systems. These vaccines consist mainly of attenuated virus strains that have lost their virulent properties but are still replicative and demonstrate the desired antigenic features. Although the vaccines can mimic the course of naturally acquired immunity, they bear the risk of reversion to virulence, which could result in infection instead of protection [44]. Moreover, chicken embryos or animal cells propagation systems carry the inherent threat for unintentional contamination because they are rich in nutrients and thus susceptible to contamination. The avian leukosis virus has been found as a contaminant in commercial Marek's disease vaccines of poultry [45]. Although the contaminated vaccines were promptly removed from the market, it was reported that routine quality assurance measures had failed to detect the contaminant virus. This has undeniably raised safety issues of vaccine production in animal-derived sources. Plants, when used as production system, have lower risks of contamination by extraneous infectious agents.

Other than the apparent advantages in terms of cost, scalability, and safety, plant expression platforms are able to carry out posttranslational modification of proteins like disulfide bonds formation and glycosylation [46]. The proteins could be targeted to and retained in the endoplasmic reticulum of the cell to allow N-glycosylation and avoid complex-type N-glycan modifications by the Golgi apparatus [43]. Being more structurally closer to those of insect cell expression system, the use of plant system, however, would require modification and harmonization should species-specific N-glycosylation be needed to produce therapeutic glycoproteins for veterinary or human purposes [47, 48]. While animal cell cultures are able to carry out posttranslational modification and reproduce glycoproteins with N-glycan structures specific to the animal species they are derived from, they are compensated by the apparent high production cost [49]. As with the insect cell and plant expression systems, the use of mammalian cell cultures from nonhuman origin for expression of glycoproteins for human use would need to be humanized [49]. Similarly, although the microbial production systems like *E. coli* and yeasts are relatively much cheaper than mammalian cell systems, they are not be able to synthesize glycosylated proteins with desired biological properties [48]. As bacteria do not glycosylate, while yeasts may hyperglycosylate, the immunogenicity of the proteins produced might be affected [46].

4. Plant-Based Expression Platforms of Recombinant Proteins

Many plants have been explored and used for the production of recombinant proteins and vaccine antigens (Table 2; [41, 50]). Generally, these can be divided into leafy crops, fruits and root vegetables, and seeds. Soybean, alfalfa, and corn are among the most efficient plant systems for production of foreign proteins from an economic point of view [41]. Preliminary studies to generate stably transformed transgenic plants expressing proteins of interest have often seen the use of model plants such as *Arabidopsis thaliana* and tobacco [39]. With the completion of sequencing on the *Arabidopsis* nuclear genomes [51], transgenic plant research is blossoming. A variety of *Arabidopsis* lines and mutants with accessible genetics information are available. Hence, transformation protocols of *Arabidopsis* are established and could be performed successfully even by nonspecialists. However, the plant is not useful for commercial production as it has a low biomass [50].

On the contrary, tobacco could achieve a relatively high biomass yield [52]. Besides, it is a nonfood and nonfeed crop; thus the risk of transgenic tobacco entering feed and human food chains is thus reduced [50]. However, the risk of crossing with nontransgenic tobacco in the open field production cannot be fully eliminated [41]. Moreover, transgenic tobacco cannot be consumed directly without downstream processing as it contains high amount of nicotine and other toxic alkaloids that must be removed completely before it could be delivered orally. Nevertheless, low-alkaloid varieties that require less processing are available. Besides, the suspension cultures of tobacco cells are devoid of these toxic metabolites and they can also be used to produce foreign proteins [53].

Other leafy crops that have been explored for molecular farming include alfalfa, clover, and lettuce [50]. Alfalfa and clover have a relatively established transformation protocols and they can be easily cultivated by clonal propagation [41]. The plant leaves can be consumed uncooked and this is particularly useful in the development of veterinary vaccines [50]. Moreover, these leafy crops contain a high protein level and they could achieve a large dry biomass yield per hectare of land [53]. Alfalfa could be harvested many times and up to nine times in a year. The N-glycosylation pattern in alfalfa is predominantly homogenous [50]. The consistency in the N-glycosylation process is of such importance particularly in the production of therapeutic proteins as the biological functions of these proteins are affected by the N-linked glycan structures [54, 55]. In contrast to the N-glycosylation in tobacco that showed a highly heterogeneous pattern, up to 75% of the monoclonal antibody expressed in alfalfa exhibited identical glycan structures suitable for downstream humanization processing [56]. However, they have the risk of outcrossing with nontransgenic plants in the open field production. Although having a deep root system reduces the need for chemical fertilizer, transgenic plants pose some difficulties for thorough cleaning from the production field [41].

Fruits and root vegetables like tomatoes and potatoes have also become preferred plant expression hosts. Potatoes have frequently been used because the transformation protocols to generate transgenic lines are established. Tuber extracts from the transgenic lines expressing the S1 glycoprotein gene of infectious bronchitis virus (IBV) have been shown to protect the chickens from clinical disease, as well as virus shedding upon challenge [57, 58]. Besides, microtuber production of potato is available for quick assay [41]. Foreign proteins produced are also stable and could be stored for longer periods in storage tissues without refrigeration [50]. The risk of outcrossing in the open field production is low as the plant could be clonally propagated. In addition, as the industrial processing of tuber is established, the cost of downstream processing can be greatly reduced. However, potato tuber contains a relatively low protein content [41] and it is not palatable although it can be eaten raw. While cooking can improve its palatability, it might lead to denaturation of the foreign protein, thus resulting in poor immunogenicity if it was used to produce vaccine antigens [59].

Therefore, tomatoes have become a more attractive alternative system [41], since they are palatable and can be eaten

TABLE 2: Comparison of different plant-based expression platforms for recombinant proteins production.

Plant hosts	Advantages	Disadvantages
Model plants		
Arabidopsis thaliana	Often used for preliminary studies. A variety of *Arabidopsis* lines and mutants with accessible genetics information are available. Small genome size and short life cycle. Self-pollinating plant that could produce numerous seeds. Exceptional ease for transformation by *Agrobacterium*-mediated approach.	Low biomass.
Tobacco	Established transformation and expression protocols. High biomass yield. Nonfood and nonfeed crop. Less risk of feed and human food chains contamination. Low-alkaloid varieties are available, which requires less processing.	Risk of crossing with nontransgenic tobacco in the open field production. Contain high nicotine and other toxic alkaloids. Direct consumption not possible.
Leafy crops		
Alfalfa Clover Lettuce	Established transformation protocols. Clonal propagation is possible. Direct consumption and useful for animal vaccines. High protein level. Large dry biomass yield. Many harvests per year. Homogenous N-linked glycan structures in alfalfa. Edible raw and useful for human vaccines. Fast growing.	Risk of outcrossing with nontransgenic plants in the open field production. Low protein stability. Perishable tissues and must be processed soon after harvest. Deep root system in alfalfa makes them difficult for thorough cleaning from the production field.
Fruits and root vegetables		
Potato	Established transformation protocols. Microtuber production is available for quick assay. Stable storage for longer periods in storage tissues without refrigeration. Clonal propagation, low risk of outcrossing in the open field production. Industrial processing of tuber is well established.	Low protein content. Raw tuber is not palatable, while cooking might cause denaturation of the foreign protein.
Tomato	Palatable in raw form. High biomass yield. Inherent high level of vitamin A may help in boosting immune responses. Industrial cultivation and processing are well established.	Low protein content. Acidic in nature and may be incompatible with some antigens or use for infants. Spoil readily.
Cereal and legume seeds		
Maize	Most widely used cereal crop for molecular farming. Large grain size and high per hectare biomass yield. In vitro manipulation and transformation of maize are well studied. Commercial production, processing, and scalability are established.	Cross-pollinating plant. Concerns for contamination of food maize crops.
Rice	High biomass yield. Commercial production, processing, and scalability are established. Self-pollinating, reduced risk of illegitimate gene flow due to pollen release.	Longer time-to-product period.
Barley	Self-pollinating.	Less widely grown. Inefficient transformation system.
Pea Soybean	Higher protein content than that of the cereals. Self-pollinating are risk of gene flow contamination are less.	Laborious and inefficient transformation procedures. Lower annual grain yield and higher production cost compared to maize and rice.

raw without cooking. Thus, vaccine antigens expressed in them do not risk to be denatured by heat treatments. The first vaccine candidate used for expression in tomatoes was the rabies virus glycoprotein [60]. Furthermore, they had been used to express the capsid proteins VP2 and VP6 of rotavirus, which were shown to be immunogenic to mice by intraperitoneal delivery [61]. The inherent high level of vitamin A in tomatoes may also help in boosting immune responses [59]. Tomatoes have a well-established industrial cultivation and processing system just like potatoes. However, the fruit are also relatively low in protein content and must be chilled after harvest in order to prevent spoilage [59]. Although freeze-drying technology is available to preserve the fruit, this adds an additional cost to the downstream processing.

Plant seeds represent another expression platform for synthesis of foreign protein and vaccine antigens, as well as their storage. In comparison to perishable plants like leafy crops and fruits, plant seeds enable long-term storage of the foreign protein produced [1]. The plant seeds are generally low in water content where most seeds have a water content of less than 10% of their total biomass, whereas in most cases the leaves contain more than 90% of water [62]. Besides, plant seeds are relatively high in protein content, which ranged from 10% to 40% of their wet weight, while in most leaves the protein percentage is less than 5% [62]. Thus, plant seeds represent a good vehicle to promote stable protein accumulation and storage. Moreover, protease activities in plant seeds are low and thus the risk of spoilage is greatly reduced as the foreign proteins produced are protected from proteolytic degradation [50]. It was demonstrated that antibodies and vaccine antigens accumulated in seeds remained stable without loss of activity for years at room temperature [63, 64]. Hence, seeds are suitable for direct consumption and useful especially for the development of animal vaccines. Industrial scale seed plantation and production are well established, beginning from cultivation, harvest, storage, distribution, and processing of the seeds [1].

Maize is the most widely used cereal crop for molecular farming [65]. The maize seeds or corn has a larger grain size and higher per hectare biomass yield compared to other cereals. The in vitro manipulation and transformation of maize have been widely studied, while its commercial production, processing, and scalability are also well established. The first commercialized corn-produced product was avidin [12] from the company ProdiGene and is available in the Sigma catalogue for diagnostic use [65]. In addition, corn has been used for the development of animal vaccines. The transmissible gastroenteritis virus (TGEV) envelope spike (S) protein expressed in corn was shown to induce protective antibodies in both piglets and gilts [66, 67]. Similarly, oral feeding of transgenic maize expressing the glycoprotein protein of NDV was shown to be immunogenic and conferred protective immunity to chicken [68].

Rice represents another leading platform for production of foreign proteins [1]. Like maize, rice has a high biomass yield, and its production, processing, and scalability have also been established. One apparent advantage of rice over maize is the reduced risk of illegitimate gene flow due to

pollen release resulting from self-pollination [62]. In an oral feeding immunization trial of 2-week-old specific-pathogen-free (SPF) chickens with rice seeds expressing the VP2 protein of infectious bursal disease virus (IBDV), challenge and protection studies showed evidence of protective immunity in the chickens [69]. Barley is another commercial platform being studied other than maize and rice. The self-pollinating trait of barley is an important advantage to be considered in its development as a foreign protein production system. For example, subcutaneous injection of the F4 fimbriae adhesin protein of enterotoxigenic E. coli produced in barley grains was shown to induce neutralizing antibodies in mice [70].

Pea and soybean are the two commonest legume platforms being studied in plant molecular farming [1]. In one study, soybean seeds were used to express enterotoxigenic E. coli LT-B protein [71]. These transgenic seeds were able to induce both systemic and mucosal immunity in mice upon oral administration and conferred partial protection upon challenge. A major advantage of legumes over cereals is that the total protein content of legume grains is relatively much higher than that of cereals. Compared to total proteins (8 to 13%) from cereal grains, the total protein content in pea and soybean can be as high as 40% [72]. However, this apparent advantage is compensated by the laborious and inefficient transformation procedures of legumes in addition to their relatively lower annual grain yield and higher production cost when compared to maize and rice. Nevertheless, both pea and soybean are self-pollinating species; thus the risk of gene flow contamination is less.

Overall, one of the major disadvantages of seed-based expression is the relatively longer time-to-product period [62]. As the expression of protein is targeted to the seeds, the transgenic plants are grown through a flowering cycle to produce seeds. The assessment for the expression of foreign proteins could only begin when the seed is set. This also makes seed-based production systems become less appropriate for expression of certain foreign proteins like the influenza viral antigens [62]. Since the influenza vaccines are revised annually, the amount of seed produced in the given time may be insufficient to supply the population. Besides, seed-based production involves a flowering cycle that might increase the risk of pollen release and gene flow contamination by pollen transfer especially in the open field production system [53]. In contrast, transgenic leafy crops can be harvested before flowering and thus the risk of outcrossing is reduced.

5. Proof of Concept Plant-Derived Veterinary Vaccines

The tremendous developments of plant-made veterinary vaccines have been mainly due to the ability to conduct challenge experiments in specific animal species of interest [4]. Key examples on the plant-produced immunogenic proteins tested against disease challenge in target animal species are shown in Table 3. One of the first demonstrations showing protective efficacy of the plant-derived vaccine was from mink enteritis virus (MEV), where a short, linear, and neutralizing epitope from the viral VP2 capsid protein was expressed in black-eyed bean [73]. Using a plant chimeric

TABLE 3: Summary of plant-derived immunogenic veterinary viral antigens tested against disease challenge in target animals.

Target animals	Disease antigens	Protein expressed	Plant host(s)	Expression approach	Findings	References
Mink	Mink enteritis virus	VP2 capsid protein	Black-eyed bean	CVPs using cowpea mosaic virus	Subcutaneous injection of 1 mg of the chimeric virus protected mink against clinical disease and challenge from the virulent virus.	[73]
Rabbit	Rabbit haemorrhagic disease virus	VP60 protein	Potato, leaf	Stable transformation	Animals primed subcutaneously with 12 μg of recombinant protein emulsified in oil adjuvant and boosted intramuscularly after 30, 60, and 90 days were protected from challenge with the virulent virus.	[74]
			Potato, tuber	Stable transformation	Rabbits fed with 500 μg of recombinant protein and boosted on 21, 42, and 63 days after primary vaccination were partially protected from challenge with the virulent virus.	[75]
Swine	Transmissible gastroenteritis virus	Envelope spike (S) protein	Maize	Stable transformation	Piglets fed with 2 mg S protein daily for 10 consecutive days prior to challenge showed fewer symptoms of infection than the control group vaccinated with commercial vaccine.	[66]
					Gilts previously primed with commercial vaccine and boosted orally two times, each with 26 mg S protein, showed a significant increase of TGEV neutralizing antibody titer in serum, colostrum, and milk.	[67]
Cloven-hoofed animals	Foot-and-mouth disease virus	VP1 capsid protein	Chenopodium quinoa	CVPs using bamboo mosaic virus	Two intramuscular injections with 5 mg of chimeric virus in SPF pigs at six weeks apart induced neutralizing antibodies and demonstrated a complete protection against challenge.	[76]
Poultry	Newcastle disease virus	Fusion protein	Maize	Stable transformation	Oral feeding of transgenic maize was shown to be immunogenic and conferred complete protection against challenge comparable to that by a commercial vaccine to the chicken.	[68]
	Infectious bronchitis virus	S1 glycoprotein	Potato, tuber	Stable transformation	Day-old chicks fed orally with 57.2 μg of recombinant protein and boosted at 7 and 14 days after were protected from clinical disease and virus shedding upon challenge.	[57]
			Rice seed	Stable transformation	Oral feeding with 10 mg of recombinant protein protected chicken from challenge with a highly virulent virus, showing a better bursal lesion score compared to chickens that received the live attenuated vaccine.	[69]
	Infectious bursal disease virus	VP2 capsid protein	Chenopodium quinoa	CVPs using bamboo mosaic virus	Intramuscular injection with 600 μg chimeric virus in oil adjuvant was shown to induce specific antibodies and protected SPF chickens upon challenge with a very virulent virus strain.	[77]
			Nicotiana benthamiana	Transient expression	Intramuscular injection with 12 μg of recombinant protein emulsified in oil adjuvant given at 22 and 35 days later was shown to produce neutralizing antibodies in chickens, with reduced T-cell infiltration into the bursa of Fabricius upon challenge.	[78]

virus particles (CVPs) approach, the short epitope was inserted into the cowpea mosaic virus and displayed on the surface of CVPs upon infection in plants. Subcutaneous injection of 1 mg of the chimeric viral particles expressing MEV peptide on the CVPs surfaces protected mink against clinical disease and challenge from the virulent MEV. In yet another study, studies showed that the VP60 protein of rabbit haemorrhagic disease virus produced from the transgenic potatoes conferred protection to rabbits against infection upon parenteral immunization [74]. It was also immunogenic and induced partial protection to the rabbits upon oral delivery of the vaccine [75].

Indeed, the most promising proof of concept for an edible plant-based animal vaccine delivered orally was against TGEV of swine [67, 79, 80]. The S protein of TGEV expressed in corn was mixed in medicated milk replacer and fed orally to 10-day-old piglets [66]. With a dose of 2 mg S protein in single feeding, the piglets were fed over a 10-day period before being challenged with a virulent TGEV orally. Compared to the control group vaccinated with the commercial vaccine, where 78% of the piglets developed diarrhoea, only 50% of the piglets fed with transgenic corn had diarrhoea. The study concluded that transgenic corn was able to confer partial protection to piglets against clinical disease and experimental challenge with virulent virus. In addition, further studies were conducted to examine vaccination with transgenic corn in gilts and the transfer of protective anti-S protein antibody to suckling piglets through colostrum [67]. In the study, all gilts were primed with a modified live TGEV vaccine orally at days 115 and 102 and intramuscularly at day 88 before farrowing. Following primary vaccination, the gilts were separated into groups and subjected to different types of booster treatments. When compared to the control group that did not receive any booster dose, gilts given a double oral booster of transgenic corn containing 26 mg of S protein at days 35 and 14 before farrowing showed a significant increase of TGEV neutralizing antibody titer in the serum, colostrum, and milk. Such responses were comparable to gilts that received modified live virus vaccine as a booster. The level of neutralizing antibody titer in milk was suggested to be adequately protective to the suckling piglets, although efficacy test was not performed in the piglets [67].

Furthermore, the possibility of conducting protective efficacy experiments in target animal has also allowed the development of plant-expressed foot-and-mouth disease virus (FMDV) vaccine for cloven-hoofed animals. The FMDV VP1 capsid protein carrying the virus neutralizing epitopes was the target of expression in various plants. Transgenic plants expressing either the complete protein or antigenic peptide of VP1 have been generated in plants like *Arabidopsis* [81], alfalfa [82, 83], and potato [84]. Earlier studies conducted in mice via intraperitoneal [81–84] and/or oral [82] delivery of the leaves extract showed the vaccine was immunogenic and protective. Moreover, the VP1 protein was also expressed with the use of plant viral display vector like the tobacco mosaic virus in tobacco leaf via the CVPs approach [85]. The entire VP1 protein expressed by the plant virus and the resulting CVPs injected intraperitoneally into mice conferred protection

against viral challenge with live FMDV. Although these studies have shown an induction of protective immunity in mice, it was only later that the protective efficacy experiments was conducted in swine, one of the natural hosts for FMDV. In a related study, expression of the immunogenic VP1 peptide encompassing amino acids 128 to 164 via the CVPs approach was successfully carried out [76]. Using the bamboo mosaic virus (BaMV) as a plant viral display vector, the VP1 peptide was genetically fused to the modified coat protein gene of BaMV. Upon infection in the leaves of *Chenopodium quinoa*, the BaMV plant host, the VP1 peptide was displayed on the surface of CVPs. Two intramuscular injections with 5 mg of VP1-displaying CVPs in two-month-old SPF pigs at six weeks apart resulted in the induction of anti-FMDV neutralizing antibodies. The vaccine demonstrated a complete protection in pigs against FMDV challenge four weeks after the booster dose was administered.

In the poultry vaccine arena, several infectious pathogens of economic importance have been the attention of development of plant-made vaccines. The NDV is one of them, and the virus surface glycoprotein fusion and/or hemagglutinin neuraminidase are the targets of expression. In addition to the first approved plant-produced NDV vaccine [21] that was made in tobacco cell culture, NDV viral proteins had been expressed in other plant systems as well. Oral feeding of transgenic maize expressing the viral fusion protein was shown to be immunogenic and conferred protective immunity to chicken [68].

Besides, the IBV S1 glycoprotein contains virus neutralizing and hemagglutination-inhibiting epitopes have been the component of interest for vaccine development. By stably transforming the S1 glycoprotein gene into the potato plant, tuber extracts from the transgenic potatoes were used for vaccination and protective efficacy studies in chicken [57, 58]. Here, day-old chicks were fed orally with either 2.5 or 5 g of tuber extracts corresponding to 28.6 or 57.2 μg of S1 glycoprotein and feeding was repeated at days 7 and 14. Virus challenge performed via intranasal route using the virulent IBV seven days after the final vaccination showed all chicks fed with 5 g of tuber extracts were protected from clinical disease and virus shedding. This result was comparable to the control group vaccinated with commercial modified live vaccine.

The IBDV, being a highly contagious and deadly virus of young chickens, is another important pathogen of poultry. It is a double stranded RNA virus with two genome segments, termed A and B [86]. The VP2 capsid protein of IBDV segment A contains the virus neutralizing epitopes and was selected as the component for the development of plant-made vaccine [69, 87]. In one study, the VP2 gene of the variant IBDV strain E was expressed in *Arabidopsis thaliana* [87], while in another study the VP2 gene of a virulent IBDV strain with attenuated segment A was expressed in rice seeds [69]. In the oral feeding immunization trial with rice seeds, 2-week-old SPF chickens were fed with transgenic rice seeds at weekly interval for four times before being challenged with the virulent IBDV strain [69]. Chickens fed with 5 g of transgenic rice seed containing 40.21 μg of VP2 protein in a grain [69], amounting to approximately 10 mg dose of VP2 protein [88], gave the best result in challenge and protection studies. Evaluation based on lesion scoring of the bursa after challenge revealed that orally immunized chickens achieved better lesion score compared to chickens that received the live attenuated vaccine. The orally immunized chickens also contained less antigen present in the bursal tissue based on immunofluorescence assay. Furthermore, the full-length VP2 gene of a classical IBDV strain has been transiently expressed in *Nicotiana benthamiana* leaves and the recombinant protein was extracted for subunit vaccination [78]. Eighteen-day-old chicks injected intramuscularly with 12 μg of VP2 protein emulsified in oil adjuvant and boosted after 22 and 35 days were shown to produce anti-IBDV antibody with neutralizing ability. Apart from VP2 protein obtained by stable or transient transformation in plants, the CVPs approach was also used to generate viable chimeric BaMV virus carrying the VP2 P domain loop P_{BC} of a very virulent IBDV [77]. Intramuscular injection with 600 μg recombinant BaMV in oil adjuvant to 3-week-old SPF chickens was shown to induce IBDV-specific antibodies and protected the chickens upon challenge with a very virulent IBDV strain 28 days after vaccination. These studies concluded that plant-made VP2 protein represents a useful vaccination strategy against IBDV in chicken.

6. Conclusions

It is indeed surprising to see that 26 years down the road only two recombinant protein products from plants had made it through the regulatory processes to be licensed: monoclonal antibody against HBsAg and poultry vaccine against NDV. The idea of plant-made vaccines as edible vaccines has received much publicity and enthusiastic development since the first proof of concept recombinant plant-derived pharmaceutical proteins was reported. However, the progress made was not without hurdles [3]. Although the reports of successful expression of target antigens of interest were numerous, many of these failed to achieve expression levels suitable for commercialization [41]. Besides, the use of food plants for production of vaccine antigens has sprouted fears of contamination of the human food chain. Worries about regulatory issues have also deterred the development of plant-made vaccines. However, the regulatory pathway for plant molecular farming of vaccine antigens for veterinary use is far shorter when compared to products intended for human use. Therefore, this represents an opportunity that warrants the pursuit of plant-made vaccines for animals. The demonstration of safety and increase usage of plant-produced recombinant protein products in animals will lead to the acceptance and recognition of plant expression technology. This will in turn encourage their use for production of plant-based biopharmaceuticals for human use. Finally, with a better understanding of plant gene expression and molecular biology, the realisation of an ideal plant-made edible vaccine will not be far. Hence, the molecular farming of vaccines, be it for veterinary or human use, will be worth the exploration.

Acknowledgments

The authors wish to appreciate Dr. Y. Abba for proofreading the paper draft. The study is funded by the Ministry of Higher Education, Malaysia.

References

[1] O. S. Lau and S. S. M. Sun, "Plant seeds as bioreactors for recombinant protein production," *Biotechnology Advances*, vol. 27, no. 6, pp. 1015–1022, 2009.

[2] A. M. Walmsley and C. J. Arntzen, "Plants for delivery of edible vaccines," *Current Opinion in Biotechnology*, vol. 11, no. 2, pp. 126–129, 2000.

[3] E. P. Rybicki, "Plant-produced vaccines: promise and reality," *Drug Discovery Today*, vol. 14, no. 1-2, pp. 16–24, 2009.

[4] L. Santi, "Plant derived veterinary vaccines," *Veterinary Research Communications*, vol. 33, no. 1, supplement, pp. S61–S66, 2009.

[5] J. J. Joensuu, V. Niklander-Teeri, and J. E. Brandle, "Transgenic plants for animal health: plant-made vaccine antigens for animal infectious disease control," *Phytochemistry Reviews*, vol. 7, no. 3, pp. 553–577, 2008.

[6] A. Spök, R. M. Twyman, R. Fischer, J. K. C. Ma, and P. A. C. Sparrow, "Evolution of a regulatory framework for pharmaceuticals derived from genetically modified plants," *Trends in Biotechnology*, vol. 26, no. 9, pp. 506–517, 2008.

[7] G. A. De Zoeten, J. R. Penswick, M. A. Horisberger, P. Ahl, M. Schultze, and T. Hohn, "The expression, localization, and effect of a human interferon in plants," *Virology*, vol. 172, no. 1, pp. 213–222, 1989.

[8] A. Hiatt, R. Cafferkey, and K. Bowdish, "Production of antibodies in transgenic plants," *Nature*, vol. 342, no. 6245, pp. 76–78, 1989.

[9] P. C. Sijmons, B. M. M. Dekker, B. Schrammeijer, T. C. Verwoerd, P. J. M. Van Den Elzen, and A. Hoekema, "Production of correctly processed human serum albumin in transgenic plants," *Nature Biotechnology*, vol. 8, no. 3, pp. 217–221, 1990.

[10] M. Pujol, N. I. Ramírez, M. Ayala et al., "An integral approach towards a practical application for a plant-made monoclonal antibody in vaccine purification," *Vaccine*, vol. 23, no. 15, pp. 1833–1837, 2005.

[11] J. K.-C. Ma, E. Barros, R. Bock et al., "Molecular farming for new drugs and vaccines. Current perspectives on the production of pharmaceuticals in transgenic plants," *EMBO Reports*, vol. 6, no. 7, pp. 593–599, 2005.

[12] E. E. Hood, D. R. Witcher, S. Maddock et al., "Commercial production of avidin from transgenic maize: characterization of transformant, production, processing, extraction and purification," *Molecular Breeding*, vol. 3, no. 4, pp. 291–306, 1997.

[13] D. R. Witcher, E. E. Hood, D. Peterson et al., "Commercial production of β-glucuronidase (GUS): a model system for the production of proteins in plants," *Molecular Breeding*, vol. 4, no. 4, pp. 301–312, 1998.

[14] S. L. Woodard, J. M. Mayor, M. R. Bailey et al., "Maize (Zea mays)-derived bovine trypsin: characterization of the first large-scale, commercial protein product from transgenic plants," *Biotechnology and Applied Biochemistry*, vol. 38, no. 2, pp. 123–130, 2003.

[15] H. S. Mason, D. M.-K. Lam, and C. J. Arntzen, "Expression of hepatitis B surface antigen in transgenic plants," *Proceedings of the National Academy of Sciences of the United States of America,* vol. 89, no. 24, pp. 11745–11749, 1992.

[16] J. Kapusta, A. Modelska, M. Figlerowicz et al., "A plant-derived edible vaccine against hepatitis B virus," *The FASEB Journal,* vol. 13, no. 13, pp. 1796–1799, 1999.

[17] Y. Thanavala, M. Mahoney, S. Pal et al., "Immunogenicity in humans of an edible vaccine for hepatitis B," *Proceedings of the National Academy of Sciences of the United States of America,* vol. 102, no. 9, pp. 3378–3382, 2005.

[18] H. S. Mason, T. A. Haq, J. D. Clements, and C. J. Arntzen, "Edible vaccine protects mice against *Escherichia coli* heat-labile enterotoxin (LT): potatoes expressing a synthetic LT-B gene," *Vaccine,* vol. 16, no. 13, pp. 1336–1343, 1998.

[19] C. O. Tacket, M. F. Pasetti, R. Edelman, J. A. Howard, and S. Streatfield, "Immunogenicity of recombinant LT-B delivered orally to humans in transgenic corn," *Vaccine,* vol. 22, no. 31-32, pp. 4385–4389, 2004.

[20] H. S. Mason, J. M. Ball, J.-J. Shi, X. Jiang, M. K. Estes, and C. J. Arntzen, "Expression of Norwalk virus capsid protein in transgenic tobacco and potato and its oral immunogenicity in mice," *Proceedings of the National Academy of Sciences of the United States of America,* vol. 93, no. 11, pp. 5335–5340, 1996.

[21] P. Vermij and E. Waltz, "USDA approves the first plant-based vaccine," *Nature Biotechnology,* vol. 24, no. 3, pp. 233–234, 2006.

[22] J. K. Ma, "The caries vaccine: a growing prospect," *Dental Update,* vol. 26, no. 9, pp. 374–380, 1999.

[23] D. W. Pascual, "Vaccines are for dinner," *Proceedings of the National Academy of Sciences of the United States of America,* vol. 104, no. 26, pp. 10757–10758, 2007.

[24] J. Tregoning, P. Maliga, G. Dougan, and P. J. Nixon, "New advances in the production of edible plant vaccines: chloroplast expression of a tetanus vaccine antigen, TetC," *Phytochemistry,* vol. 65, no. 8, pp. 989–994, 2004.

[25] G. J. O'Brien, C. J. Bryant, C. Voogd, H. B. Greenberg, R. C. Gardner, and A. R. Bellamy, "Rotavirus VP6 expressed by PVX vectors in *Nicotiana benthamiana* coats PVX rods and also assembles into viruslike particles," *Virology,* vol. 270, no. 2, pp. 444–453, 2000.

[26] Z. Huang, I. Dry, D. Webster, R. Strugnell, and S. Wesselingh, "Plant-derived measles virus hemagglutinin protein induces neutralizing antibodies in mice," *Vaccine,* vol. 19, no. 15-16, pp. 2163–2171, 2001.

[27] D. E. Webster, M. L. Cooney, Z. Huang et al., "Successful boosting of a DNA measles immunization with an oral plant-derived measles virus vaccine," *Journal of Virology,* vol. 76, no. 15, pp. 7910–7912, 2002.

[28] L. McLain, Z. Durrani, L. A. Wisniewski, C. Porta, G. P. Lomonossoff, and N. J. Dimmock, "Stimulation of neutralizing antibodies to human immunodeficiency virus type 1 in three strains of mice immunized with a 22 amino acid peptide of gp41 expressed on the surface of a plant virus," *Vaccine,* vol. 14, no. 8, pp. 799–810, 1996.

[29] G. G. Zhang, L. Rodrigues, B. Rovinski, and K. A. White, "Production of HIV-1 p24 protein in transgenic tobacco plants," *Applied Biochemistry and Biotechnology—Part B Molecular Biotechnology,* vol. 20, no. 2, pp. 131–136, 2002.

[30] A. Meyers, E. Chakauya, E. Shephard et al., "Expression of HIV-1 antigens in plants as potential subunit vaccines," *BMC Biotechnology,* vol. 8, no. 1, article 53, 2008.

[31] E. S. Tackaberry, A. K. Dudani, F. Prior et al., "Development of biopharmaceuticals in plant expression systems: cloning, expression and immunological reactivity of human cytomegalovirus glycoprotein B (UL55) in seeds of transgenic tobacco," *Vaccine,* vol. 17, no. 23-24, pp. 3020–3029, 1999.

[32] H. Belanger, N. Fleysh, C. O. X. Shannon et al., "Human respiratory syncytial virus vaccine antigen produced in plants," *The FASEB Journal,* vol. 14, no. 14, pp. 2323–2328, 2000.

[33] J. S. Sandhu, S. F. Krasnyanski, L. L. Domier, S. S. Korban, M. D. Osadjan, and D. E. Buetow, "Oral immunization of mice with transgenic tomato fruit expressing respiratory syncytial virus-F protein induces a systemic immune response," *Transgenic Research,* vol. 9, no. 2, pp. 127–135, 2000.

[34] F. R. Brennan, T. D. Jones, M. Longstaff et al., "Immunogenicity of peptides derived from a fibronectin-binding protein of *S. aureus* expressed on two different plant viruses," *Vaccine,* vol. 17, no. 15-16, pp. 1846–1857, 1999.

[35] F. R. Brennan, T. D. Jones, L. B. Gilleland et al., "Pseudomonas aeruginosa outer-membrane protein F epitopes are highly immunogenic in mice when expressed on a plant virus," *Microbiology,* vol. 145, no. 1, pp. 211–220, 1999.

[36] J. Staczek, M. Bendahmane, L. B. Gilleland, R. N. Beachy, and H. E. Gilleland Jr., "Immunization with a chimeric tobacco mosaic virus containing an epitope of outer membrane protein F of *Pseudomonas aeruginosa* provides protection against challenge with *P. aeruginosa,*" *Vaccine,* vol. 18, no. 21, pp. 2266–2274, 2000.

[37] T. H. Turpen, S. J. Reinl, Y. Charoenvit, S. L. Hoffman, V. Fallarme, and L. K. Grill, "Malaria epitopes expressed on the surface of recombinant tobacco mosaic virus," *Nature Biotechnology,* vol. 13, no. 1, pp. 53–57, 1995.

[38] F. Sala, M. M. Rigano, A. Barbante, B. Basso, A. M. Walmsley, and S. Castiglione, "Vaccine antigen production in transgenic plants: strategies, gene constructs and perspectives," *Vaccine,* vol. 21, no. 7-8, pp. 803–808, 2003.

[39] D. M. Floss, D. Falkenburg, and U. Conrad, "Production of vaccines and therapeutic antibodies for veterinary applications in transgenic plants: an overview," *Transgenic Research,* vol. 16, no. 3, pp. 315–332, 2007.

[40] M. M. Rigano and A. M. Walmsley, "Expression systems and developments in plant-made vaccines," *Immunology and Cell Biology,* vol. 83, no. 3, pp. 271–277, 2005.

[41] H. S. Mason, H. Warzecha, T. Mor, and C. J. Arntzen, "Edible plant vaccines: applications for prophylactic and therapeutic molecular medicine," *Trends in Molecular Medicine,* vol. 8, no. 7, pp. 324–329, 2002.

[42] G. Giddings, "Transgenic plants as protein factories," *Current Opinion in Biotechnology,* vol. 12, no. 5, pp. 450–454, 2001.

[43] V. Mett, C. E. Farrance, B. J. Green, and V. Yusibov, "Plants as biofactories," *Biologicals,* vol. 36, no. 6, pp. 354–358, 2008.

[44] J. C. Muskett, N. E. Reed, and D. H. Thornton, "Increased virulence of an infectious bursal disease live virus vaccine after passage in chicks," *Vaccine,* vol. 3, no. 4, pp. 309–312, 1985.

[45] G. Zavala and S. Cheng, "Detection and characterization of avian leukosis virus in Marek's disease vaccines," *Avian Diseases,* vol. 50, no. 2, pp. 209–215, 2006.

[46] S. J. Streatfield and J. A. Howard, "Plant-based vaccines," *International Journal for Parasitology,* vol. 33, no. 5-6, pp. 479–493, 2003.

[47] I. B. H. Wilson, "Glycosylation of proteins in plants and invertebrates," *Current Opinion in Structural Biology,* vol. 12, no. 5, pp. 569–577, 2002.

[48] S. A. Brooks, "Appropriate glycosylation of recombinant proteins for human use," *Molecular Biotechnology*, vol. 28, no. 3, pp. 241–255, 2004.

[49] C. Saint-Jore-Dupas, L. Faye, and V. Gomord, "From planta to pharma with glycosylation in the toolbox," *Trends in Biotechnology*, vol. 25, no. 7, pp. 317–323, 2007.

[50] R. Fischer, E. Stoger, S. Schillberg, P. Christou, and R. M. Twyman, "Plant-based production of biopharmaceuticals," *Current Opinion in Plant Biology*, vol. 7, no. 2, pp. 152–158, 2004.

[51] Arabidopsis Genome Initiative, "Analysis of the genome sequence of the flowering plant *Arabidopsis thaliana*," *Nature*, vol. 408, pp. 796–815, 2000.

[52] H. Daniell, S. J. Streatfield, and K. Wycoff, "Medical molecular farming: production of antibodies, biopharmaceuticals and edible vaccines in plants," *Trends in Plant Science*, vol. 6, no. 5, pp. 219–226, 2001.

[53] R. M. Twyman, E. Stoger, S. Schillberg, P. Christou, and R. Fischer, "Molecular farming in plants: host systems and expression technology," *Trends in Biotechnology*, vol. 21, no. 12, pp. 570–578, 2003.

[54] P. Lerouge, M. Cabanes-Macheteau, C. Rayon, A.-C. Fischette-Lainé, V. Gomord, and L. Faye, "N-glycoprotein biosynthesis in plants: recent developments and future trends," *Plant Molecular Biology*, vol. 38, no. 1-2, pp. 31–48, 1998.

[55] V. Gomord, A.-C. Fitchette, L. Menu-Bouaouiche et al., "Plant-specific glycosylation patterns in the context of therapeutic protein production," *Plant Biotechnology Journal*, vol. 8, no. 5, pp. 564–587, 2010.

[56] M. Bardor, C. Loutelier-Bourhis, T. Paccalet et al., "Monoclonal C5-1 antibody produced in transgenic alfalfa plants exhibits a *N*-glycosylation that is homogenous and suitable for glyco-engineering into human-compatible structures," *Plant Biotechnology Journal*, vol. 1, no. 6, pp. 451–462, 2003.

[57] J.-Y. Zhou, J.-X. Wu, L.-Q. Cheng et al., "Expression of immunogenic S1 glycoprotein of infectious bronchitis virus in transgenic potatoes," *Journal of Virology*, vol. 77, no. 16, pp. 9090–9093, 2003.

[58] J.-Y. Zhou, L.-Q. Cheng, X.-J. Zheng et al., "Generation of the transgenic potato expressing full-length spike protein of infectious bronchitis virus," *Journal of Biotechnology*, vol. 111, no. 2, pp. 121–130, 2004.

[59] K. S. Gunn, N. Singh, J. Giambrone, and H. Wu, "Using transgenic plants as bioreactors to produce edible vaccines," *Journal of Biotech Research*, vol. 4, no. 1, pp. 92–99, 2012.

[60] P. B. McGarvey, J. Hammond, M. M. Dienelt et al., "Expression of the rabies virus glycoprotein in transgenic tomatoes," *Nature Biotechnology*, vol. 13, no. 13, pp. 1484–1487, 1995.

[61] S. Saldaña, F. E. Guadarrama, T. D. J. Olivera Flores et al., "Production of rotavirus-like particles in tomato (*Lycopersicon esculentum* L.) fruit by expression of capsid proteins VP2 and VP6 and immunological studies," *Viral Immunology*, vol. 19, no. 1, pp. 42–53, 2006.

[62] J. Boothe, C. Nykiforuk, Y. Shen et al., "Seed-based expression systems for plant molecular farming," *Plant Biotechnology Journal*, vol. 8, no. 5, pp. 588–606, 2010.

[63] E. Stöger, C. Vaquero, E. Torres et al., "Cereal crops as viable production and storage systems for pharmaceutical scFv antibodies," *Plant Molecular Biology*, vol. 42, no. 4, pp. 583–590, 2000.

[64] T. Nochi, H. Takagi, Y. Yuki et al., "Rice-based mucosal vaccine as a global strategy for cold-chain- and needle-free vaccination," *Proceedings of the National Academy of Sciences of the United States of America*, vol. 104, no. 26, pp. 10986–10991, 2007.

[65] K. Ramessar, M. Sabalza, T. Capell, and P. Christou, "Maize plants: an ideal production platform for effective and safe molecular pharming," *Plant Science*, vol. 174, no. 4, pp. 409–419, 2008.

[66] S. J. Streatfield, J. M. Jilka, E. E. Hood et al., "Plant-based vaccines: unique advantages," *Vaccine*, vol. 19, no. 17–19, pp. 2742–2748, 2001.

[67] B. J. Lamphear, J. M. Jilka, L. Kesl, M. Welter, J. A. Howard, and S. J. Streatfield, "A corn-based delivery system for animal vaccines: an oral transmissible gastroenteritis virus vaccine boosts lactogenic immunity in swine," *Vaccine*, vol. 22, no. 19, pp. 2420–2424, 2004.

[68] O. Guerrero-Andrade, E. Loza-Rubio, T. Olivera-Flores, T. Fehérvári-Bone, and M. A. Gómez-Lim, "Expression of the Newcastle disease virus fusion protein in transgenic maize and immunological studies," *Transgenic Research*, vol. 15, no. 4, pp. 455–463, 2006.

[69] J. Wu, L. Yu, L. Li, J. Hu, J. Zhou, and X. Zhou, "Oral immunization with transgenic rice seeds expressing VP2 protein of infectious bursal disease virus induces protective immune responses in chickens," *Plant Biotechnology Journal*, vol. 5, no. 5, pp. 570–578, 2007.

[70] J. J. Joensuu, M. Kotiaho, T. H. Teeri et al., "Glycosylated F4 (K88) fimbrial adhesin FaeG expressed in barley endosperm induces ETEC-neutralizing antibodies in mice," *Transgenic Research*, vol. 15, no. 3, pp. 359–373, 2006.

[71] T. Moravec, M. A. Schmidt, E. M. Herman, and T. Woodford-Thomas, "Production of *Escherichia coli* heat labile toxin (LT) B subunit in soybean seed and analysis of its immunogenicity as an oral vaccine," *Vaccine*, vol. 25, no. 9, pp. 1647–1657, 2007.

[72] E. Stoger, J. K.-C. Ma, R. Fischer, and P. Christou, "Sowing the seeds of success: pharmaceutical proteins from plants," *Current Opinion in Biotechnology*, vol. 16, no. 2, pp. 167–173, 2005.

[73] K. Dalsgaard, Å. Uttentha, T. D. Jones et al., "Plant-derived vaccine protects target animals against a viral disease," *Nature Biotechnology*, vol. 15, no. 3, pp. 248–252, 1997.

[74] S. Castañón, M. S. Marín, J. M. Martín-Alonso et al., "Immunization with potato plants expressing VP60 protein protects against rabbit hemorrhagic disease virus," *Journal of Virology*, vol. 73, no. 5, pp. 4452–4455, 1999.

[75] J. M. Martín-Alonso, S. Castañón, P. Alonso, F. Parra, and R. Ordás, "Oral immunization using tuber extracts from transgenic potato plants expressing rabbit hemorrhagic disease virus capsid protein," *Transgenic Research*, vol. 12, no. 1, pp. 127–130, 2003.

[76] C.-D. Yang, J.-T. Liao, C.-Y. Lai et al., "Induction of protective immunity in swine by recombinant bamboo mosaic virus expressing foot-and-mouth disease virus epitopes," *BMC Biotechnology*, vol. 7, no. 1, article 62, 2007.

[77] T.-H. Chen, T.-H. Chen, C.-C. Hu et al., "Induction of protective immunity in chickens immunized with plant-made chimeric bamboo mosaic virus particles expressing very virulent Infectious bursal disease virus antigen," *Virus Research*, vol. 166, no. 1-2, pp. 109–115, 2012.

[78] E. Gómez, M. S. Lucero, S. Chimeno Zoth, J. M. Carballeda, M. J. Gravisaco, and A. Berinstein, "Transient expression of VP2

in *Nicotiana benthamiana* and its use as a plant-based vaccine against infectious bursal disease virus," *Vaccine*, vol. 31, no. 23, pp. 2623–2627, 2013.

[79] B. J. Lamphear, S. J. Streatfield, J. M. Jilka et al., "Delivery of subunit vaccines in maize seed," *Journal of Controlled Release*, vol. 85, no. 1–3, pp. 169–180, 2002.

[80] J. A. Howard, "Commercialization of plant-based vaccines from research and development to manufacturing.," *Animal Health Research Reviews*, vol. 5, no. 2, pp. 243–245, 2004.

[81] C. Carrillo, A. Wigdorovitz, J. C. Oliveros et al., "Protective immune response to foot-and-mouth disease virus with VP1 expressed in transgenic plants," *Journal of Virology*, vol. 72, no. 2, pp. 1688–1690, 1998.

[82] A. Wigdorovitz, C. Carrillo, M. J. Dus Santos et al., "Induction of a protective antibody response to foot and mouth disease virus in mice following oral or parenteral immunization with alfalfa transgenic plants expressing the viral structural protein VP1," *Virology*, vol. 255, no. 2, pp. 347–353, 1999.

[83] M. J. D. Santos, A. Wigdorovitz, K. Trono et al., "A novel methodology to develop a foot and mouth disease virus (FMDV) peptide-based vaccine in transgenic plants," *Vaccine*, vol. 20, no. 7-8, pp. 1141–1147, 2002.

[84] C. Carrillo, A. Wigdorovitz, K. Trono et al., "Induction of a virus-specific antibody response to foot and mouth disease virus using the structural protein VP1 expressed in transgenic potato plants," *Viral Immunology*, vol. 14, no. 1, pp. 49–57, 2001.

[85] A. Wigdorovitz, D. M. Pérez Filgueira, N. Robertson et al., "Protection of mice against challenge with foot and mouth disease virus (FMDV) by immunization with foliar extracts from plants infected with recombinant tobacco mosaic virus expressing the FMDV structural protein VP1," *Virology*, vol. 264, no. 1, pp. 85–91, 1999.

[86] H. Nick, D. Cursiefen, and H. Becht, "Structural and growth characteristics of infectious bursal disease virus," *Journal of Virology*, vol. 18, no. 1, pp. 227–234, 1976.

[87] H. Wu, N. K. Singh, R. D. Locy, K. Scissum-Gunn, and J. J. Giambrone, "Expression of immunogenic VP2 protein of infectious bursal disease virus in *Arabidopsis thaliana*," *Biotechnology Letters*, vol. 26, no. 10, pp. 787–792, 2004.

[88] H. S. Mason and M. M. Herbst-Kralovetz, "Plant-derived antigens as mucosal vaccines," *Current Topics in Microbiology and Immunology*, vol. 354, no. 1, pp. 101–120, 2012.

15

Genotype Diversity of Newcastle Disease Virus in Nigeria: Disease Control Challenges and Future Outlook

Muhammad Bashir Bello ⓘ,[1,2] **Khatijah Mohd Yusoff** ⓘ,[2,3]
Aini Ideris ⓘ,[2,4] **Mohd Hair-Bejo**,[2,4] **Ben P. H. Peeters**,[5] **Abdurrahman Hassan Jibril**,[1]
Farouk Muhammad Tambuwal,[1] **and Abdul Rahman Omar** ⓘ[2,4]

[1]Faculty of Veterinary Medicine, Usmanu Danfodiyo University, PMB 2346, Sokoto, Nigeria
[2]Laboratory of Vaccines and Immunotherapeutics, Institute of Bioscience, Universiti Putra Malaysia, 43400 Serdang, Selangor, Malaysia
[3]Faculty of Biotechnology and Biomolecular Sciences, Universiti Putra Malaysia, 43400, Selangor, Malaysia
[4]Faculty of Veterinary Medicine, Universiti Putra Malaysia, 43400 Serdang, Selangor, Malaysia
[5]Division of Virology, Central Veterinary Institute, Wageningen University, P.O. Box 65, NL8200 Lelystad, Netherlands

Correspondence should be addressed to Abdul Rahman Omar; aro@upm.edu.my

Academic Editor: Binod Kumar

Newcastle disease (ND) is one of the most important avian diseases with considerable threat to the productivity of poultry all over the world. The disease is associated with severe respiratory, gastrointestinal, and neurological lesions in chicken leading to high mortality and several other production related losses. The aetiology of the disease is an avian paramyxovirus type-1 or Newcastle disease virus (NDV), whose isolates are serologically grouped into a single serotype but genetically classified into a total of 19 genotypes, owing to the continuous emergence and evolution of the virus. In Nigeria, molecular characterization of NDV is generally very scanty and majorly focuses on the amplification of the partial F gene for genotype assignment. However, with the introduction of the most objective NDV genotyping criteria which utilize complete fusion protein coding sequences in phylogenetic taxonomy, the enormous genetic diversity of the virus in Nigeria became very conspicuous. In this review, we examine the current ecological distribution of various NDV genotypes in Nigeria based on the available complete fusion protein nucleotide sequences (1662 bp) in the NCBI database. We then discuss the challenges of ND control as a result of the wide genetic distance between the currently circulating NDV isolates and the commonest vaccines used to combat the disease in the country. Finally, we suggest future directions in the war against the economically devastating ND in Nigeria.

1. Introduction

Poultry production is globally threatened by a highly devastating disease of birds called Newcastle disease (ND). The disease was named after a place known as Newcastle Upon Tyne, in England where it was reported for the first time in 1926 [1]. The disease was also reported around the same time in Java, Indonesia [2]. Amazingly, its geographic distribution slowly expanded, leading to a well-established pandemic of the disease barely two decades after its novel emergence [3]. Subsequently in the late 1960s, the second pandemic of the disease occurred with an incredibly high speed, taking only four years to spread throughout the world, probably due

to extensive commercialization of poultry production and the improvement of air transport systems which facilitated the exchange of exotic birds into new areas [4]. Although this pandemic was quickly placed under control with the then available ND vaccines, the third pandemic still occurred around the early 1980s among the racing pigeons [5, 6]. This particular pandemic proved to be difficult to control because of the nature of racing pigeon husbandry system. Eventually, the pandemic virus spilt over to the domesticated chicken and caused serious economic losses in the poultry subsector [7]. The fourth pandemic, which started around the mid-1980s in the South-Eastern Asia, is currently believed to be on-going and has so far spread extensively to the Middle

East, Europe, America, and Africa [8–11]. In Nigeria, the first official documentation of ND was in 1952 (Hill et al. 1953) and at present, the disease has been reported in all the ago-ecological zones of the country [12–15].

The aetiology of ND is an avian paramyxovirus type-1, which is a member of the genus *Avulavirus* in the family Paramyxoviridae [16]. The genetic material of the virus is a negative sense RNA made up of six genes encoding six structural proteins in the order $3'$NP-P-M-F-HN-L$5'$ [17, 18]. Pathogenicity indices such as the mean death time (MDT) in 9-10-day-old embryonated chicken eggs and the intracerebral pathogenicity index (ICPI) in 1-day-old chicks are often used to classify the virus isolates into velogenic, mesogenic, and lentogenic strains [19]. The velogenic strains (neurotrophic or viscerotropic) are highly fatal and therefore demonstrate the severest clinical form of the disease, causing haemorrhagic gastroenteritis, pneumonia, and/or encephalitis [20, 21]. The mesogenic strains which are moderately pathogenic cause respiratory and neurological symptoms but with significantly low mortality [22, 23]. On the other hand, the lentogenic pathotypes are of extremely low virulence, causing only mild respiratory or asymptomatic enteric disease in the affected chicken [23, 24]. Interestingly, the major determinant of NDV virulence has been traced to be the amino acid composition of its fusion protein cleavage site [25]. All virulent strains have multiple basic amino acid residues at positions 112-116 and a phenyl alanine at position 117, making them cleavable by most of the ubiquitously distributed intracellular furin-like proteases in various chicken tissues [26]. In contrast, the F cleavage site of the avirulent strains is normally composed of monobasic amino acid residues at positions 112-116 and a leucine residue at position 117 [27]. Thus the chemistry of Fo cleavage site can be used as a good index for rapid pathotyping of NDV using molecular based assays.

In Nigeria, molecular characterization of ND outbreaks was until recently very scanty and largely focused on the partial F gene sequences for phylogenetic grouping of isolates [29, 30]. With the introduction of more objective criteria that utilizes the complete F gene coding sequences for assigning new genotypes [31], the genetic diversity of NDV in Nigeria has become more apparent [32–34]. Unfortunately to date, the consequences of this genetic diversity on disease control using the available vaccines in the country remain poorly addressed. Therefore in this review, we analyze the current ecological distribution of NDV genotypes in various parts of Nigeria and discuss the implication of the genotype mismatch between the circulating field strains and the vaccine strains to ND control in the country.

2. Taxonomy and Global Distribution of Newcastle Disease Virus Isolates

Although all NDV strains are classified under one serotype [35], their genetic diversity is enormous [36–39]. In the past, various schemes have been concurrently used to classify NDV based on their genetic information. The first classification system proposed by the Aldous group divides all the isolates into six lineages and 13 sublineages [40]. An additional

lineage and seven more sublineages were later proposed [41, 42]. The other scheme of NDV taxonomy proposed by Ballagi-Pordány et al. [3] and later substantiated by Czeglédi et al. [43] groups the NDV isolates into various genotypes and subgenotypes. Conflicts and confusion generated by these schemes of classification necessitated the need to develop unified criteria for NDV taxonomy. After analyzing the two systems extensively, Diel et al. [31] proposed the adoption of the genotype based classification not only because it is the most widely used, but also because it gives a stronger correlation between the intergenetic groups evolutionary distances and their phylogenetic relationships. Therefore, a unified nomenclature system was proposed for the then existing isolates and more comprehensive criteria for the assignment of newly emerged genotypes were proposed [31]. According to the criteria, classification of a new genotype will be based on the phylogenetic topology using the complete, not partial F gene coding sequences. Furthermore, at least four isolates obtained from epidemiologically distinct events must form a phylogenetic cluster with a bootstrap value of nothing less than 60%. In addition, the isolates should have an average interpopulation evolutionary distance of ≥ 10. However, a mean evolutionary distance of 3-10% shall be used to designate a new subgenotype within a group [31].

Using these objective criteria, NDV isolates have been broadly classified into class I and class II [44–46]. The class I isolates are all grouped into a single genotype and three subgenotypes because of their high genetic relatedness which is nearly 96% [47]. They are mostly isolated from wild and domesticated birds found in Africa, Asia, Europe, and America [36, 48, 49]. With the exception of one isolate that caused serious disease outbreak in the Northern Ireland around the early 1990s [50], all members of this class are considered of low virulence in chicken. On the contrary, the class II isolates are a mixture of viruses with diverse virulence potentials ranging from the most popular vaccine strains used for disease control to the highly virulent strains that cause outbreaks in different parts of the world (Table 1). According to the recent literatures, class II isolates are classified into genotypes I-XVIII, with majority of the genotypes being further subdivided into various subgenotypes [51–53]. For instance, genotype I isolates which are globally distributed are composed of three subgenotypes: 1a, 1b, and 1c most of which are considered lentogenic. Indeed, the widely reported Queensland V4 and Ulster/chicken/Ireland/1967 vaccine strains are all grouped under this genotype [52, 53]. However, Gould et al. [54] reported the occurrence of virulent genotype I isolates in Australia. Similarly, the genotype II isolates are a mixture of velogenic [37, 38] and lentogenic viruses such as LaSota and B1 strains used globally for disease control [55]. Isolates in this genotype have been majorly recovered from domestic fowl, chicken, and wild birds found in North and South America, Africa, Asia, and Europe [44, 45].

Isolates belonging to genotypes III, IV, V, and VI are all predicted or pathotyped to be virulent in chicken. The genotype III isolates which include the popular mesogenic Mukteshwar strain used as a vaccine strain were recovered from birds in Japan as early as 1930s and also in Pakistan

TABLE 1: Current classification and distribution of class II NDV genotypes.

Genotypes	Subgenotypes	Geographic distribution	Remarks
I	Ia, Ib, Ic	Australia, Africa, Europe, US, Asia	Low virulence, Ulster, V4
II	-	North and South America, Africa, Asia and Europe	Avirulent, lentogenic, Lasota, B1
III	-	Japan and Australia, Taiwan, Zimbabwe	Ancient strains but still emerging, mesogenic Mukteshwar
IV	-	Europe, Africa, Asia	Virulent, Herts/33 (UK)
V	Va, Vb, Vc, Vd	South America, Europe and Africa	Virulent, Anhinga (US)
VI	VIa, VIb, VIc, VId, VIe, VIf, VIg, VIh, VIi, VIj, VIk	Europe, Asia, Africa, South America	Pigeon paramyxoviruses
VII	VIIa, VIIb, VIIc,, VIId, VIIe, VIIf, VIIg, VIIh, VIIi	Emerged in Far East in 1990, spread to Europe and Asia, Africa.	Virulent, 4th ND panzootic virus, 5th panzootic virus
VIII	-	South Africa, Asia	Highly virulent, AF22440
IX	-	First isolated in China in 1948	Highly virulent
X	-	Taiwan, Argentina, USA	Virulent
XI	-	Madagascar	Virulent, restricted distribution
XII	-	South America and China	Virulent
XIII	XIIIa, XIIIb, XIIIc	Asia, Europe and Africa	Virulent, continuously emerging
XIV	XIVa, XIVb	West Africa	Highly virulent, recovered from domestic birds only
XV	-	China	Originated from mixed virulent and vaccine viruses
XVI	-	Europe in 1940s, Africa and Asia in 1980s	Highly related to genotype IV
XVII	XVIIa, XVIIb	West and Central Africa	Highly virulent, continuously emerging evolving
XVIII	XVIIIa, XVIIIb	West Africa	Highly virulent

around the mid 1970s before they subsequently resurge in China less than two decades ago [56, 57]. Likewise, the genotype IV isolates occurred among the European poultry before the 1940s and include the extensively characterized Herts/33 strain [3, 58]. However, isolates in this genotype are currently thought to be extinct [44, 45] due to the absence of their recent genetic information in the GenBank database. As for the genotype V isolates that emerged for the first time around the 1970s in America and spread to the European continent in 1980s [43, 59], their recovery from poultry has recently been reported in East Africa, suggesting the expansion of their geographic distribution [60] and their continuous evolution. So far, isolates in this genotype are divided into four distinct subgenotypes (Va, Vb, Vc, and Vd) because of their within-the-group heterogeneity. However, the genotype VI isolates which are cosmopolitan in distribution are much more heterogeneous genetically. They are currently divided into subgenotypes VIa-k [37, 38, 51]

because of their enormous genetic diversity. In addition, they are mainly found in wild birds, chicken, and more frequently in domestic pigeons, hence the name pigeon paramyxoviruses [6, 52, 61].

Genotype VII isolates are arguably the most important group of NDV reported in the 21st century. From the year 2000 to date, these viruses have been incriminated in several economically important disease outbreaks in Asia, the Middle East, and some parts of America and South Africa [62–65]. Because of their extensive genetic diversity and continuous emergence, they are currently grouped into twelve subgenotypes (VIIa-l) [66] and are believed to be associated with the ongoing fourth pandemic of the disease. As a matter of fact, some of these subgenotypes are predicted to be the potential fifth ND pandemic viruses because of the recent expansion of their host range and geographic distribution as well as their increased virulence among the vaccinated birds [67–70]. In particular, subgenotype VIIi isolates have recently replaced the predominant VIIa isolates in countries such as Pakistan since 2011 [71]. Similarly, subgenotype VIIj isolates believed to have emerged from viruses circulating in China and Ukraine are increasingly isolated in several countries including Iran [72]. This complex genetic diversity of genotype VII NDV highlights the need to monitor the epidemiological dynamics of the emerging viruses so that effective vaccination program can be designed. Unlike the genotype VII isolates, members of genotype VIII taxon are less diverse both genetically and in terms of spatial distribution. Apart from the report on their occurrence in Malaysia, Singapore, China, Turkey, Argentina, and South Africa between the 1960s and 1990s [8, 17], no report exists on their emergence in other parts of the world in the recent times. Hence they are thought to currently cease circulation in domestic birds. In contrast, the genotype IX isolates are still evolving in wild birds and domesticated poultry since survey of NDV between 2008 and 2011 revealed their presence in China [73, 74]. Nevertheless, they are still considered to be among the early genotypes, having been isolated as early as 1940s [3]. However, unlike members of this genotype (genotype IX) which are mostly virulent in chicken, genotype X isolates are all predicted to be in the lentogenic class. Despite their restricted geographic distribution, they are still maintained between the turkeys and wild birds in Argentina and the United States of America [75, 76]. They are however among the less genetically diverse groups of NDV.

Perhaps the most geographically restricted group of NDV are the genotype XI isolates. They have only been reported from Madagascar, where they are believed to circulate between the wild birds and domestic chicken [35, 58]. Although they are all predicted to be virulent based on the chemistry of their F cleavage site, there are reports of their isolation from apparently normal unvaccinated birds in Madagascar [35]. Meanwhile the genotype XII isolates, which are all predicted to be virulent, have been reported from both China and America in geese and chicken, respectively [44, 45, 77]. The epidemiological connection between the isolates in America and those in China is however still not clear, since migratory birds have not so far been incriminated in carrying these viruses [31, 44, 45]. Genotype XIII isolates which have been recovered from birds in Europe, Asia, and Africa are all predicted to be virulent based on the amino acid composition of their F cleavage site [78]. They are thought to be continuously evolving especially in Asia and the Middle East. Currently, they are divided into subgenotypes XIIIa, XIIIb, and XIIIc [79, 80].

The rest of the NDV genotypes are all predicted to be virulent in chicken. Isolates belonging to genotypes XIV, XVII, and XVIII have been recovered mainly from domesticated birds such as chicken, turkeys, and guinea fowls. Each of these genotypes is currently divided into two subgenotypes, a and b [53]. Because their geographic distribution is restricted to the west and central Africa, they are often referred to as regional NDV genotypes. On the other hand, members of the genotype XV group are considered to be recombinant isolates that might have emerged from the suboptimally vaccinated poultry in China some two decades ago [44, 45]. However, it is doubtful if they are still maintained in the poultry due

to the absence of report on their occurrence in the last 15 years. Finally, genotype XVI isolates which were isolated from the Mexican chicken as early the 1940s [81] are believed to have been maintained in either the vaccinated or wild birds unnoticed for quite several years. They were also isolated in the Caribbean islands between 1986 and 2008 [43].

3. Ecology of NDV Genotypes in Nigeria

Analysis of the complete F gene coding sequences (1662bp) for Nigerian strains of NDV available in the NCBI database reveals the occurrence of genetically distinct strains in various species of birds across the lengths and breadths of Nigeria (Table 2). Based on phylogenetic relationships and evolutionary distances, those isolates were grouped into class II genotypes I, VI, XIV, XVII, and XVIII. Except the genotype I isolates with GRQGRL amino acid motifs at positions 112-117 of the F gene, all other isolates considered in this study are predicted to be virulent in chicken based on the presence of multiple basic amino acid residues in their F cleavage sites (Table 1). Notably, among those virulent cleavage sites, the "RRQKRF" is the most diverse, being possessed by all the analyzed sequences except those from genotypes I and VIh. Furthermore, some strains from subgenotypes XVIIa, XIVb, and VIh display "RRRKRF" at their cleavage sites whereas only one isolate from subgenotype VIg, another one from subgenotype XVIIb, and four isolates from subgenotype VIh possess "KRQKRF", "RRQRRF", and "RRKKRF" cleavage sites, respectively. Interestingly, recent studies on amino acid composition of NDV F cleavage site revealed that strains with Q at the third position in the cleavage site are predicted to have an enhanced cell-cell spreading ability [27]. Thus, in future development of vaccines based on indigenous NDV isolates in Nigeria, special consideration should be given to those isolates with Q at the third position of their F cleavage site.

Isolates of NDV belonging to the genotype VI group have been recovered from pigeons, doves, and chicken in the Northern (Kano and Jigawa) as well as the Southern (Oyo and Lagos) parts of Nigeria (Table 2). They are classified into subgenotypes VIg, VIh, and VIi with the overall average evolutionary divergence among the three subgenotypes being 7.3%. The highest genetic distance among these groups occurs between the subgenotypes VIh and VIi (Table 2). Surprisingly, the Nigerian genotype VIg isolates share a high degree of phylogenetic relationship with the Russian, Egyptian, and Ukrainian isolates whereas the genotype VIh isolates are more related to the pigeon paramyxovirus isolated from wild birds in Kenya (Figure 1(a)). On the other hand, the isolates grouped under subgenotypes VIi form the same phylogenetic cluster with the Italian strains. These close genetic relationships among the isolates could be of epidemiological significance and certainly suggest a recent common ancestry during their evolution [52, 53]. Given that these viruses can easily be transmitted from pigeons and doves to domesticated chicken especially at ecological contact surfaces [82–84] and that some of them have been shown to dramatically gain virulence upon a few passages in chicken

TABLE 2: Some features of the Newcastle disease virus subgenotypes found in Nigeria.

Subgenotype	Strain Identity	Year of isolation	Cleavage site	Location
VIg	JQ039385.1 dove/Nigeria/VRD07-163/2007	2007	RRQKRF	Kano
	JQ039389.1 pigeon/Nigeria/VRD07-369/2007	2007	KRQKRF	Jigawa
	HG326601.1 pigeon/Nigeria/NIE07-061/2007	2007	RRKKRF	Oyo
	HG326602.1 pigeon/Nigeria/NIE07-062/2007	2007	RRKKRF	Oyo
	HG326603.1 pigeon/Nigeria/NIE07-063/2007	2007	RRKKRF	Oyo
	HG326604.1 pigeon/Nigeria/NIE09-1898/2009	2009	RRKKRF	Lagos
VIh	HG424627.1 pigeon/Nigeria/NIE13-092/2013	2013	RRRKRF	Oyo
	HG424628.1 pigeon/Nigeria/NIE13-093/2013	2013	RRRKRF	Oyo
	JQ039387.1 Nigeria/VRD08-37BRpe(7-9)/2008	2008	RRRKRF	Jigawa
	JQ039388.1 Nigeria/VRD08-37(10-11-13)/2008	2007	RRRKRF	Jigawa
	JQ039391.1 Nigeria/VRD07-231/2007	2007	RRRKRF	Jigawa
VIi	HG424625.1 pigeon/Nigeria/NIE13-005/2013	2013	RRQKRF	Oyo
	HG424626.1 pigeon/Nigeria/NIE13-008/2013	2013	RRQKRF	Oyo
	HF969131.1 chicken/Nigeria/NIE08-2117/2009	2009	RRQKRF	Sokoto
	HF969136.1 chicken/Nigeria/NIE08-2194/2009	2009	RRQKRF	Sokoto
	HF969139.1 chicken/Nigeria/NIE08-2280/2009	2009	RRQKRF	Sokoto
	HF969144.1 chicken/Nigeria/NIE09-2009/2009	2009	RRQKRF	Yobe
	HF969150.1 chicken/Nigeria/NIE09-2044/2009	2009	RRQKRF	Yobe
	HF969153.1 chicken/Nigeria/NIE09-2079/2009	2009	RRQKRF	Yobe
	HF969155.1 chicken/Nigeria/NIE09-2087/2009	2009	RRQKRF	Yobe
XIVa	HF969167.1 turkey/Nigeria/NIE10-082/2011	2011	RRQKRF	Sokoto
	HF969186.1 chicken/Nigeria/NIE07-125/2007	2007	RRQKRF	Lagos
	HF969193.1 chicken/Nigeria/NIE08-2150/2009	2009	RRQKRF	Sokoto
	HF969200.1 chicken/Nigeria/NIE08-2362/2009	2009	RRQKRF	Sokoto
	HF969205.1 turkey/Nigeria/NIE09-2071/2009	2009	RRQKRF	Yobe
	HF969206.1 chicken/Nigeria/NIE09-2101/2009	2009	RRQKRF	Yobe
	JQ039386.1 VRD08-36/2008	2008	RRQKRF	Taraba
	HF969158.1 avian/Nigeria/NIE09-2168/2009	2009	RRQKRF	Yobe

TABLE 2: Continued.

Subgenotype	Strain Identity	Year of isolation	Cleavage site	Location
	HF969133.1 chicken/Nigeria/NIE08-2159/2009	2009	RRRKRF	Sokoto
	HF969141.1 chicken/Nigeria/NIE08-2359/2009	2009	RRRKRF	Sokoto
	HF969142.1 chicken/Nigeria/NIE09-1596/2009	2009	RRQKRF	Benue
	HF969143.1 chicken/Nigeria/NIE09-1597/2009	2009	RRQKRF	Benue
	HF969145.1 chicken/Nigeria/NIE09-2014/2009	2009	RRRKRF	Yobe
	HF969146.1 chicken/Nigeria/NIE09-2017/2009	2009	RRRKRF	Yobe
	HF969149.1 chicken/Nigeria/NIE09-2041/2009	2009	RRRKRF	Yobe
	HF969151.1 chicken/Nigeria/NIE09-2053/2009	2009	RRRKRF	Yobe
	HF969157.1 chicken/Nigeria/NIE09-2166/2009	2009	RRRKRF	Yobe
	HF969161.1 chicken/Nigeria/NIE10-024/2011	2011	RRRKRF	Sokoto
	HF969162.1 chicken/Nigeria/NIE10-032/2011	2011	RRRKRF	Sokoto
	HF969163.1 chicken/Nigeria/NIE10-034/2011	2011	RRQKRF	Sokoto
	HF969164.1 chicken/Nigeria/NIE10-041/2011	2011	RRRKRF	Sokoto
	HF969165.1 chicken/Nigeria/NIE10-043/2011	2011	RRRKRF	Sokoto
	HF969166.1 chicken/Nigeria/NIE10-076/2011	2011	RRRKRF	Sokoto
	HF969169.1 chicken/Nigeria/NIE10-150/2011	2011	RRRKRF	Sokoto
	HF969170.1 chicken/Nigeria/NIE10-160/2011	2011	RRRKRF	Sokoto
	HF969172.1 chicken/Nigeria/NIE10-258/2011	2011	RRQKRF	Sokoto
	HF969173.1 chicken/Nigeria/NIE10-302/2011	2011	RRRKRF	Sokoto
	HF969177.1 chicken/Nigeria/NIE10-409/2011	2011	RRRKRF	Sokoto
XIVb	HF969178.1 chicken/Nigeria/NIE08-2270/2009	2009	RRRKRF	Sokoto
	HF969187.1 chicken/Nigeria/NIE08-0453/2008	2008	RRRKRF	Yobe
	HF969190.1 chicken/Nigeria/NIE08-2032/2009	2009	RRRKRF	Sokoto
	HF969198.1 chicken/Nigeria/NIE08-2279/2009	2009	RRQKRF	Yobe
	HF969201.1 chicken/Nigeria/NIE09-1599/2009	2009	RRRKRF	Benue
	HF969202.1 chicken/Nigeria/NIE09-2013/2009	2009	RRRKRF	Yobe
	HF969203.1 turkey/Nigeria/NIE09-2021/2009	2009	RRRKRF	Yobe
	HF969208.1 chicken/Nigeria/NIE10-122/2011	2011	RRRKRF	Sokoto
	HF969210.1 chicken/Nigeria/NIE10-139/2011	2011	RRQKRF	Sokoto
	HF969211.1 chicken/Nigeria/NIE10-263/2011	2011	RRRKRF	Sokoto
	HF969212.1 chicken/Nigeria/NIE10-318/2011	2011	RRRKRF	Sokoto
	HF969213.1 chicken/Nigeria/NIE10-325/2011	2011	RRQKRF	Sokoto
	HF969214.1 chicken/Nigeria/NIE10-333/2011	2011	RRRKRF	Sokoto
	JQ039390.1 chicken/Nigeria/VRD07-233/2007	2007	RRRKRF	-
	KC568205.1 NG-705/KD.TW.7C	2009	RRQKRF	Kaduna
	KC568206.1 NG-706/JG.KZ.14T	2009	RRRKRF	Jigawa
	KC568209.1 NG-720/KD.TW.03T	2009	RRQKRF	Kaduna
	KT948996.1 duck/Nigeria/NG-695/KG.LOM.11-16/2009	2009	RRRKRF	Kogi
	KY171989.1 chicken/Nigeria/VRD10/143/N68/913/2010	2010	RRRKRF	-
	KY171990.1 chicken/Nigeria/KD/TW/03T/N45/720/2009	2009	RRQKRF	Kaduna
	KY171993.1 chicken/Nigeria/VRD09/03I/N23/715/2009	2009	RRRKRF	-
	KY171994.1 chicken/Nigeria/VRD09/001/N19/714/2009	2009	RRRKRF	-

Table 2: Continued.

Subgenotype	Strain Identity	Year of isolation	Cleavage site	Location
Unassigned	KC568207.1 NG-707/GM.GMM.17-18T	2009	RRRKRF	Gombe
	KU058680.1 duck/Nigeria/903/KUDU-113/1992	1992	RRQKRF	-
	FJ772449.1 avian-913-33-Nigeria-2006	2006	RRQKRF	-
	FJ772486.1 avian-3724-6-Nigeria-2008	2008	RRQKRF	-
	HF969129.1 chicken/Nigeria/NIE08-1363/2008	2008	RRQKRF	Plateau
	HF969130.1 guinea fowl/Nigeria/NIE08-2004/2009	2009	RRQKRF	Sokoto
	HF969132.1 chicken/Nigeria/NIE08-2149/2009	2009	RRQKRF	Sokoto
	HF969134.1 chicken/Nigeria/NIE08-2168/2009	2009	RRQKRF	Sokoto
	HF969135.1 chicken/Nigeria/NIE08-2187/2009	2009	RRQKRF	Sokoto
	HF969137.1 chicken/Nigeria/NIE08-2208/2009	2009	RRQKRF	Sokoto
	HF969138.1 chicken/Nigeria/NIE08-2224/2009	2009	RRQKRF	Sokoto
	HF969140.1 chicken/Nigeria/NIE08-2340/2009	2009	RRQKRF	Sokoto
	HF969147.1 chicken/Nigeria/NIE09-2031/2009	2009	RRQKRF	Yobe
	HF969148.1 chicken/Nigeria/NIE09-2034/2009	2009	RRQKRF	Yobe
	HF969152.1 chicken/Nigeria/NIE09-2072/2009	2009	RRQKRF	Yobe
	HF969154.1 chicken/Nigeria/NIE09-2083/2009	2009	RRQKRF	Yobe
	HF969156.1 chicken/Nigeria/NIE09-2128/2009	2009	RRQKRF	Yobe
	HF969168.1 chicken/Nigeria/NIE10-124/2011	2011	RRRKRF	Sokoto
	HF969174.1 chicken/Nigeria/NIE10-304/2011	2011	RRRKRF	Sokoto
	HF969175.1 chicken/Nigeria/NIE10-306/2011	2011	RRRKRF	Sokoto
XVIIa	HF969176.1 chicken/Nigeria/NIE10-310/2011	2011	RRRKRF	Sokoto
	HF969188.1 chicken/Nigeria/NIE08-1365/2008	2008	RRQKRF	Plateau
	HF969189.1 chicken/Nigeria/NIE08-1366/2008	2008	RRQKRF	Plateau
	HF969191.1 chicken/Nigeria/NIE08-2042/2009	2009	RRQKRF	Sokoto
	HF969192.1 chicken/Nigeria/NIE08-2119/2009	2009	RRQKRF	Sokoto
	HF969195.1 chicken/Nigeria/NIE08-2247/2009	2009	RRQKRF	Sokoto
	HF969197.1 chicken/Nigeria/NIE08-2267/2009	2009	RRQKRF	Sokoto
	HF969199.1 chicken/Nigeria/NIE08-2349/2009	2009	RRQKRF	Sokoto
	HF969204.1 chicken/Nigeria/NIE09-2028/2009	2009	RRQKRF	Yobe
	HF969207.1 avian/Nigeria/NIE09-2167/2009	2009	RRQKRF	Yobe
	HF969209.1 chicken/Nigeria/NIE10-123/2011	2011	RRRKRF	Sokoto
	HF969215.1 chicken/Nigeria/NIE10-335/2011	2011	RRRKRF	Sokoto
	JQ039392.1 avian/Nigeria/VRD07-733/2007	2007	RRQKRF	-
	JQ039393.1 chicken/Nigeria/VRD07-141/2007	2007	RRQKRF	Sokoto
	JQ039394.1 chicken/Nigeria/VRD07-410/2007	2007	RRQKRF	Jigawa
	KC568204.1 pigeon/Nigeria/ZM/KN/PG01/N1/688/2009	2009	RRQKRF	Zamfara
	KC568208.1 NG-710/GM.PLBM.10-12T	2009	RRQKRF	Gombe
	KY171991.1 Nigeria/VRD17/04/N2/861/2004	2004	RRQKRF	-
	KY171992.1 chicken/Nigeria/JN/469/N44/892/2009	2009	RRQKRF	Plateau
	KY171995.1 chicken/Nigeria/VRD124/06/N11/867/2006	2006	RRQKRF	Plateau

TABLE 2: Continued.

Subgenotype	Strain Identity	Year of isolation	Cleavage site	Location
	FJ772446.1 avian-913-1-Nigeria-2006	2006	RRQKRF	-
	HF969128.1 avian/Nigeria/NIE07-216/2007	2007	RRQKRF	-
XVIIb	HF969171.1 chicken/Nigeria/NIE10-182/2011	2011	RRQKRF	Sokoto
	HF969194.1 chicken/Nigeria/NIE08-2199/2009	2009	RRQKRF	Sokoto
	HF969196.1 chicken/Nigeria/NIE08-2261/2009	2009	RRQKRF	Sokoto
	KF442614.1 Nigeria/228-7/2006	2006	RRQRRF	-
XVIIIb	HF969216.1 chicken/Nigeria/NIE11-1286/2011	2011	RRQKRF	Oyo
	HF969217.1 chicken/Nigeria/NIE10-171/2011	2011	RRQKRF	Sokoto
	HG326605.1 Spur-winged goose/Nigeria/ NIE-08-0121/2008	2008	GKQGRL	Yobe
Class I	HG326606.1 Spur-winged goose/Nigeria/ NIE-08-0121/2008	2008	GKQGRL	Yobe
	HG326607.1 Spur-winged goose/Nigeria/ NIE-08-0121/2008	2008	GKQGRL	Yobe
	HG326608.1 Spur-winged goose/Nigeria/ NIE-08-0121/2008	2008	GKQGRL	Yobe

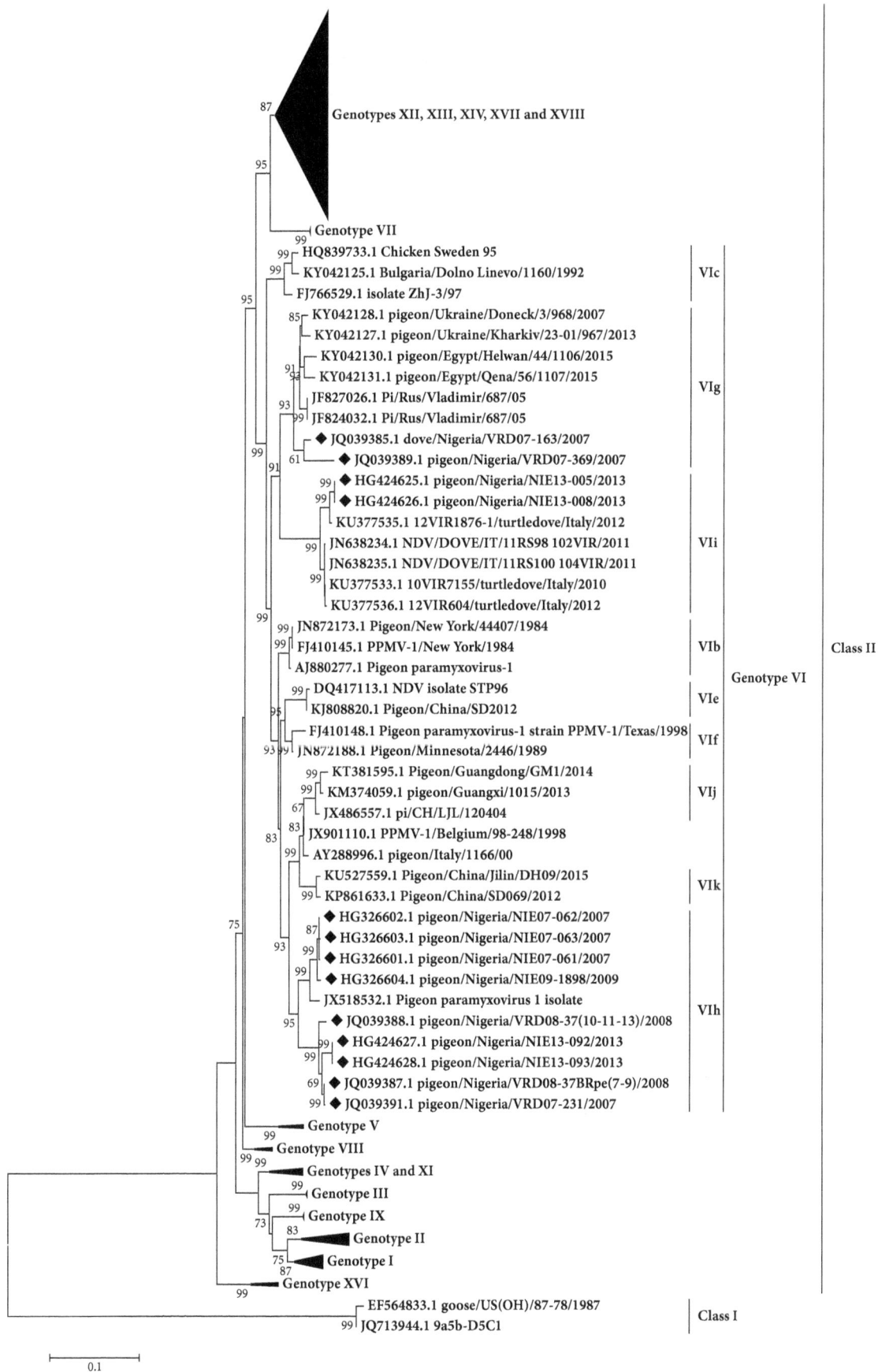

(a)

FIGURE 1: Continued.

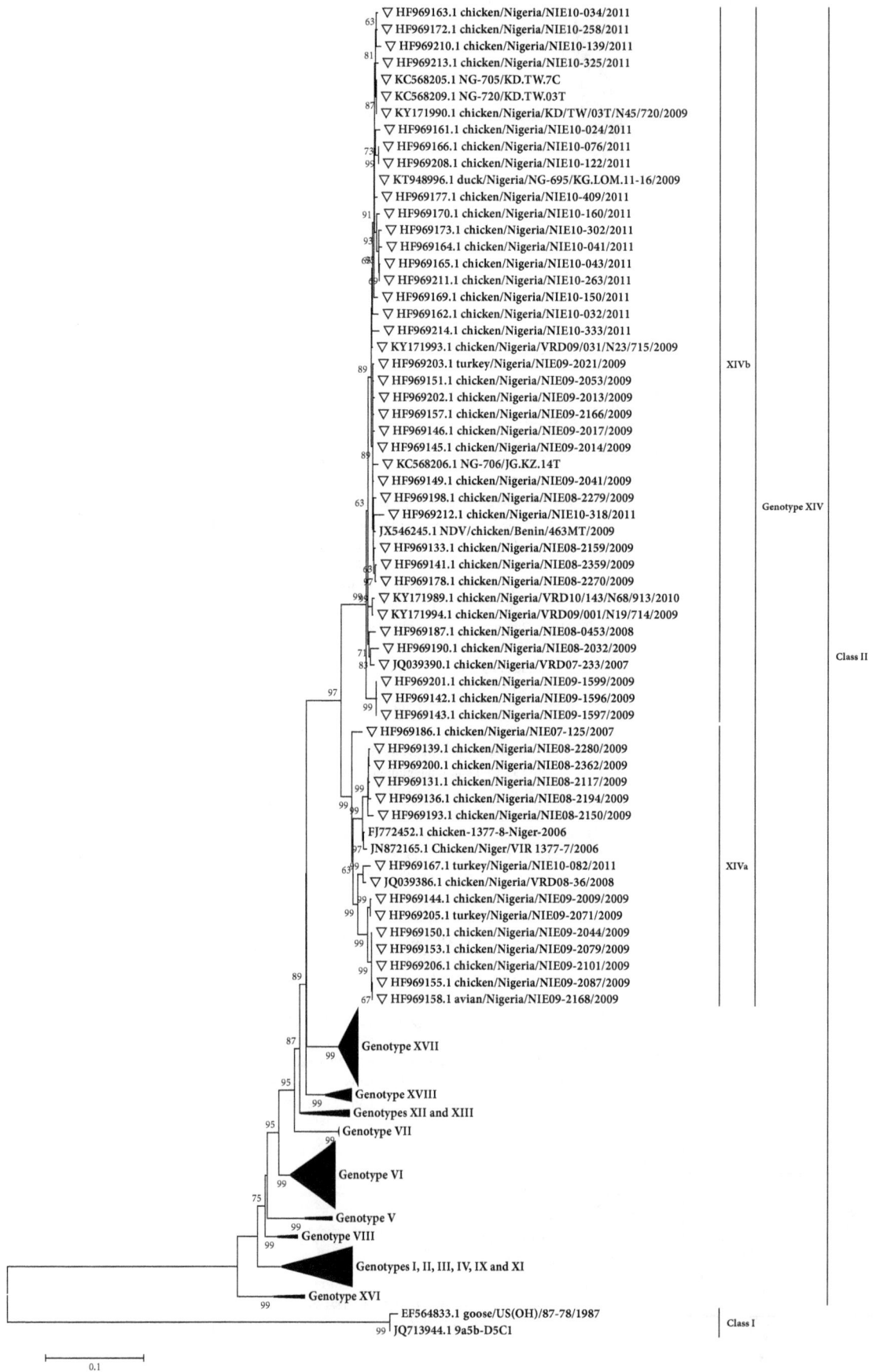

(b)

FIGURE 1: Continued.

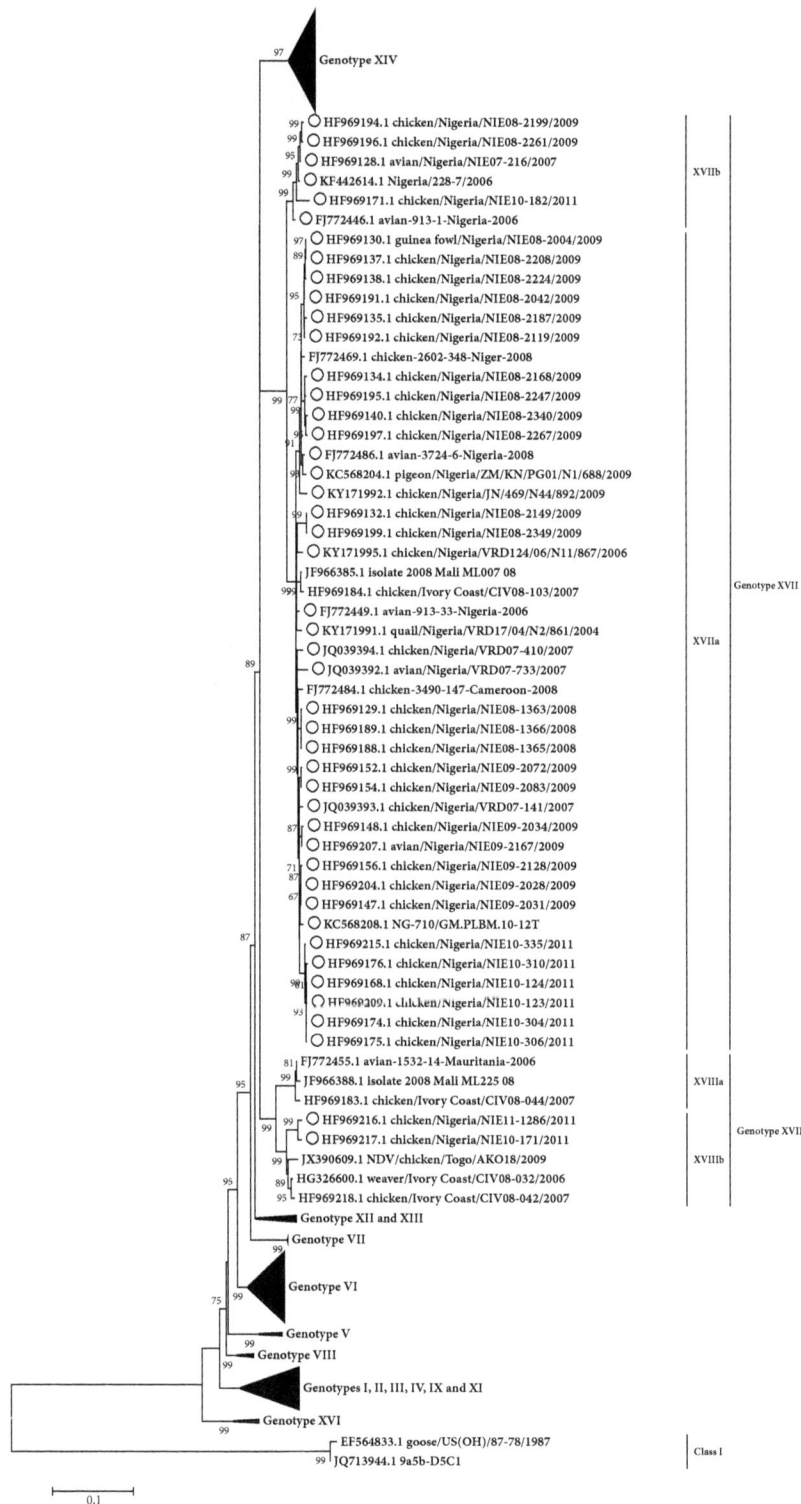

(c)

FIGURE 1: **Molecular phylogenetic analysis of complete F coding regions (1662bp) for Nigerian Newcastle disease virus isolates**. (a) Zoomed view of prevalent genotype VI isolates is shown. The coloured taxa indicate the subgenotypes with isolates prevalent in Nigeria (indicated with black icons at the node). (b) Relationship of Nigerian genotype XIV isolates with other reference strains is shown (all isolates prevalent in Nigeria are labelled with inverted triangle). (c) Expanded view of Nigerian genotype XVII and XVIII isolates (labelled with circles at the node). The evolutionary history was inferred using the maximum likelihood method based on the Tamura 3-parameter model. The tree with the highest log likelihood (-22231.3479) is shown. The percentage of trees in which the associated taxa clustered together is shown next to the branches. Initial tree(s) for the heuristic search were obtained by applying the neighbor-joining method to a matrix of pairwise distances estimated using the maximum composite likelihood (MCL) approach. A discrete Gamma distribution was used to model evolutionary rate differences among sites (5 categories (+G, parameter = 0.6931)). The tree is drawn to scale, with branch lengths measured in the number of substitutions per site. The analysis involved 195 nucleotide sequences. Codon positions included were 1st+2nd+3rd+Noncoding. All positions containing gaps and missing data were eliminated. Evolutionary analyses were conducted in MEGA6 [28].

TABLE 3: Estimates of evolutionary divergence among the virulent NDV genotypes circulating in Nigeria.

	VIg	VIh	VIi	XIVa	XIVb	XVIIa	XVIIb	XVIIIb
VIg		(0.005)	(0.006)	(0.007)	(0.008)	(0.007)	(0.007)	(0.008)
VIh	0.081		(0.007)	(0.007)	(0.007)	(0.007)	(0.007)	(0.007)
VIi	0.099	0.113		(0.008)	(0.009)	(0.008)	(0.008)	(0.008)
XIVa	0.127	0.128	0.149		(0.004)	(0.005)	(0.006)	(0.006)
XIVb	0.132	0.135	0.146	0.067		(0.007)	(0.007)	(0.007)
XVIIa	0.124	0.128	0.136	0.106	0.109		(0.004)	(0.006)
XVIIb	0.122	0.126	0.135	0.104	0.105	0.041		(0.007)
XVIIIb	0.118	0.120	0.132	0.112	0.114	0.093	0.095	

The table shows number of base differences per site from averaging over all sequence pairs between groups. Standard error estimate(s) are shown above the diagonal and were obtained by a bootstrap procedure (500 replicates). The analysis involved 120 nucleotide sequences. Codon positions included were 1st+2nd+3rd+Noncoding. All positions containing gaps and missing data were eliminated. Evolutionary analyses were conducted in MEGA6 [28].

[85, 86], their occurrence in Nigerian pigeon population economically threatens the poultry subsector in the country. Thus, there is a need to intensify disease surveillance in live birds markets, households, and commercial poultry farms, so that disease epidemics due to these isolates can be quickly detected and contained.

Isolates belonging to genotype XIV are the most predominantly isolated strains of NDV in Nigeria. Both subgenotypes, XIVa and XIVb, have been recovered from domestic birds found in the North-West (Sokoto, Kaduna, Jigawa), North-Central (Benue, Kogi), North-East (Taraba and Yobe), and South-Western parts of the country (Lagos) (Table 1). The intergroup genetic distance between the two subgenotypes averages at 6.7% (Table 3). Meanwhile, subgenotype XIVa isolates appear to be more genetically diverse, having an average intragenotype evolutionary divergence of 2.6%. On the other hand, isolates in the subgenotype XIVb are less divergent with about 98.6% overall mean similarity among themselves (data not shown). Phylogenetically, the genotype XIVa isolates form a cluster with some strains in Niger Republic while the Nigerian genotype XIVb isolates tend to be more closely related to the 2009 isolates from Benin Republic (Figure 1(b)). Interestingly, the isolates in genotype XIVa that share the highest nucleotide similarity with those from Niger Republic were all obtained from Sokoto State which shares a direct international border with Niger Republic. Their intimate phylogenetic relationship could therefore be partially explained by the cross border movements between the two countries which may facilitate the spread of the virus from one place to another. Notably, all genotype XIV isolates are so far restricted in distribution to only the West African subregion where they cause havoc in the regional poultry industry [11]. However, their emergence in other parts of the continent within the next few years would not be unexpected given the poor transboundary biosecurity measures in most of the African countries.

Several strains of NDV isolated in Nigeria from 2006-2011 belong to either subgenotype XVIIa or XVIIb, with the mean evolutionary divergence between the two subgenotypes being 4.1% (Table 3). Members of the subgenotypes XVIIa are highly similar, with an average nucleotide sequence similarity of 98.1% at the level of F protein gene. Surprisingly, despite their extensive spatial distribution in the northern states

(Sokoto, Zamfara, Plateau, Gombe, and Yobe states), none of these isolates was recovered from the southern parts of the country. It is however not clear whether this is due to sampling bias or they truly do not exist in those areas. On the basis of phylogenetic analysis, genotype XVIIa isolates from Nigeria are closely related to those from Niger Republic, Cameroun, Burkina Faso, and Mali whereas the genotype XVIIb isolates, whose mean intrasubgenotype distance was estimated to be 1.5%, are so far exclusively composed of Nigerian strains (Figure 1(c)). Importantly, the ecological distribution of genotype XVII isolates is to date restricted to the West and Central Africa [32, 53] where they are believed to considerably militate against poultry production. Indeed, representatives of these isolates have recently been shown to cause a typical velogenic viscerotropic ND [87] characterized by end stage morbidity and high mortality in chicken. There is therefore need to intensify the ongoing passive and active surveillance for ND in various parts of the country in order to avert the potential economic losses due to outbreaks with these strains.

Two highly similar sequences (99%) obtained from Nigerian NDV strains in the NCBI database were categorised under the subgenotype XVIIIb. They were obtained from Sokoto State in the North and Oyo State from the South. Based on the phylogenetic tree analysis, the two strains are quite related to the isolates from Togo and Ivory-Coast (Figure 1(c)) as earlier reported by Shittu et al. [32]. On the contrary, subgenotype XVIIIa isolates are yet to be encountered in Nigeria. Surprisingly, the interpopulation evolutionary distance between the two isolates in the subgenotype XVIIIb and those in either subgenotype XVIIa or XVIIb is slightly lower than the 10% cut-off for differentiating new genotypes (Table 2). This discrepancy was earlier observed by [88] who wondered if genotype XVIII isolates could be another subgroup of genotype XVII. However, Snoeck and Muller (2016) maintained that the two genotypes (XVII and XVIII) still stand and that the parameter used by Desingu et al. to challenge the existence of genotype XVIII was incorrect. Therefore, it is possible that the slightly lower than the threshold interpopulation distance observed in this study was due to the small number of genotype XVIII sequences from Nigeria (n=2) used in the analysis. As all the known genotype XVIII isolates are predicted to be virulent

TABLE 4: Genetic distances between the common vaccine strains and the prevalent virulent NDV subgenotypes in Nigeria.

Vaccine	Prevalent subgenotype							
	VIg	VIh	VIi	XIVa	XIVb	XVIIa	XVIIb	XVIIIb
B1	0.156	0.155	0.162	0.173	0.185	0.165	0.173	0.16
Komarov	0.155	0.155	0.161	0.169	0.180	0.157	0.165	0.159
Lasota	0.159	0.157	0.166	0.174	0.186	0.165	0.173	0.162
V4	0.147	0.151	0.156	0.165	0.175	0.153	0.16	0.152
VGGA	0.162	0.162	0.169	0.179	0.191	0.17	0.178	0.166
I2	0.145	0.153	0.155	0.163	0.173	0.151	0.149	0.156

The table shows number of base substitutions per site of the complete F gene sequence pairs between vaccine strains and NDV subgenotypes in Nigeria. The analysis involved 126 nucleotide sequences. Codon positions included were 1st+2nd+3rd+Noncoding. All positions containing gaps and missing data were eliminated. Evolutionary analyses were conducted in MEGA6 [28].

in chicken, their emergence in other parts of the country should be carefully monitored as part of the usual disease surveillance programme in the country.

4. Challenges for Newcastle Disease Control in Nigeria

Vaccination remains the most practical method of disease control in poultry and therefore plays a major role in strengthening the modern poultry industry [89, 90]. The ultimate goal of any vaccination program is the induction of sterilising immunity in the vaccinated host [91]. However, this is hardly achievable in poultry [89], owing to numerous factors that may adversely affect the efficacy of vaccination. The fact that all NDV strains are grouped into one serotype [92] suggests that immunity developed against one strain should offer cross protection against challenge with any other strains. Unfortunately to date, outbreaks of ND are frequently reported among farms that have vaccinated using the available vaccines [32, 52, 53]. The cause of these disease outbreaks among the vaccinated birds is still controversial in the literature. While some researchers hold the view that the poor vaccine induced immunity is due to the suboptimal vaccine intake following its mass administration in poultry [93], others believe that the genetic variation between the vaccine and the circulating field strains might be the major factor responsible for the incomplete protective efficacy of the current vaccines [94, 95]. Although the currently used vaccines, when correctly administered, are known to fully protect birds against clinical disease and mortality [95, 96], they cannot block the replication of the virulent virus post challenge [44, 45]. Thus, the vaccinated birds may look apparently healthy but still excrete a large amount of the virulent virus, which can in turn cause disease among unprotected birds. Since it is an established fact that ND vaccines are more effective in reducing virus shedding when the vaccine strains are genetically closer to the challenge strain [57, 97], the evolutionary distance between the vaccine strains and the circulating field strain represents an important factor in effective disease control, since it explains the continuous occurrence of ND outbreaks despite the extensive poultry vaccination programs in the country.

Based on the evolutionary analysis of the complete F coding sequences performed in this study, all the virulent NDV genotypes circulating in Nigeria are shown to be distantly related to the currently available vaccine strains in the country (Table 4). LaSota which is the most widely used live attenuated ND vaccine in Nigeria and indeed many parts of the world has an average nucleotide sequence divergence of 15.7-18.6% when compared with all the existing virulent class II subgenotypes in Nigeria (Table 4). Similarly, the very popular Komarov inactivated NDV vaccine differs from the circulating NDV subgenotypes in the country with an average evolutionary distance of 15.5-18% (Table 4). Recently in Indonesia, sequence divergence between the field and the vaccine strains has been implicated in a severe disease outbreak that led to 70% mortality among the vaccinated birds [95]. Furthermore, in Malaysia where the prevalent isolates are genotype VII strains that considerably diverge from the LaSota strain, the frequency of ND outbreaks among the vaccinated farms has steadily increased from 2009 to date [62, 98]. Therefore, the wide genetic divergence between the Nigerian NDV strains and vaccine strains used in the country should be a source of a serious concern to the national poultry industry and requires urgent attention. These problems collectively highlight the possible limitations of the current vaccines in offering a complete protection against the circulating strains of NDV in Nigeria. The need to improve the current disease control strategies is therefore imperative.

5. Way Forward

The panacea for all these ND control challenges in Nigeria is the maintenance of strict biosecurity and the development of rationally designed vaccines based on the currently circulating isolates in the country. With the advent of reverse genetics technology that allows the recovery of recombinant NDV from their cloned cDNA [99], genotype-matched live attenuated vaccines can be easily generated. Since the complete genome sequence of some biologically well-characterized viruses in the country has already been obtained [33, 34], efforts should be intensified towards rescuing their attenuated counterparts by simply engineering their F cleavage site to encode monobasic amino acid residues instead of the poly basic motifs [100]. By developing a reverse genetics system for one prevalent strain in the country, vaccine candidates against all the circulating strains can easily be obtained by F gene swapping in the full length infectious clone followed by the recovery of the chimeric viruses by reverse genetics techniques. Alternatively, recombinant viral vectors such as herpesvirus of turkey [101] (HVT) expressing surface glycoproteins (F and/or HN) of the circulating NDV can be developed as an effective genotype-matched vaccine against the prevailing genotypes in the country.

6. Conclusion

In summary, a comprehensive distribution of NDV genotypes in various regions of Nigeria has been provided. Apparently, multiple genetically distinct strains of NDV are cocirculating in some states of the federation, an important factor that may favour the emergence of novel virulent isolates in the country. In particular, apart from genotype VI isolates, all the virulent NDV genotypes prevalent in Nigeria have been isolated in Sokoto State between 2007 and 2011, making the State a potential hotspot of different NDV genotypes in Nigeria. It is interesting to know that genotype VII isolates responsible for the on-going fourth and the imminent fifth ND panzootic [102, 103] have not been reported in Nigeria despite their recent emergence in some African countries [104, 105]. Since these panzootic viruses have a high potential for international spread, there is a need to intensify disease surveillance activities and strengthen biosecurity barriers so as to avoid their introduction into the country. Finally, given the wide evolutionary divergence between the commonly used vaccines and the circulating NDV strains in the country, there is a need to revise the current ND control strategies in Nigeria. Genotype-matched vaccines with improved protective efficacy and virus shedding blocking ability should be designed to specifically target the currently circulating NDV genotypes in the country.

Acknowledgments

This is a review article and does not require any substantial funding. However, the cost of open access publication will be covered by the Transdisciplinary Research Grant Scheme (TRGS) of the Ministry of Higher Education Malaysia with the grant number 5535402.

References

[1] D. J. Alexander, "Newcastle disease," *British Poultry Science*, vol. 42, no. 1, pp. 5–22, 2001.

[2] D. J. Alexander, "Ecology and Epidemiology of Newcastle Disease," *Avian Influenza and Newcastle Disease: A Field and Laboratory Manual*, pp. 19–26, 2009.

[3] A. Ballagi-Pordány, E. Wehmann, J. Herczeg, S. Belák, and B. Lomniczi, "Identification and grouping of Newcastle disease virus strains by restriction site analysis of a region from the F gene," *Archives of Virology*, vol. 141, pp. 243–261, 1996.

[4] D. J. Alexander, E. W. Aldous, and C. M. Fuller, "The long view: a selective review of 40 years of Newcastle disease research," *Avian Pathology*, vol. 41, no. 4, pp. 329–335, 2012.

[5] D. J. Alexander, G. Parsons, and R. Marshall, "Avian paramyxovirus type 1 infections of racing pigeons: 4 laboratory assessment of vaccination.," *Veterinary Record*, vol. 118, no. 10, pp. 262–266, 1986.

[6] J. T. Lumeij and J. W. E. Stam, "Paramyxovirus disease in racing pigeons," *Veterinary Quarterly*, vol. 7, no. 1, Article ID 9693954, pp. 60–65, 1985.

[7] G. Cross, "Paramyxovirus-1 infection (Newcastle disease) of pigeons," *Seminars in Avian and Exotic Pet Medicine*, vol. 4, no. 2, pp. 92–95, 1995.

[8] J. Herczeg, E. Wehmann, R. R. Bragg et al., "Two novel genetic groups (VIIb and VIII) responsible for recent Newcastle disease outbreaks in Southern Africa, one (VIIb) of which reached Southern Europe," *Archives of Virology*, vol. 144, no. 11, pp. 2087–2099, 1999.

[9] E. K. Lee, W. J. Jeon, J. H. Kwon, C. B. Yang, and K. S. Choi, "Molecular epidemiological investigation of Newcastle disease virus from domestic ducks in Korea," *Veterinary Microbiology*, vol. 134, no. 3, pp. 241–248, 2009.

[10] H. Liu, Z. Wang, Y. Wang, C. Sun, D. Zheng, and Y. Wu, "Characterization of Newcastle disease virus isolated from waterfowl in China," *Avian Diseases*, vol. 52, no. 1, pp. 150–155, 2008.

[11] A. Samuel, B. Nayak, A. Paldurai et al., "Phylogenetic and pathotypic characterization of newcastle disease viruses circulating in west africa and efficacy of a current vaccine," *Journal of Clinical Microbiology*, vol. 51, no. 3, pp. 771–781, 2013.

[12] O. J. Ibu, J. O. A. Okoye, E. P. Adulugba et al., "Prevalence of newcastle disease viruses in wild and captive birds in central Nigeria," *International Journal of Poultry Science*, vol. 8, no. 6, pp. 574–578, 2009.

[13] A. H. Jibril, J. U. Umoh, J. Kabir et al., "Newcastle Disease in Local Chickens of Live Bird Markets and Households in Zamfara State, Nigeria," *ISRN Epidemiology*, vol. 2014, Article ID 513961, 4 pages, 2014.

[14] A. H. Jibril, J. U. Umoh, J. Kabir, M. M. Gashua, and M. B. Bello, "Application of participatory epidemiology techniques to investigate Newcastle disease among rural farmers in Zamfara state, Nigeria," *Journal of Applied Poultry Research*, vol. 24, no. 2, pp. 233–239, 2015.

[15] L. Sa'idu, L. B. Tekdek, and P. A. Abdu, "Prevalence of Newcastle disease antibodies in domestic and semi-domestic birds in Zaria, Nigeria," *Veterinarski Arhiv*, vol. 74, no. 4, pp. 309–317, 2004.

[16] P. Gogoi, K. Ganar, and S. Kumar, "Avian paramyxovirus: a brief review," *Transboundary and Emerging Diseases*, vol. 64, no. 1, pp. 53–67, 2017.

[17] K. Murulitharan, K. Yusoff, A. R. Omar, and A. Molouki, "Characterization of Malaysian velogenic NDV strain AF2240-I genomic sequence: A comparative study," *Virus Genes*, vol. 46, no. 3, pp. 431–440, 2013.

[18] D. A. Satharasinghe, K. Murulitharan, S. W. Tan et al., "Detection of inter-lineage natural recombination in avian paramyxovirus serotype 1 using simplified deep sequencing platform," *Frontiers in Microbiology*, vol. 7, pp. 1–14, 2016.

[19] OIE, "Newcastle Disease (Infection with Newcastle Disease Virus)," in *Manual of Diagnostic Tests and Vaccines for Terrestrial Animals: (Mammals, Birds and Bees)*, vol. 1, pp. 555–574, 2012.

[20] M. Banerjee, W. M. Reed, S. D. Fitzgerald, and B. Panigraphy, "Neurotropic velogenic Newcastle disease in cormorants in Michigan: pathology and virus characterization," *Avian Diseases*, vol. 38, no. 4, pp. 873–878, 1994.

[21] A. M. Piacenti, D. J. King, B. S. Seal, J. Zhang, and C. C. Brown, "Pathogenesis of Newcastle disease in commercial and specific pathogen-free turkeys experimentally infected with isolates of different virulence," *Veterinary Pathology*, vol. 43, no. 2, pp. 168–178, 2006.

[22] W. Fan, Y. Wang, S. Wang et al., "Virulence in Newcastle disease virus: A genotyping and molecular evolution spectrum perspective," *Research in Veterinary Science*, vol. 111, pp. 49–54, 2017.

[23] V. M. B. D. Moura, L. Susta, S. Cardenas-Garcia et al., "Neuropathogenic capacity of lentogenic, mesogenic, and velogenic newcastle disease virus strains in day-old chickens," *Veterinary Pathology*, vol. 53, no. 1, pp. 53–64, 2016.

[24] H. Hamid, R. S. F. Campbell, and C. Lamichhane, "The Pathology of infection of chickens with the lentogenic V4 strain of newcastle disease virus," *Avian Pathology*, vol. 19, no. 4, pp. 687–696, 1990.

[25] O. S. de Leeuw, L. Hartog, G. Koch, and B. P. H. Peeters, "Effect of fusion protein cleavage site mutations on virulence of Newcastle disease virus: Non-virulent cleavage site mutants revert to virulence after one passage in chicken brain," *Journal of General Virology*, vol. 84, pp. 475–484, 2003.

[26] A. Panda, Z. Huang, S. Elankumaran, D. D. Rockemann, and S. K. Samal, "Role of fusion protein cleavage site in the virulence of Newcastle disease virus," *Microbial Pathogenesis*, vol. 36, no. 1, pp. 1–10, 2004.

[27] Y. Wang, W. Yu, N. Huo et al., "Comprehensive analysis of amino acid sequence diversity at the F protein cleavage site of Newcastle disease virus in fusogenic activity," *PLoS ONE*, vol. 12, no. 9, Article ID e0183923, 2017.

[28] K. Tamura, G. Stecher, D. Peterson, A. Filipski, and S. Kumar, "MEGA6: molecular evolutionary genetics analysis version 6.0," *Molecular Biology and Evolution*, vol. 30, no. 12, pp. 2725–2729, 2013.

[29] T. Hamisu, H. Kazeem, K. Majiyagbe et al., "Molecular screening and isolation of Newcastle disease virus from live poultry markets and chickens from commercial poultry farms in Zaria, Kaduna state, Nigeria," *Sokoto Journal of Veterinary Sciences*, vol. 14, no. 3, pp. 18–25, 2017.

[30] P. Solomon, C. Abolnik, T. M. Joannis, and S. Bisschop, "Virulent Newcastle disease virus in Nigeria: Identification of a new clade of sub-lineage 5f from livebird markets," *Virus Genes*, vol. 44, no. 1, pp. 98–103, 2012.

[31] D. G. Diel, L. H. A. da Silva, H. Liu, Z. Wang, P. J. Miller, and C. L. Afonso, "Genetic diversity of avian paramyxovirus type 1: Proposal for a unified nomenclature and classification system of Newcastle disease virus genotypes," *Infection, Genetics and Evolution*, vol. 12, no. 8, pp. 1770–1779, 2012.

[32] I. Shittu, T. M. Joannis, G. N. Odaibo, and O. D. Olaleye, "Newcastle disease in Nigeria: epizootiology and current knowledge of circulating genotypes," *VirusDisease*, vol. 27, no. 4, pp. 329–339, 2016.

[33] I. Shittu, P. Sharma, T. M. Joannis et al., "Complete genome sequence of a genotype XVII newcastle disease virus, isolated from an apparently healthy domestic duck in nigeria," *Genome Announcements*, vol. 4, no. 1, Article ID e01716-15, 2016.

[34] I. Shittu, P. Sharma, J. D. Volkening et al., "Identification and complete genome sequence analysis of a genotype XIV newcastle disease virus from Nigeria," *Genome Announcements*, vol. 4, no. 1, Article ID e01581-15, 2016.

[35] R. S. de Almeida, S. Hammoumi, P. Gil et al., "New avian paramyxoviruses type I strains identified in Africa provide new outcomes for phylogeny reconstruction and genotype classification," *PLoS ONE*, vol. 8, no. 10, Article ID e76413, 2013.

[36] L. M. Kim, D. J. King, P. E. Curry et al., "Phylogenetic diversity among low-virulence newcastle disease viruses from waterfowl and shorebirds and comparison of genotype distributions to those of poultry-origin isolates," *Journal of Virology*, vol. 81, no. 22, pp. 12641–12653, 2007.

[37] L. M. Kim, D. J. King, H. Guzman et al., "Biological and phylogenetic characterization of pigeon paramyxovirus serotype 1 circulating in wild North American pigeons and doves," *Journal of Clinical Microbiology*, vol. 46, no. 10, pp. 3303–3310, 2008.

[38] L. M. Kim, D. L. Suarez, and C. L. Afonso, "Detection of a broad range of class I and II Newcastle disease viruses using multiplex real-time reverse transcription polymerase chain reaction assay," *Journal of Veterinary Diagnostic Investigation*, vol. 20, no. 4, pp. 414–425, 2008.

[39] H. Liu, P. Zhang, P. Wu et al., "Phylogenetic characterization and virulence of two Newcastle disease viruses isolated from wild birds in China," *Infection, Genetics and Evolution*, vol. 20, pp. 215–224, 2013.

[40] E. W. Aldous, J. K. Mynn, J. Banks, and D. J. Alexander, "A molecular epidemiological study of avian paramyxovirus type 1 (Newcastle disease virus) isolates by phylogenetic analysis of a partial nucleotide sequence of the fusion protein gene," *Avian Pathology*, vol. 32, pp. 237–255, 2003.

[41] G. Cattoli, A. Fusaro, I. Monne et al., "Emergence of a new genetic lineage of Newcastle disease virus in West and Central Africa-Implications for diagnosis and control," *Veterinary Microbiology*, vol. 142, no. 3-4, pp. 168–176, 2010.

[42] C. J. Snoeck, M. F. Ducatez, A. A. Owoade et al., "Newcastle disease virus in West Africa: New virulent strains identified in non-commercial farms," *Archives of Virology*, vol. 154, no. 1, pp. 47–54, 2009.

[43] A. Czeglédi, D. Ujvári, E. Somogyi, E. Wehmann, O. Werner, and B. Lomniczi, "Third genome size category of avian paramyxovirus serotype 1 (Newcastle disease virus) and evolutionary implications," *Virus Research*, vol. 120, no. 1-2, pp. 36–48, 2006.

[44] K. M. Dimitrov, C. L. Afonso, Q. Yu, and P. J. Miller, "Newcastle disease vaccines—A solved problem or a continuous challenge?" *Veterinary Microbiology*, vol. 206, pp. 126–136, 2016.

[45] K. M. Dimitrov, A. M. Ramey, X. Qiu, J. Bahl, and C. L. Afonso, "Infection, Genetics and Evolution Temporal, geographic, and host distribution of avian paramyxovirus 1 (Newcastle disease virus)," *Infection, Genetics and Evolution*, vol. 39, pp. 22–34, 2016.

[46] Y. Kang, Y. Li, R. Yuan et al., "Phylogenetic relationships and pathogenicity variation of two Newcastle disease viruses isolated from domestic ducks in Southern China," *Virology Journal*, vol. 11, no. 1, article 147, 2014.

[47] S. Ren, X. Xie, Y. Wang et al., "Molecular characterization of a Class I Newcastle disease virus strain isolated from a pigeon in China," *Avian Pathology*, vol. 45, no. 4, pp. 408–417, 2016.

[48] M. A. Hoque, G. W. Burgess, D. Karo-Karo, A. L. Cheam, and L. F. Skerratt, "Monitoring of wild birds for Newcastle disease virus in north Queensland, Australia," *Preventive Veterinary Medicine*, vol. 103, no. 1, pp. 49–62, 2012.

[49] H. Liu, F. Chen, Y. Zhao et al., "Genomic characterization of the first class I Newcastle disease virus isolated from the mainland of China," *Virus Genes*, vol. 40, no. 3, pp. 365–371, 2010.

[50] D. J. Alexander, G. Campbell, R. J. Manvell, M. S. Collins, G. Parsons, and M. S. McNulty, "Characterisation of an antigenically unusual virus responsible for two outbreaks of Newcastle disease in the Republic of Ireland in 1990," *Veterinary Record*, vol. 130, no. 4, pp. 65–68, 1992.

[51] Y. He, T. L. Taylor, K. M. Dimitrov et al., "Whole-genome sequencing of genotype VI Newcastle disease viruses from formalin-fixed paraffin-embedded tissues from wild pigeons reveals continuous evolution and previously unrecognized genetic diversity in the U.S.," *Virology Journal*, vol. 15, no. 1, 2018.

[52] C. J. Snoeck, A. T. Adeyanju, A. a. Owoade et al., "Genetic diversity of newcastle disease virus in wild birds and pigeons in West Africa," *Applied and Environmental Microbiology*, vol. 79, no. 24, pp. 7867–7874, 2013.

[53] C. J. Snoeck, A. A. Owoade, E. Couacy-Hymann et al., "High genetic diversity of newcastle disease virus in poultry in west and central Africa: Cocirculation of genotype XIV and newly defined genotypes XVII and XVIII," *Journal of Clinical Microbiology*, vol. 51, no. 7, pp. 2250–2260, 2013.

[54] A. R. Gould, J. A. Kattenbelt, P. Selleck, E. Hansson, A. Della-Porta, and H. A. Westbury, "Virulent Newcastle disease in Australia: Molecular epidemiological analysis of viruses isolated prior to and during the outbreaks of 1998-2000," *Virus Research*, vol. 77, no. 1, pp. 51–60, 2001.

[55] B. S. Seal, M. G. Wise, J. C. Pedersen et al., "Genomic sequences of low-virulence avian paramyxovirus-1 (Newcastle disease virus) isolates obtained from live-bird markets in North America not related to commonly utilized commercial vaccine strains," *Veterinary Microbiology*, vol. 106, no. 1-2, pp. 7–16, 2005.

[56] A. Czeglédi, E. Wehmann, and B. Lomniczi, "On the origins and relationships of Newcastle disease virus vaccine strains Hertfordshire and Mukteswar, and virulent strain Herts'33," *Avian Pathology*, vol. 32, no. 3, pp. 271–276, 2003.

[57] P. J. Miller, E. L. Decanini, and C. L. Afonso, "Newcastle disease: evolution of genotypes and the related diagnostic challenges," *Infection, Genetics and Evolution: Journal of Molecular Epidemiology and Evolutionary Genetics in Infectious Diseases*, vol. 10, no. 1, pp. 26–35, 2010.

[58] O. F. Maminiaina, P. Gil, F. Briand et al., "Newcastle Disease Virus in Madagascar: Identification of an Original Genotype Possibly Deriving from a Died Out Ancestor of Genotype IV," *PLoS ONE*, vol. 5, no. 11, Article ID e13987, 2010.

[59] L. Susta, K. R. Hamal, P. J. Miller et al., "Separate evolution of virulent Newcastle disease viruses from Mexico and Central America," *Journal of Clinical Microbiology*, vol. 52, no. 5, pp. 1382–1390, 2014.

[60] M. Sabra, K. M. Dimitrov, I. V. Goraichuk et al., "Phylogenetic assessment reveals continuous evolution and circulation of pigeon-derived virulent avian avulaviruses 1 in Eastern Europe, Asia, and Africa," *BMC Veterinary Research*, vol. 13, no. 1, 2017.

[61] C. Terregino, G. Cattoli, B. Grossele, E. Bertoli, E. Tisato, and I. Capua, "Characterization of Newcastle disease virus isolates obtained from Eurasian collared doves (Streptopelia decaocto) in Italy," *Avian Pathology*, vol. 32, no. 1, pp. 63–68, 2003.

[62] O. A. Aljumaili, S. K. Yeap, A. R. Omar, and I. Aini, "Isolation and characterization of genotype VII newcastle disease virus from NDV vaccinated farms in Malaysia," *Pertanika Journal of Tropical Agricultural Science*, vol. 40, no. 4, pp. 677–690, 2017.

[63] S. A. Shohaimi, R. A. Raus, O. G. Huai, B. M. Asmayatim, N. Nayan, and A. M. Yusuf, "Sequence and phylogenetic analysis of newcastle disease virus genotype VII isolated in Malaysia during 1999-2012," *Jurnal Teknologi*, vol. 77, no. 25, pp. 159–164, 2015.

[64] J. Wang, Y. Cong, R. Yin et al., "Generation and evaluation of a recombinant genotype VII Newcastle disease virus expressing VP3 protein of Goose parvovirus as a bivalent vaccine in goslings," *Virus Research*, vol. 203, pp. 77–83, 2015.

[65] Y. Zhang, yuan. Shao, M. yu, X. Yu, J. Zhao, and G. Zhang, "Molecular characterization of chicken-derived genotype VIId Newcastle disease virus isolates in China during 2005-2012 reveals a new length in hemagglutinin-neuraminidase," *Infection, Genetics and Evolution*, vol. 21, pp. 359–366, 2014.

[66] F. Sabouri, M. Vasfi Marandi, and M. Bashashati, "Characterization of a novel VIII sub-genotype of Newcastle disease virus circulating in Iran," *Avian Pathology*, vol. 47, no. 1, 2017.

[67] M. M. Ebrahimi, S. Shahsavandi, G. Moazenijula, and M. Shamsara, "Phylogeny and evolution of Newcastle disease virus genotypes isolated in Asia during 2008-2011," *Virus Genes*, vol. 45, no. 1, pp. 63–68, 2012.

[68] M. Esmaelizad, V. Mayahi, M. Pashaei, and H. Goudarzi, "Identification of novel Newcastle disease virus sub-genotype VII-(j) based on the fusion protein," *Archives of Virology*, vol. 162, no. 4, pp. 971–978, 2017.

[69] N. Siddique, K. Naeem, M. A. Abbas et al., "Sequence and phylogenetic analysis of virulent Newcastle disease virus isolates from Pakistan during 2009-2013 reveals circulation of new sub genotype," *Virology*, vol. 444, no. 1-2, pp. 37–40, 2013.

[70] S. W. Tan, A. Ideris, A. R. Omar, K. Yusoff, and M. Hair-Bejo, "Sequence and phylogenetic analysis of Newcastle disease virus genotypes isolated in Malaysia between," *Archives of Virology*, vol. 155, no. 1, pp. 63–70, 2010.

[71] S. Umar, "Emergence of new sub-genotypes of Newcastle disease virus in Pakistan," *World's Poultry Science Journal*, vol. 73, no. 3, pp. 567–580, 2017.

[72] C. Xue, Y. Cong, R. Yin et al., "Genetic diversity of the genotype VII Newcastle disease virus: identification of a novel VIIj sub-genotype," *Virus Genes*, vol. 53, no. 1, pp. 63–70, 2017.

[73] X. Duan, P. Zhang, M. Jing et al., "Characterization of genotype IX Newcastle disease virus strains isolated from wild birds in the northern Qinling Mountains, China," *Virus Genes*, vol. 48, no. 1, pp. 48–55, 2014.

[74] X. Qiu, Q. Sun, S. Wu et al., "Entire genome sequence analysis of genotype IX Newcastle disease viruses reveals their early-genotype phylogenetic position and recent-genotype genome size," *Virology Journal*, vol. 8, article no. 117, 2011.

[75] N. L. Hines, M. L. Killian, J. C. Pedersen et al., "An rRT-PCR Assay to Detect the Matrix Gene of a Broad Range of Avian Paramyxovirus Serotype-1 Strains," *Avian Diseases*, vol. 56, no. 2, pp. 387–395, 2012.

[76] R. Maqbool, S. A. Wani, A. Wali et al., "Avian paramyxovirus serotype-1 detection from chicken reared in Kashmir valley," *Journal of Pure and Applied Microbiology*, vol. 11, no. 1, pp. 355–357, 2017.

[77] A. Chumbe, R. Izquierdo-Lara, L. Tataje-Lavanda et al., "Characterization and sequencing of a genotype XII Newcastle

disease virus isolated from a peacock (Pavo cristatus) in Peru," *Genome Announcements*, vol. 3, no. 4, pp. 3-4, 2015.

[78] V. Gowthaman, S. D. Singh, K. Dhama et al., "Isolation and characterization of genotype XIII Newcastle disease virus from Emu in India," *VirusDisease*, vol. 27, no. 3, pp. 315–318, 2016.

[79] M. Das and S. Kumar, "Evidence of independent evolution of genotype XIII Newcastle disease viruses in India," *Archives of Virology*, vol. 162, no. 4, pp. 997–1007, 2017.

[80] B. Nath and S. Kumar, "Emerging variant of genotype XIII Newcastle disease virus from Northeast India," *Acta Tropica*, vol. 172, pp. 64–69, 2017.

[81] S. C. Courtney, L. Susta, D. Gomez et al., "Highly divergent virulent isolates of newcastle disease virus from the dominican republic are members of a new genotype that may have evolved unnoticed for over 2 decades," *Journal of Clinical Microbiology*, vol. 51, no. 2, pp. 508–517, 2013.

[82] S. Akhtar, M. A. Muneer, K. Muhammad et al., "Genetic characterization and phylogeny of pigeon paramyxovirus isolate (PPMV-1) from Pakistan," *SpringerPlus*, vol. 5, no. 1, article 1295, 2016.

[83] T. Munir, A. Aslam, B. Zahid, I. Ahmed, M. S. Imran, and M. Ijaz, "Potential of commonly resident wild birds towards newcastle disease virus transmission," *Pakistan Veterinary Journal*, vol. 35, no. 1, pp. 106-107, 2015.

[84] P. Zhang, G. Xie, X. Liu et al., "High genetic diversity of Newcastle disease virus in wild and domestic birds in northeastern China from 2013 to 2015 reveals potential epidemic trends," *Applied and Environmental Microbiology*, vol. 82, no. 5, pp. 1530–1536, 2016.

[85] J. C. F. M. Dortmans, P. J. M. Rottier, G. Koch, and B. P. H. Peeters, "Passaging of a newcastle disease virus pigeon variant in chickens results in selection of viruses with mutations in the polymerase complex enhancing virus replication and virulence," *Journal of General Virology*, vol. 92, no. 2, pp. 336–345, 2011.

[86] C. Meng, X. Qiu, S. Yu et al., "Evolution of newcastle disease virus quasispecies diversity and enhanced virulence after passage through chicken air sacs," *Journal of Virology*, vol. 90, no. 4, pp. 2052–2063, 2016.

[87] L. Susta, M. E. B. Jones, G. Cattoli et al., "Pathologic Characterization of Genotypes XIV and XVII Newcastle Disease Viruses and Efficacy of Classical Vaccination on Specific Pathogen-Free Birds," *Veterinary Pathology*, vol. 52, no. 1, pp. 120–131, 2015.

[88] P. A. Desingu, K. Dhama, Y. S. Malik, and R. K. Singh, "May newly defined genotypes XVII and XVIII of newcastle disease virus in poultry from west and central Africa be considered a single genotype (XVII)?" *Journal of Clinical Microbiology*, vol. 54, no. 9, article 2399, 2016.

[89] S. Marangon and L. Busani, "The use of vaccination in poultry production," *Revue Scientifique et Technique*, vol. 26, no. 1, pp. 265–274, 2006.

[90] W. I. Muir, W. L. Bryden, and A. J. Husband, "Immunity, vaccination and the avian intestinal tract," *Developmental and Comparative Immunology*, vol. 24, no. 2-3, pp. 325–342, 2000.

[91] H. W. Doerr and A. Berger, "Vaccination against infectious diseases: What is promising?" *Medical Microbiology and Immunology*, vol. 203, no. 6, pp. 365–371, 2014.

[92] D. R. Kapczynski, C. L. Afonso, and P. J. Miller, "Immune responses of poultry to Newcastle disease virus," *Developmental and Comparative Immunology*, vol. 41, no. 3, pp. 447–453, 2013.

[93] J. C. F. M. Dortmans, B. P. H. Peeters, and G. Koch, "Newcastle disease virus outbreaks: Vaccine mismatch or inadequate application?" *Veterinary Microbiology*, vol. 160, no. 1-2, pp. 17–22, 2012.

[94] Z. Hu, S. Hu, C. Meng, X. Wang, J. Zhu, and X. Liu, "Generation of a genotype VII Newcastle disease virus vaccine candidate with high yield in embryonated chicken eggs," *Avian Diseases*, vol. 55, no. 3, pp. 391–397, 2011.

[95] S. Xiao, B. Nayak, A. Samuel et al., "Generation by Reverse Genetics of an Effective, Stable, Live-Attenuated Newcastle Disease Virus Vaccine Based on a Currently Circulating, Highly Virulent Indonesian Strain," *PLoS ONE*, vol. 7, no. 12, Article ID e52751, 2012.

[96] M. B. Bello, K. Yusoff, A. Ideris, M. Hair-bejo, B. P. H. Peeters, and A. R. Omar, "Diagnostic and vaccination approaches for newcastle disease virus in poultry: the current and emerging perspectives," *Biomed Research International*, vol. 2018, Article ID 7278459, 18 pages, 2018.

[97] P. J. Miller, C. L. Afonso, J. El Attrache et al., "Effects of Newcastle disease virus vaccine antibodies on the shedding and transmission of challenge viruses," *Developmental and Comparative Immunology*, vol. 41, no. 4, pp. 505–513, 2013.

[98] K. Roohani, S. W. Tan, S. K. Yeap, A. Ideris, M. H. Bejo, and A. R. Omar, "Characterisation of genotype VII Newcastle disease virus (NDV) isolated from NDV vaccinated chickens, and the efficacy of LaSota and recombinant genotype VII vaccines against challenge with velogenic NDV," *Journal of Veterinary Science*, vol. 16, no. 4, pp. 447–457, 2015.

[99] B. P. H. Peeters, O. S. De Leeuw, G. Koch, and A. L. J. Gielkens, "Rescue of Newcastle disease virus from cloned cDNA: Evidence that cleavability of the fusion protein is a major determinant for virulence," *Journal of Virology*, vol. 73, no. 6, pp. 5001–5009, 1999.

[100] O. S. de Leeuw, G. Koch, L. Hartog, N. Ravenshorst, and B. P. H. Peeters, "Virulence of Newcastle disease virus is determined by the cleavage site of the fusion protein and by both the stem region and globular head of the haemagglutinin-neuraminidase protein," *Journal of General Virology*, vol. 86, no. 6, pp. 1759–1769, 2005.

[101] V. Palya, I. Kiss, T. Tatár-Kis, T. Mató, B. Felföldi, and Y. Gardin, "Advancement in vaccination against newcastle disease: Recombinant HVT NDV provides high clinical protection and reduces challenge virus shedding with the absence of vaccine reactions," *Avian Diseases*, vol. 56, no. 2, pp. 282–287, 2012.

[102] P. J. Miller, R. Haddas, L. Simanov et al., "Identification of new sub-genotypes of virulent Newcastle disease virus with potential panzootic features," *Infection, Genetics and Evolution*, vol. 29, pp. 216–229, 2015.

[103] F. Perozo, R. Marcano, and C. L. Afonso, "Biological and phylogenetic characterization of a genotype VII Newcastle disease virus from Venezuela: Efficacy of field vaccination," *Journal of Clinical Microbiology*, vol. 50, no. 4, pp. 1204–1208, 2012.

[104] S. S. Ewies, A. Ali, S. M. Tamam, and H. M. Madbouly, "Molecular characterization of Newcastle disease virus (genotype VII) from broiler chickens in Egypt," *Beni-Suef University Journal of Basic and Applied Sciences*, vol. 6, no. 3, pp. 232–237, 2017.

[105] S.-H. Kim, S. Nayak, A. Paldurai et al., "Complete genome sequence of a novel newcastle disease virus: Strain isolated from a chicken in West Africa," *Journal of Virology*, vol. 86, no. 20, pp. 11394-11395, 2012.

16

Incidence and Molecular Characterization of Hepatitis E Virus from Swine in Eastern Cape, South Africa

Olusesan Adeyemi Adelabu,[1,2] Benson Chuks Iweriebor,[1,2] U. U. Nwodo,[1,2]
Larry Chikwelu Obi,[3] and Anthony Ifeanyi Okoh[1,2]

[1]SAMRC Microbial Water Quality Monitoring Centre, University of Fort Hare, Private Bag X1314, Alice,
 Eastern Cape Province 5700, South Africa
[2]Applied and Environmental Microbiology Research Group (AEMREG), Department of Biochemistry and Microbiology,
 University of Fort Hare, Private Bag X1314, Alice, Eastern Cape Province 5700, South Africa
[3]Academic and Research Division, University of Fort Hare, Private Bag X1314, Alice, Eastern Cape Province, South Africa

Correspondence should be addressed to Olusesan Adeyemi Adelabu; 201409080@ufh.ac.za

Academic Editor: Finn S. Pedersen

Hepatitis E virus-mediated infection is a serious public health concern in economically developing nations of the world. Globally, four major genotypes of HEV have been documented. Hepatitis E has been suggested to be zoonotic owing to the increase of evidence through various studies. Thus far, this paper reports on prevalence of hepatitis E virus among swine herd in selected communal and commercial farms in the Eastern Cape Province of South Africa. A total of 160 faecal samples were collected from swine herds in Amathole and Chris Hani District Municipalities of Eastern Cape Province for the presence of HEV. Of the 160 faecal samples screened, only seven were positive (4.4%) for HEV. The nucleotide sequences analyses revealed the isolates as sharing 82% to 99% identities with other strains (KX896664, KX896665, KX896666, KX896667, KX896668, KX896669, and KX896670) from different regions of the world. We conclude that HEV is present among swine in the Eastern Cape Province, albeit in low incidence, and this does have public health implications. There is a need for maintenance of high hygienic standards in order to prevent human infections through swine faecal materials and appropriate cooking of pork is highly advised.

1. Introduction

In many developing countries in Asia, Middle East, and Africa, Hepatitis E has become a significant public health concern [1, 2], as well as sporadic cases of acute hepatitis in developed countries [3]. It is a generic term symbolising infection of the liver which is caused by different viruses such as hepatitis A to hepatitis E [4].

Hepatitis E virus is still considered an emerging pathogen in developing countries, owing to the scarcity of information on its infection especially in animals which have arisen from few studies and neglect of the disease and its public health problem [5]. Although most of available information describe human HEV outbreaks in Kenya, Sudan, Uganda, Democratic Republic of Congo (DRC), and Central African Republic [6, 7], information on HEV infection in animals in developing countries of Africa remains underreported.

The widespread HEV infection has been reported in Nigeria, with prevalence rate of 76.7% of genotype 3, and also in Cameroon, Republic of Congo, and Tunisia [8]. The causative agent of the infection known as hepatitis E virus, is a nonenveloped, single-stranded, and positive sense RNA virus, with nearly 7.2 kb genome which encodes three open reading frames (ORFs), translated into ORFs 1–3, with a short 59 untranslated region (UTR). Open reading frame 1 encodes for nonstructural protein while ORF 2 and ORF 3 encode for viral capsid protein and multifunctional small proteins, respectively [9]. It was classified as the only member of the genus *Hepevirus* [10]. However, a new taxonomic division within the family Hepeviridae, due to contradictions in respect to the designation of species and genotypes, has been proposed by Smith et al. (2014), in which the family Hepeviridae is divided to genera *Orthohepevirus* (all mammalian and avian HEV isolates) and *Piscihepevirus* (cutthroat trout virus) while species within the genus *Orthohepevirus* are assigned *Orthohepevirus* A-D [11, 12].

Several studies have reported HEV to be transmitted via faecal-oral routes, usually via contaminated water in developing countries [13–15], while, in the developed countries, direct contacts with infected animals and consumption of poorly cooked/contaminated pork meat and its products, among others, have been reported as routes of transmission and are probable means of zoonotic HEV transmission [16, 17]. The recent identification of other various genetically diverse *hepatitis E virus* strains from different animal species poses additional potential concerns for HEV zoonotic infection [12, 18]

HEV is a single serotype virus with four distinct genotypes which have the potential of infecting man (genotypes I–4). Genotypes 1 and 2 are primarily classified to infect only human population, while genotypes 3 and 4 are said to be zoonotic in developing and developed nations [19–22].

Though it is a slight to temperate disease in severity with mortality rate of <1–4%, among young adults but greater in infected pregnant women, where high mortality rate is progressive in each succeeding trimester to approximately 40%, about 90% of children aged <10 years infected with HEV living in HEV endemic areas have been reported [23].

Several decades into the documentation of the Hepatitis E virus genome, medical virology research is still advancing in knowledge acquisition sequel to the amplified alertness and apparent prominence of hepatitis E as a significant public health concern [16]. Analyses of HEV from animal reservoirs have also confirmed that the strains circulating among domestic and wild pigs are genetically related to the strains identified in human cases [12, 24]. In this paper, we report on the prevalence of swine HEV isolates in selected swine herds in Eastern Cape, South Africa, using the highly conserved capsid protein.

2. Materials and Methods

2.1. Description of the Study Areas. Both commercial and communal swine herds from Amathole and Chris Hani Districts Municipalities were selected for this study, and, for the purpose of confidentiality, these herds will be referred to as swine herds A and B.

Swine herd A is located along the geographical coordinates of 31°34′0″S and 28°46′0″E. It has about 1000 pigs penned in groups of 8 to 10 according to sizes and age.

Swine herd B is located along the geographical coordinates of 32°30′0″S and 27°30′0″E, with capacity of approximately 400 pigs, ranging from nursery to finisher pigs in different pens.

3. Sample Collection

One hundred and sixty faecal samples from 3–5-month-old pigs in selected swine herds were collected with sterile swab for this study. Ten (10 grams) of the samples were each separately suspended in 1x Phosphate buffered saline (PBS) followed by vigorous shaking with vortex machine, centrifuged at 5000 rpm for 5 min, and the supernatants were separated and stored at −80°C until further use as source of HEV genomic RNA.

4. Viral RNA Extraction

The Viral RNA was purified from 160 μl of the swine faecal samples using Quick-RNA Miniprep kit (Zymo research, USA), the manufacturer's protocol was adhered to. The Viral RNA was eluted from the spin column with 50 μl of the elution buffer and frozen at −80°C until further use.

5. Nested Reverse-Transcriptase Polymerase Chain Reaction (RT-PCR)

Two sets of degenerated primers flanking a segment of the ORF 2 gene encoding the structural capsid protein were used: external primers [Forward 5′-AGCTCCTGTACCTGATGT-TGACTC-3′], [Reverse 5′-CTACAGAGCGCCAGC-CTTGATTGC-3′] with expected RT-PCR product size of 427 bp and internal primers [Forward, 5′-GCTCAC-GTCATCTGTCGCTGCTGG-3′], [Reverse, 5′-GGGCTG-AACCAAAATCCTGACATC-3′] with expected RT-PCR product size of 289 bp.

The RNA was reverse transcribed using 5 μl of total RNA, 1 μl each of both forward and reverse primers (external primers), 12 μl of master-mix, 5.6 μl of RNase-free water, and 0.4 μl of reverse transcriptase (Thermo-Fisher, Scientific), at 50°C for 60 min to generate complementary DNA (cDNA), followed by a conventional PCR using 5 μl of cDNA as template with master-mix: 12 μl, forward and reverse primers: 1 μl each, and RNase-free water: 6 μl to make a final reaction volume of 25 μl, for the detection of low level of virus and confirmation of the first round PCR product. PCR was carried out for 40 cycles which includes the initial denaturation and denaturation at 95°C for 3 minutes and 94°C for 1 min, respectively, followed by annealing for 1 min at 58°C, elongation for 1 min at 72°C, and final elongation at 72°C for 7 min.

Subsequently, a nested PCR was carried out by using the following: 3 μl of RT-PCR product, master-mix: 14 μl, forward and reverse primers: 1 μl each, and RNase-free water: 6 μl to make a final volume of 25 μl.

The nested PCR products were examined by electrophoresis on a 1.5% agarose gel (product), stained with 10 mg/ml ethidium bromide, at 100 V for 60 mins. The 427 base pair (bp) was viewed under ultraviolet illumination. The positive PCR products were sent to DNA sequencing facility centre for sequencing, using Sanger sequencing method.

6. Results

A total of one hundred and sixty faecal samples from 3–5-month-old pigs collected from swine herds, one hundred and thirty from a commercial farm (UFT) located at Nkonkobe Local Municipality, under Amathole District Municipality,

TABLE 1: Age-dependent prevalence of HEV RNA in the faeces of swine in Eastern Cape Province.

Age (months)	Type of farm	Number of pigs tested	Number of pigs with HEV
3–5	Commercial	130	3 (2.3%)
3–5	Communal	30	4 (13%)
Total		160	7 (4.4%)

and thirty samples from a communal farm (UMCF) located at Mhlontlo Local Municipality, under Chris Hani District Municipality, were analysed. All the samples collected from both farms were screened for the presence of HEV: three (3) samples were positive from the samples collected from commercial farm while four (4) were positive from the samples from communal farm (Table 1).

For the seven swine HEV isolates generated from this study, nucleotide sequences of ORF 2 RT-PCR products were obtained after sequence editing, using Chromas software (version 2.5). Nucleotide sequence comparison by BLAST as implemented in the NCBI database (https://www.ncbi.nlm.nih.gov/) showed UMCF01-04 having 87% to 99% homology with the 440 bp fragments of ORF 2 of swine HEV isolates from Japan, Netherlands, and France, respectively, while isolates UFT01-03 showed about 82% to 93% nucleic acid identity in the 440 bp section of ORF 2 among swine and human isolates from US and Japan.

Subsequently, phylogenetic analysis of the seven isolates of swine HEV was carried out by comparing the highly preserved 300 bp of OFR 2 to other swine and human HEV strains from different geographical regions. The GenBank accession numbers of the swine and human HEV reference strains used in the phylogenetic analysis in this study are as follows: Japan: LC073306, LC022740, AB986280, AB434138, AB671034, AB671046, LC037975, AB094207, AB073911, AB094211, AB476429, AB671052, AB607892, AB094209AB112743, AB290039, AB298181, AB683185, AB607888, and AB607890; Netherlands: AF336290, AY032756, AF332620, AF336290, and AY032758; USA: AF110387, AF110388, AF466681, AF466660, and AF020497; United Kingdom: AJ344190 and AJ428851; Canada: KP255948, DQ860005, KF956531, and KP255925; Taiwan: AF117275 and KP255922; France: JQ763611; Venezuela: KJ645943; India: FJ230850; Argentina: AF264010; China: DQ445498; Philippines: HM366941; Nigeria: KJ451629 and KJ451633; South Africa: KT833800 and KU178916; Cameroun: KC012634.

Phylogenetic analysis of the swine HEV isolates was evaluated using Geneious R9.1.5 (Biomatters Limited). Phylogenetic analysis showed that all seven isolates from this study clustered with both human and swine HEV from different geographical regions of the world especially with Japan human and swine strains, Netherland swine HEV strains (AY032758, AF332620), and human HEV strain from France (JQ763611) (Figure 1). Isolates designated with UFT01-UFT03, recovered from commercial farm, formed a distinct cluster with swine HEV strain from United States of America (AF466681).

Isolate UMCF01 formed a distinct cluster with the swine HEV strains from Japan (AB671046) and UMCF02 clustered with swine HEV strains isolated from a blood donor in Japan (AB094207 and AB094211), belonging to genotype 3, while isolates UMCF03 and UMCF04 phylogenetically formed distinct clusters with both human and swine HEV strains from Japan, respectively. Sequences reported in this study have been deposited to GenBank database under the accession numbers KX896664, KX896665, KX896666, KX896667, KX896668, KX896669, and KX896670.

7. Discussion

Globally, large proportion of swine have been acknowledged to be infected with HEV while its recovery from the faeces of 2- to 6-month-old pigs have been reported [25, 26], and, as an emerging pathogen, several novel strains of human HEV have also been detected from patients with severe hepatitis in both developing and developed geographical regions of the world [27–29].

Various studies have reported the incidence of swine HEV from different parts of the world [30–33]. In the United Kingdom, China, Japan, and Canada, over 20% of swine faecal samples have been confirmed positive for HEV RNA [34–37], depending on the region sampled. Also, the widespread distribution of HEV has been reported in Nigeria, with prevalence rate of 76.7% of genotype 3 as well as in Cameroon, Republic of Congo, and Tunisia [8, 38]. All these are pointing to increased responsiveness and surveillance and prevalent nature of this virus in the environment. In this study, a total of 7/160 (4.4%) HEV strains, belonging to genotype 3, were recovered from swine for the first time in the Eastern Cape Province of South Africa.

In developed countries, hepatitis E virus is considered a rare infection and most hepatitis E cases are linked with travelling to endemic regions. However, in recent years, cumulative numbers of sporadic cases have been reported among adults, especially in patients with unknown epidemiological risk factor [39–41]. Also, zoonotic transmission of HEV from wild boars has recently been reported in Italy [42], as well as in Germany, where the consumption of wild deer meat was associated with indigenous HEV infection [43], and genomic sequence recovered from wild boar in Sweden showed a very high percentage of relatedness to human and domestic pigs in the same environment [44].

Besides infections in swine, the report of HEV infection in other animals is rapidly increasing. Genotypes 2, 3, and 4 strains of HEV have also been recovered in other nonhuman hosts, including mongoose, rats, birds, rabbits, bats and fish macaque, sheep, chicken, yak, and cattle [45–47]. Thus, swine has been primarily suspected as a source of zoonotic transmission owing to the fact that other animals are not closely related to human life [12, 48, 49]

Furthermore, cross-species infection has been reported in China and Korea [49], due to traditional mixed farming system whereby various domestic animals are reared together in a close range [50] and this may hypothetically proliferate the zoonotic sources which could facilitate the transmission of HEV to humans. In the study area, especially in the

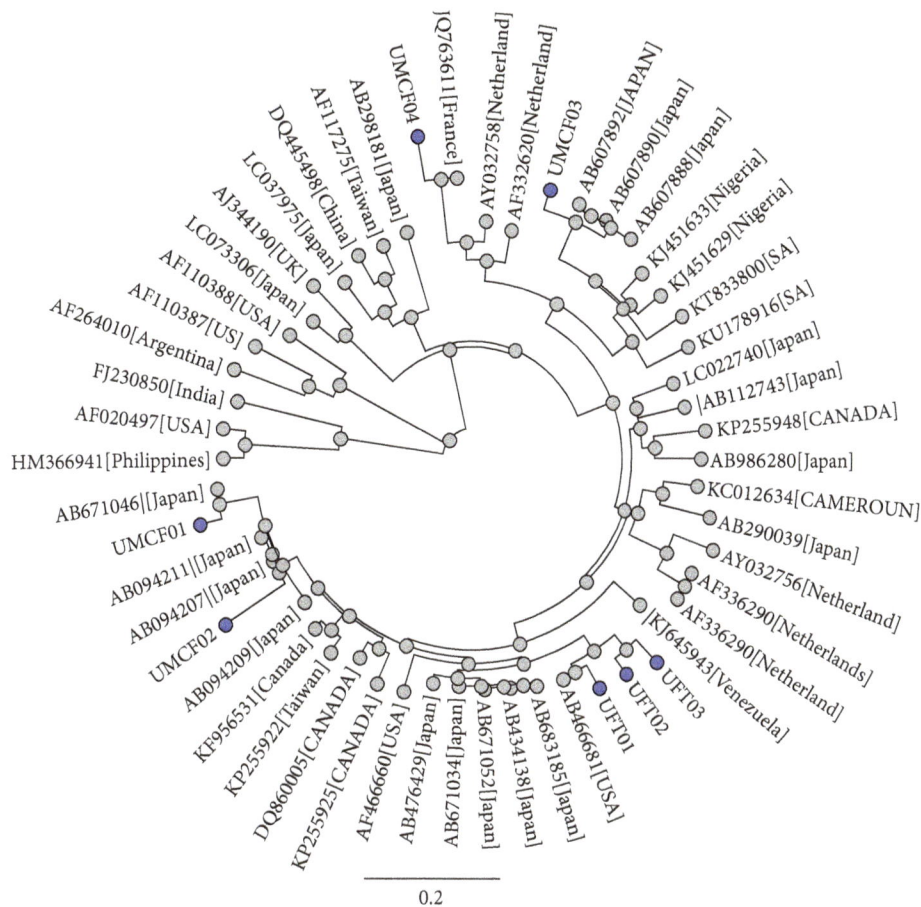

FIGURE 1: Phylogenetic relationships of HEV isolates obtained in this study. Phylogenetic analysis was based on 300 bp of the ORF 2 gene of the swine HEV isolates obtained in this study along reference sequences of other swine and human HEV strains from different geographical regions of the world that were obtained from the GenBank. Tree was drawn with Geneious R9.1.5 (Biomatters Limited). Sequences obtained in this study are given in blue dots.

communal farm, it was observed that pigs are being reared with other domestic animals, including cattle, chickens, ducks, and sheep. As such, the traditional farming system portends an increased risk of zoonosis in the study area.

In South Africa, the first case of HEV genotype 3 from a 50-year-old transplant patient with a preexisting medical condition has been reported [51]. This suggests that HEV is underdiagnosed and underdocumented in this region; hence molecular HEV testing needs to be encouraged to support the management of immunocompromised patients.

The data generated from this study raises a concern about a possible zoonosis of HEV strains circulating in the study area, as farming is the occupation of majority of the populace in the study area and the use of swine waste as manure to improve the farm yields has been a common practise. Also, most of the people living in the rural parts in the study area depend on water from dams and rivers for both drinking and domestic activities, and, for this reason, transmission of HEV from animal to man is anticipated. This is consistent with the findings of [52, 53]. It is, therefore, imperative to safeguard the public against HEV infection, especially children (<10 years), the aged people (≥50 years), immune-comprised

individuals, and pregnant women. In addition, information on human HEV seroprevalence is required among the people living in the study area to establish their exposure to the virus.

The result from this study is also supported by a seroprevalence study conducted among selected group of people in relation to pork consumption in the Western Cape Province, South Africa, which revealed HEV IgG seroprevalence of 29.7% [54], suggesting swine as reservoirs of the virus.

Within respect to the sequence comparison, genetic relatedness, and phylogeny analysis of the 300 bp of ORF 2, all swine HEV strains from this study are mostly clustered with previously reported human and swine strains from USA, Netherlands, Japan, Nigeria, France, and South Africa [37, 38, 55–57].

Similar to other reports in Africa, Hepatitis E virus genotype 3 was identified and the strains characterized in this study presented a higher nucleotide homology with the strains from Japan and Netherland than the ones from Africa [38, 58–60]. The transmission of swine HEV between countries via international trade has been documented in Africa, Asia, and America [61, 62]; hence the HEV genotype 3 obtained from this study could be linked to Europe, Asia, and America, although more scientific information is required to establish this.

Swine production in South Africa, like any other countries, is practiced either on a large scale (commercial) or small scale (communal). In communal system where pigs are allowed to roam about in sourcing for food and water, they visit flowing or stagnant waterbodies, thereby contaminating it with their faeces and urine, and consequently creating a route of transmission to humans, especially in an environment where there is a close association between pigs and humans, resulting in zoonosis of HEV infection.

Subsequently, to public health concern of zoonosis, xenozoonosis is another concern among patients undergoing organ-transplant; hence as a result of adaptation in immunecompromised individuals, quasispecies, or recombination, a nonpathogenic strain of swine HEV may become pathogenic.

With the similarities of the sequences detected among the strains of the isolates from this study and the strains from Japan, Netherlands, US, and Taiwan, and from other reports from different parts of the world, it can be deduced that HEV genotype 3 is a zoonotic virus.

As it was recently reported that HEV infection is underdiagnosed, [51] had suggested that it should be included in diagnoses as it may be the cause of non-A, non-B, or non-C hepatitis case [63]. Biosafety measures should also be encouraged in surroundings near the swine herds so as to prevent the spread of swine HEV strains outside the herds, as different strains of swine HEV in circulation are observed in this study.

The present study establishes that phylogeny can be a valuable tool in determining the source of HEV infections and geographical origin of hepatitis E virus, genotype 3 strains, infecting humans. In addition, the effectiveness of this tool for tracing human infections is dependent on regular screenings of swine and other domestic animals implicated to be reservoirs of HEV. It is reasonable to assume that if more information regarding HEV strains circulating in the study was available, it would significantly increase the reliability and precision of this model for tracing infections.

Conclusively, the detection of swine HEV strains in this study linked to human HEV isolates from Japan, America, and Netherlands points toward a significant innovative track for hepatitis E virus research. From the public health perspective, priority should be given to the development of techniques for the detection of interspecies transmission at early stage. Swine HEV-mediated infection could make an animal model for hepatitis E virus studies available. It might as well prove worthwhile for vaccine development against HEV infection in humans.

In addition, molecular-based analysis of HEV occurrence in swine herds, waterbodies, and hospitals, on a regular basis, is hereby encouraged to bring about appropriate control strategies and to prevent imminent outbreak of the virus.

Acknowledgments

The authors are grateful to the South Africa Medical Research Council for financial support.

References

[1] F. Cainelli, "Liver diseases in developing countries," *World Journal of Hepatology*, vol. 4, no. 3, pp. 66–67, 2012.

[2] N. Kamar, H. R. Dalton, F. Abravanel, and J. Izopet, "Hepatitis E virus infection," *Clinical Microbiology Reviews*, vol. 27, no. 1, pp. 116–138, 2014.

[3] G. Reuter, D. Fodor, P. Forgách, A. Kátai, and G. Szucs, "Characterization and zoonotic potential of endemic hepatitis E virus (HEV) strains in humans and animals in Hungary," *Journal of Clinical Virology*, vol. 44, no. 4, pp. 277–281, 2009.

[4] E. E. Mast, M. A. Purdy, and K. Krawczynski, "Hepatitis E," *Bailliere's Clinical Gastroenterology*, vol. 10, no. 2, pp. 227–242, 1996.

[5] B. Kmush, T. Wierzba, L. Krain, K. Nelson, and A. B. Labrique, "Epidemiology of hepatitis E in low-and middle-income countries of Asia and Africa," in *Seminars in Liver Disease*, vol. 33, no. 1, pp. 15–29, Thieme Medical, 2013.

[6] M. Kaba, P. Colson, J.-P. Musongela, L. Tshilolo, and B. Davoust, "Detection of hepatitis E virus of genotype 3 in a farm pig in Kinshasa (Democratic Republic of the Congo)," *Infection, Genetics and Evolution*, vol. 10, no. 1, pp. 154–157, 2010.

[7] V. S. de Paula, M. Wiele, A. H. Mbunkah, A. M. Daniel, M. T. Kingsley, and J. Schmidt-Chanasit, "Hepatitis E virus genotype 3 strains in domestic pigs, Cameroon," *Emerging Infectious Diseases*, vol. 19, no. 4, pp. 666–668, 2013.

[8] Y. Buisson, M. Grandadam, E. Nicand et al., "Identification of a novel hepatitis E virus in Nigeria," *Journal of General Virology*, vol. 81, no. 4, pp. 903–909, 2000.

[9] M. Monini, I. Di Bartolo, G. Ianiro et al., "Detection and molecular characterization of zoonotic viruses in swine fecal samples in Italian pig herds," *Archives of Virology*, vol. 160, no. 10, pp. 2547–2556, 2015.

[10] K. Cooper, F. F. Huang, L. Batista et al., "Identification of genotype 3 hepatitis E virus (HEV) in serum and fecal samples from pigs in Thailand and Mexico, where genotype 1 and 2 HEV strains are prevalent in the respective human populations," *Journal of Clinical Microbiology*, vol. 43, no. 4, pp. 1684–1688, 2005.

[11] D. B. Smith, P. Simmonds, S. Jameel et al., "Consensus proposals for classification of the family *Hepeviridae*," *Journal of General Virology*, vol. 95, no. 10, pp. 2223–2232, 2014.

[12] Y. Debing, D. Moradpour, J. Neyts, and J. Gouttenoire, "Update on hepatitis E virology: implications for clinical practice," *Journal of Hepatology*, vol. 65, no. 1, pp. 200–212, 2016.

[13] M. C. Donati, E. A. Fagan, and T. J. Harrison, "Sequence analysis of full length HEV clones derived directly from liver in fulminant hepatitis E," in *Proceedings of the IX Triennial International Symposium on Viral Hepatitis and Liver Disease*, 1997.

[14] R. Aggarwal and K. Krawczynski, "Hepatitis E: an overview and recent advances in clinical and laboratory research," *Journal of Gastroenterology and Hepatology*, vol. 15, no. 1, pp. 9–20, 2000.

[15] L. J. Krain, J. E. Atwell, K. E. Nelson, and A. B. Labrique, "Fetal and neonatal health consequences of vertically transmitted hepatitis E virus infection," *The American Journal of Tropical Medicine and Hygiene*, vol. 90, no. 2, pp. 365–370, 2014.

[16] S. Pischke, A. Heim, B. Bremer et al., "Hepatitis E: an emerging infectious disease in Germany?" *Zeitschrift fur Gastroenterologie*, vol. 49, no. 9, pp. 1255–1257, 2011.

[17] N. Kamar, R. Bendall, F. Legrand-Abravanel et al., "Hepatitis E," *The Lancet*, vol. 379, no. 9835, pp. 2477–2488, 2012.

[18] P. Behrendt, E. Steinmann, M. P. Manns, and H. Wedemeyer, "The impact of hepatitis e in the liver transplant setting," *Journal of Hepatology*, vol. 61, no. 6, pp. 1418–1429, 2014.

[19] L. Lu, C. Li, and C. H. Hagedorn, "Phylogenetic analysis of global hepatitis E virus sequences: genetic diversity, subtypes and zoonosis," *Reviews in Medical Virology*, vol. 16, no. 1, pp. 5–36, 2006.

[20] Y. Sato, H. Sato, K. Naka et al., "A nationwide survey of hepatitis E virus (HEV) infection in wild boars in Japan: identification of boar HEV strains of genotypes 3 and 4 and unrecognized genotypes," *Archives of Virology*, vol. 156, no. 8, pp. 1345–1358, 2011.

[21] I. Monne, L. Ceglie, G. Di Martino et al., "Hepatitis E virus genotype 4 in a pig farm, Italy, 2013," *Epidemiology and Infection*, vol. 143, no. 3, pp. 529–533, 2015.

[22] S. Pischke, P. Behrendt, C.-T. Bock, W. Jilg, M. P. Manns, and H. Wedemeyer, "Hepatitis e in Germany-an under-reported infectious disease," *Deutsches Arzteblatt International*, vol. 111, no. 35-36, pp. 577–8, 2014.

[23] J. W. Ward, F. M. Averhoff, and H. K. Koh, "World Hepatitis Day: a new era for hepatitis control," *The Lancet*, vol. 378, no. 9791, pp. 552–553, 2011.

[24] A. Berto, S. Grierson, R. Hakze-van der Honing et al., "Hepatitis E virus in pork liver sausage, France," *Emerging Infectious Diseases*, vol. 19, no. 2, pp. 264–266, 2013.

[25] P. Colson, P. Saint-Jacques, A. Ferretti, and B. Davoust, "Hepatitis E virus of subtype 3a in a pig farm, south-eastern France," *Zoonoses and Public Health*, vol. 62, no. 8, pp. 593–598, 2015.

[26] T. Merino-Ramos, M. A. Martín-Acebes, J. Casal, J.-C. Saiz, and E. Loza-Rubio, "Prevalence of Hepatitis E Virus (HEV) antibodies in Mexican pigs," *Food and Environmental Virology*, vol. 8, no. 2, pp. 156–159, 2016.

[27] Y. Kabrane-Lazizi, M. Zhang, R. H. Purcell, K. D. Miller, R. T. Davey, and S. U. Emerson, "Acute hepatitis caused by a novel strain of hepatitis E virus most closely related to United States strains," *Journal of General Virology*, vol. 82, no. 7, pp. 1687–1693, 2001.

[28] J. M. Hughes, M. E. Wilson, E. H. Teshale, D. J. Hu, and S. D. Holmberg, "The two faces of hepatitis E virus," *Clinical Infectious Diseases*, vol. 51, no. 3, pp. 328–334, 2010.

[29] C. Wu, Y. Nan, and Y.-J. Zhang, "New insights into hepatitis E virus virus-host interaction: interplay with host interferon induction," *Future Virology*, vol. 10, no. 4, pp. 439–448, 2015.

[30] S. Oncu, S. Oncu, P. Okyay, S. Ertug, and S. Sakarya, "Prevalence and risk factors for HEV infection in pregnant women," *Medical Science Monitor*, vol. 12, no. 1, pp. CR36–CR39, 2006.

[31] S. Mathew, M. Pericleous, M. Atkins, M. Nicholls, and A. Ala, "PTU-114 Prevalence rates of acute hepatitis a (HAV) and hepatitis e (HEV) in surrey, South East England: how many HAV cases are being missed?" *Gut*, vol. 64, supplement 1, p. A112, 2015.

[32] C. Crossan, S. Grierson, J. Thomson et al., "Prevalence of hepatitis e virus in slaughter-age pigs in Scotland," *Epidemiology and Infection*, vol. 143, no. 10, pp. 2237–2240, 2015.

[33] D. Žele, A. F. Barry, R. W. Hakze-Van Der Honing, G. Vengušt, and W. H. M. Van Der Poel, "Prevalence of anti-hepatitis E virus antibodies and first detection of hepatitis E virus in wild boar in Slovenia," *Vector-Borne and Zoonotic Diseases*, vol. 16, no. 1, pp. 71–74, 2016.

[34] M. Banks, G. S. Heath, S. S. Grierson et al., "Evidence for the presence of hepatitis E virus in pigs in the United Kingdom," *Veterinary Record*, vol. 154, no. 8, pp. 223–227, 2004.

[35] Y. Yan, W. Zhang, Q. Shen, L. Cui, and X. Hua, "Prevalence of four different subgenotypes of genotype 4 hepatitis E virus among swine in the Shanghai area of China," *Acta Veterinaria Scandinavica*, vol. 50, no. 1, article 12, 2008.

[36] P. Ward, P. Müller, A. Letellier et al., "Molecular characterization of Hepatitis E virus detected in swine farms in the province of Quebec," *Canadian Journal of Veterinary Research*, vol. 72, no. 1, pp. 27–31, 2008.

[37] N. Nantel-Fortier, A. Letellier, V. Lachapelle, P. Fravalo, Y. L'Homme, and J. Brassard, "Detection and Phylogenetic analysis of the hepatitis E virus in a Canadian swine production network," *Food and Environmental Virology*, vol. 8, no. 4, pp. 296–304, 2016.

[38] O. A. Owolodun, P. F. Gerber, L. G. Giménez-Lirola, J. K. P. Kwaga, and T. Opriessnig, "First report of hepatitis E virus circulation in domestic pigs in Nigeria," *The American Journal of Tropical Medicine and Hygiene*, vol. 91, no. 4, pp. 699–704, 2014.

[39] M.-A. Widdowson, W. J. M. Jaspers, W. H. M. Van Der Poel et al., "Cluster of cases of acute hepatitis associated with hepatitis E virus infection acquired in The Netherlands," *Clinical Infectious Diseases*, vol. 36, no. 1, pp. 29–33, 2003.

[40] H. R. Dalton, R. Bendall, S. Ijaz, and M. Banks, "Hepatitis E: an emerging infection in developed countries," *The Lancet Infectious Diseases*, vol. 8, no. 11, pp. 698–709, 2008.

[41] P. Manka, L. P. Bechmann, J. D. Coombes et al., "Hepatitis E virus infection as a possible cause of acute liver failure in Europe," *Clinical Gastroenterology and Hepatology*, vol. 13, no. 10, Article ID 54351, pp. 1836.e2–1842.e2, 2015.

[42] N. Martinelli, E. Pavoni, D. Filogari et al., "Hepatitis E virus in wild boar in the central northern part of Italy," *Transboundary and Emerging Diseases*, vol. 62, no. 2, pp. 217–222, 2015.

[43] O. Wichmann, S. Schimanski, J. Koch et al., "Phylogenetic and case-control study on hepatitis E virus infection in Germany," *Journal of Infectious Diseases*, vol. 198, no. 12, pp. 1732–1741, 2008.

[44] F. Widén, L. Sundqvist, A. Matyi-Toth et al., "Molecular epidemiology of hepatitis E virus in humans, pigs and wild boars in Sweden," *Epidemiology and Infection*, vol. 139, no. 3, pp. 361–371, 2011.

[45] J.-B. Geng, H.-W. Fu, L. Wang et al., "Hepatitis E virus (HEV) genotype and the prevalence of anti-HEV in 8 species of animals in the suburbs of Beijing," *Zhonghua Liuxingbingxue Zazhi*, vol. 31, no. 1, pp. 47–50, 2010.

[46] D. Thiry, A. Mauroy, N. Pavio et al., "Hepatitis E virus and related viruses in animals," *Transboundary and Emerging Diseases*, vol. 64, no. 1, pp. 37–52, 2017.

[47] D. Rodríguez-Lázaro, M. Diez-Valcarce, R. Montes-Briones, D. Gallego, M. Hernández, and J. Rovira, "Presence of pathogenic enteric viruses in illegally imported meat and meat products to EU by international air travelers," *International Journal of Food Microbiology*, vol. 209, pp. 39–43, 2015.

[48] W.-J. Park, B.-J. Park, H.-S. Ahn et al., "Hepatitis E virus as an emerging zoonotic pathogen," *Journal of Veterinary Science*, vol. 17, no. 1, pp. 1–11, 2016.

[49] H.-W. Moon, B.-W. Lee, H. W. Sung, B.-I. Yoon, and H. M. Kwon, "Identification and characterization of avian hepatitis E virus genotype 2 from chickens with hepatitis-splenomegaly syndrome in Korea," *Virus Genes*, vol. 52, no. 5, pp. 738–742, 2016.

[50] F. Huang, Y. Li, W. Yu et al., "Excretion of infectious hepatitis E virus into milk in cows imposes high risks of zoonosis," *Hepatology*, vol. 64, no. 2, pp. 350–359, 2016.

[51] M. I. Andersson, P. A. Stead, T. Maponga, H. van der Plas, and W. Preiser, "Hepatitis E virus infection: an underdiagnosed infection in transplant patients in Southern Africa?" *Journal of Clinical Virology*, vol. 70, pp. 23–25, 2015.

[52] A. Idolo, F. Serio, F. Lugoli et al., "Identification of HEV in symptom-free migrants and environmental samples in Italy," *Journal of Viral Hepatitis*, vol. 20, no. 6, pp. 438–443, 2013.

[53] C. Caruso, S. Peletto, A. Rosamilia et al., "Hepatitis E virus: a cross-sectional serological and virological study in pigs and humans at zoonotic risk within a high-density pig farming area," *Transboundary and Emerging Diseases*, 2016.

[54] R. G. Madden, S. Wallace, M. Sonderup et al., Western Cape, South Africa, 2015.

[55] W. H. M. Van der Poel, F. Verschoor, R. van der Heide et al., "Hepatitis E virus sequences in swine related to sequences in humans, the Netherlands," *Emerging Infectious Diseases*, vol. 7, no. 6, pp. 970–976, 2001.

[56] N. Chotun, E. Nel, M. F. Cotton, W. Preiser, and M. I. Andersson, "Hepatitis B virus infection in HIV-exposed infants in the Western Cape, South Africa," *Vaccine*, vol. 33, no. 36, pp. 4618–4622, 2015.

[57] T. Matsui, J.-H. Kang, K. Matsubayashi et al., "Rare case of transfusion-transmitted hepatitis E from the blood of a donor infected with the hepatitis E virus genotype 3 indigenous to Japan: viral dynamics from onset to recovery," *Hepatology Research*, vol. 45, no. 6, pp. 698–704, 2015.

[58] N. Pavio, X.-J. Meng, and V. Doceul, "Zoonotic origin of hepatitis E," *Current Opinion in Virology*, vol. 10, pp. 34–41, 2015.

[59] Y. Inagaki, Y. Oshiro, N. Hasegawa et al., "Clinical features of hepatitis E virus infection in Ibaraki, Japan: autochthonous hepatitis E and acute-on-chronic liver failure," *Tohoku Journal of Experimental Medicine*, vol. 235, no. 4, pp. 275–282, 2015.

[60] C. M. Cossaboom, C. L. Heffron, D. Cao et al., "Risk factors and sources of foodborne hepatitis E virus infection in the United States," *Journal of Medical Virology*, vol. 88, no. 9, pp. 1641–1645, 2016.

[61] J.-C. Wu, C. M. Chen, T. Y. Chiang et al., "Spread of hepatitis E virus among different-aged pigs: two-year survey in Taiwan," *Journal of Medical Virology*, vol. 66, no. 4, pp. 488–492, 2002.

[62] M. S. Munné, S. Vladimirsky, L. Otegui et al., "Identification of the first strain of swine hepatitis E virus in South America and prevalence of anti-HEV antibodies in swine in Argentina," *Journal of Medical Virology*, vol. 78, no. 12, pp. 1579–1583, 2006.

[63] H. Koot, B. M. Hogema, M. Koot, M. Molier, and H. L. Zaaijer, "Frequent hepatitis E in the Netherlands without traveling or immunosuppression," *Journal of Clinical Virology*, vol. 62, pp. 38–40, 2015.

17

Isolation and Metagenomic Identification of Avian Leukosis Virus Associated with Mortality in Broiler Chicken

Faruku Bande,[1,2] Siti Suri Arshad,[1] and Abdul Rahman Omar[1,3]

[1]*Department of Veterinary Pathology and Microbiology, Faculty of Veterinary Medicine, Universiti Putra Malaysia (UPM), 43400 Serdang, Selangor Darul Ehsan, Malaysia*

[2]*Department of Veterinary Services, Ministry of Animal Health and Fisheries Development, PMB 2109, Usman Faruk Secretariat, Sokoto 840221, Sokoto State, Nigeria*

[3]*Laboratory of Vaccine and Immunotherapeutic, Institute of Bioscience, Universiti Putra Malaysia (UPM), 43400 Serdang, Selangor Darul Ehsan, Malaysia*

Correspondence should be addressed to Siti Suri Arshad; suri@upm.edu.my and Abdul Rahman Omar; aro@upm.edu.my

Academic Editor: Finn S. Pedersen

Avian leukosis virus (ALV) belongs to the family Retroviridae and causes considerable economic losses to the poultry industry. Following an outbreak associated with high mortality in a broiler flock in northern part of Malaysia, kidney tissues from affected chickens were submitted for virus isolation and identification in chicken embryonated egg and MDCK cells. Evidence of virus growth was indicated by haemorrhage and embryo mortality in egg culture. While viral growth in cell culture was evidenced by the development of cytopathic effects. The isolated virus was purified by sucrose gradient and identified using negative staining transmission electron microscopy. Further confirmation was achieved through next-generation sequencing and nucleotide sequence homology search. Analysis of the viral sequences using the NCBI BLAST tool revealed 99-100% sequence homology with exogenous ALV viral envelope protein. Phylogenetic analysis based on partial envelope sequences showed the Malaysian isolate clustered with Taiwanese and Japanese ALV strains, which were closer to ALV subgroup J, ALV subgroup E, and recombinant A/E isolates. Based on these findings, ALV was concluded to be associated with the present outbreak. It was recommended that further studies should be conducted on the molecular epidemiology and pathogenicity of the identified virus isolate.

1. Introduction

Avian leukosis virus (ALV) is an economically important retrovirus affecting meat and egg-type chicken. The virus belongs to an *Alpharetrovirus* genus in the family Retroviridae. Based on the envelope glycoprotein (gp85) it was possible to classify exogenous ALV into different subgroups, namely, A, B, C, D, E, and J. Particularly, the viral envelope glycoprotein is responsible for attachment and receptor specificity as well as the production of neutralizing antibodies [1, 2]. Of the viral subgroups so far identified, subgroups A, B, and J are considered most prevalent and more economically important [3]. Subgroup J was first isolated in meat-type chicken in the United Kingdom in 1989 but currently is causing devastation to poultry industry worldwide [4]. Apart from its immunosuppressive effect, ALV is commonly associated with lymphoid leukosis, myelocytic myeloid leukosis, and renal as well as other forms of tumours [5]. This study reports some virological and molecular sequencing approaches used to identify the viral cause of mortality in a broiler flock in Malaysia.

2. Materials and Methods

Following a suspected outbreak in a broiler chicken farm with capacity of about 10,000 birds, tissue samples, including trachea, kidney, and proventriculus, were submitted to the virology laboratory, Universiti Putra Malaysia, for virus isolation and identification. The mortality rate was reported to reach about 10% in the 27-day-old flock ($n = 6000$) and more than 20% in the 30-day-old flock ($n = 4000$). The chickens

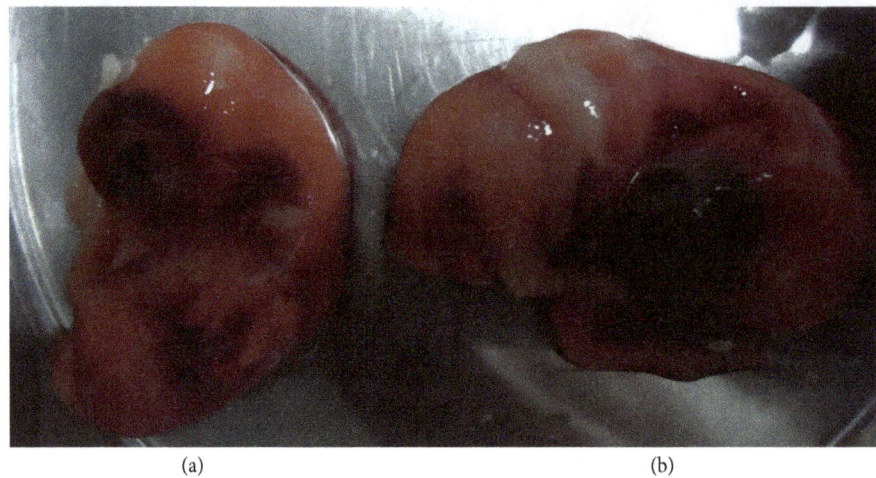

(a)   (b)

FIGURE 1: Inoculation of viral suspension in 9-day old embryonated chicken egg showing evidence of severe haemorrhage in infected embryo (a) as compared with negative control (b) after 24 hours pi.

flock health programme consisted of vaccination against NDV, IBD, and IBV. Postmortem findings revealed mild petechial haemorrhage on the proventriculus and markedly swollen kidney (figures not shown). Samples were processed and inoculated in a 9-day-old embryonated chicken egg as well as MDCK cells and then monitored for the evidences of virus growth. Identification of the virus was carried out by electron microscopy using the negative staining methods while confirmation was done by next-generation sequencing using the MiSeq illumina sequencing platform. A ScriptSeq v2 RNA-Seq library preparation kit was employed and used according to manufacturer's guidelines (epicenter, USA).

3. Results and Discussion

Avian leukosis, specifically of subgroup J origins, has been reported previously in Malaysia [6]. This study investigated a viral cause of mortality observed in a broiler farm in northern Malaysia in 2013. Due to the involvement of kidney, initial tentative diagnosis focused on avian infectious bronchitis [7]; however inoculation of kidney suspension in chicken's embryonated egg revealed evidence of virus growth characterized by severe haemorrhage and embryo mortality (Figure 1). Embryo mortality was observed to increase as the passaging of virus increases to passage 3. Specifically, at passage 2, there was about 70%–100% mortality of embryos starting from day 2 to day 3 postinoculation (pi). Avian leukosis virus has been reported to cause severe haemorrhage and death of the embryo within 4 to 5 days following infection of egg embryo [5].

Similarly, inoculation of MDCK cells with kidney derived suspension showed evidence of virus growth characterized by the presence of cytopathic effects including cell ballooning, granulation, rounding, giant cells formations, and cell detachment starting from day 3 pi (Figure 2). Although most ALVs produce no visible morphological changes in cell culture, infection of chicken embryo fibroblast cells with

cytopathic ALVs strains such as the RAV-2 was reported to cause CPE and detachment of cells 3 days after infection [8]. Other studies confirmed the tropism and growth of ALVs in chicken embryo fibroblast cells based on the presence of CPE [9, 10]. It is also generally known that MDCK cells express receptors for some avian viruses such as avian influenza [11].

Virus identification carried out using negative staining electron microscopy revealed a spherically rounded, virus-like particle with characteristic projections resembling spike structures (Figure 3). Subsequent analysis by comparison revealed that the virus morphology observed in this study was similar to that reported by Tsang et al. [12].

Despite evidence of virus growth in egg embryo and cell culture, attempts to detect common viral diseases using specific primers against NDV, AI, and IBV were unsuccessful [7]; hence, a next-generation RNA sequencing approach was employed. Following sequencing, analysis of the generated sequences (Genbank accession number: KX061539) using NCBI BLAST revealed high sequence homology with exogenous ALV viral envelope protein region. Furthermore, phylogenetic characterization using the entire envelope sequences (1230 bp) revealed close identity with exogenous ALV-TW-3593 from Taiwan (100%), ALV-Hkd-026 strains from Japan (99%), and a putative endogeneous ALV sequence designated ALVE-B11 (99%). In terms of virus subgroup, the identified local ALV sequences demonstrated closeness to ALV J, ALV E, and recombinant ALV A/E as well as an endogenous ALV of chicken (Figure 4).

In terms of protein sequences, which comprise the receptor binding SU domain (gp85) and transmembrane protein TM domain (gp37), Malaysian ALV isolate also phylogenetically clustered with Taiwanese isolate (TW3593) and Chinese isolate (WB11008e) as well as Japanese isolate (Hkd026) (figure not shown).

In view of the nature of retroviruses, it is usual that mutation and recombination in ALV may influence virus diversity and tissue tropism as well as the severity of infection they

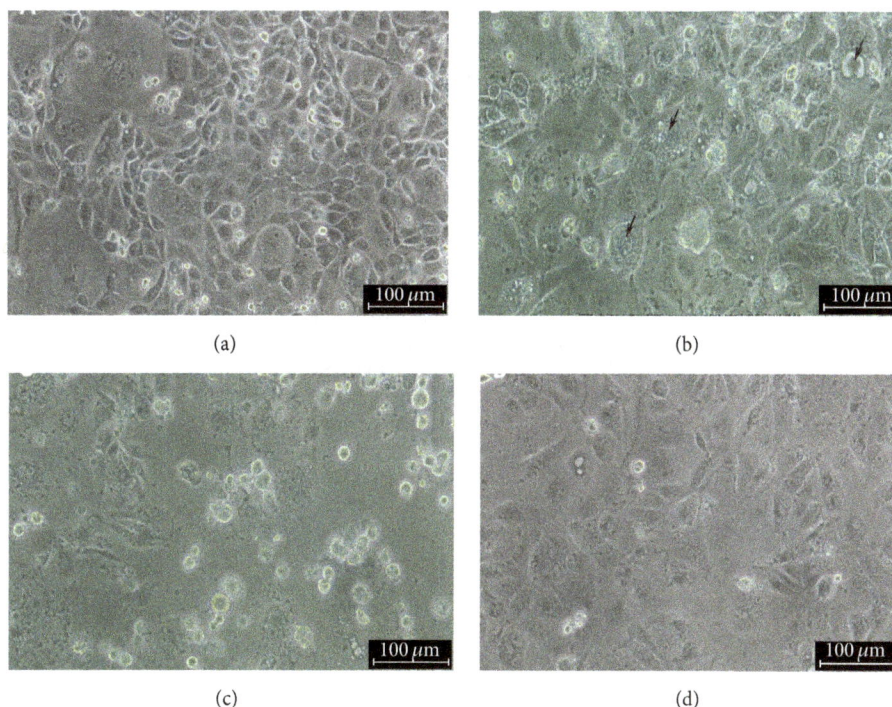

(a)   (b)

(c)   (d)

FIGURE 2: Infection of MDCK cells with virus suspension revealed evidences of virus growth as demonstrated by CPE which is characterized by cell ballooning, granulation, formation of giant cells (arrow), rounding, and cell detachment as infection progresses 3 dpi (a); 5 dpi (b) and 7 dpi (c); (d) control uninfected cells. Mag ×20 and 100 μm.

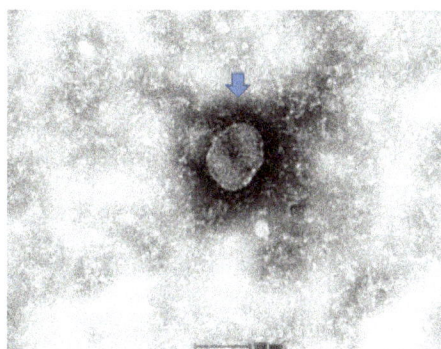

FIGURE 3: Negative staining electron microscopy showing the morphological appearance of the isolated virus. Note: presence of spike projections surrounding the viral particle (arrow) whose diameter ranges from 80 to 120 nm. Mag ×100 μm.

cause [13]. These factors might probably account for the reported high mortality rate observed in the farm as well as during passaging of virus in embryo.

4. Conclusion

Based on the findings observed in this report, it was concluded that the present outbreak was associated with ALV. The study further demonstrates that ALV continues to circulate among poultry in Malaysia though it might be underdiagnosed. There is the need for flock monitoring against ALV and the possibility of including ALV infection as one of the differentials in related outbreaks. It is recommended to further study the molecular epidemiology and pathogenesis of the present local ALV strain in Malaysia.

Authors' Contributions

All authors have contributed equally.

Acknowledgments

The authors would like to acknowledge support from the Laboratory of Vaccine and Immunotherapeutics, Institute of

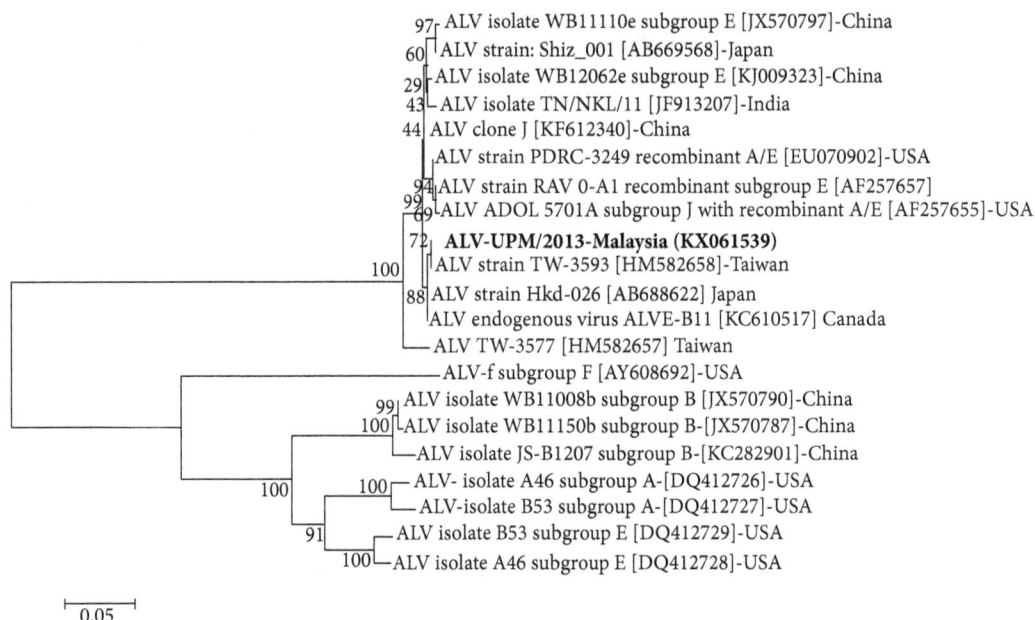

FIGURE 4: Neighbor-joining phylogenetic analysis using partial nucleotide sequences of the ALV envelope gp85 glycoprotein gene. Malaysian ALV isolate is presented in bold red ink. The confidence level of the inferred tree was determined using 1000 bootstrap. Evolutionary analysis was conducted in MEGA6 software.

Bio Sciences, UPM. Similar appreciation goes to Dr. Dilan Satharasinghe for technical assistance in sequencing.

References

[1] J. M. Coffin, "Structure and classification of retroviruses," in *The Retroviridae*, J. A. Levy, Ed., vol. 1, pp. 19–49, Plenum Press, New York, NY, USA, 1992.

[2] L. N. Payne, K. Howes, A. M. Gillespie, and L. M. Smith, "Host range of Rous sarcoma virus pseudotype RSV(HPRS-103) in 12 avian species: support for a new avian retrovirus envelope subgroup, designated," *Journal of General Virology*, vol. 73, no. 11, pp. 2995–2997, 1992.

[3] M. Dai, M. Feng, D. Liu, W. Cao, and M. Liao, "Development and application of SYBR Green i real-time PCR assay for the separate detection of subgroup J Avian leukosis virus and multiplex detection of avian leukosis virus subgroups A and B," *Virology Journal*, vol. 12, no. 1, article 52, 2015.

[4] L. N. Payne, S. R. Brown, N. Bumstead, K. Howes, J. A. Frazier, and M. E. Thouless, "A novel subgroup of exogenous avian leukosis virus in chickens," *Journal of General Virology*, vol. 72, no. 4, pp. 801–807, 1991.

[5] L. N. Payne and A. M. Fadly, *Leukosis/Sarcoma Group*, Iowa State University Press, Ames, Iowa, USA, 1997.

[6] B. R. Thapa, A. R. Omar, S. S. Arshad, and M. Hair-Bejo, "Detection of avian leukosis virus subgroup J in chicken flocks from Malaysia and their molecular characterization," *Avian Pathology*, vol. 33, no. 3, pp. 359–363, 2004.

[7] F. Bande, S. S. Arshad, A. R. Omar, M. H. Bejo, M. S. Abubakar, and Y. Abba, "Pathogenesis and diagnostic approaches of avian infectious bronchitis," *Advances in Virology*, vol. 2016, Article ID 4621659, 11 pages, 2016.

[8] S. K. Weller and H. M. Temin, "Cell killing by avian leukosis viruses," *Journal of Virology*, vol. 39, no. 3, pp. 713–721, 1981.

[9] A. M. Fadly, "Isolation and identification of avian leukosis viruses: A review," *Avian Pathology*, vol. 29, no. 6, pp. 529–535, 2000.

[10] B. Lupiani, H. Hunt, R. Silva, and A. Fadly, "Identification and characterization of recombinant subgroup J avian leukosis viruses (ALV) expressing subgroup A ALV envelope," *Virology*, vol. 276, no. 1, pp. 37–43, 2000.

[11] C.-W. Lee, K. Jung, S. J. Jadhao, and D. L. Suarez, "Evaluation of chicken-origin (DF-1) and quail-origin (QT-6) fibroblast cell lines for replication of avian influenza viruses," *Journal of Virological Methods*, vol. 153, no. 1, pp. 22–28, 2008.

[12] S. X. Tsang, W. M. Switzer, V. Shanmugam et al., "Evidence of avian leukosis virus subgroup E and endogenous avian virus in measles and mumps vaccines derived from chicken cells: investigation of transmission to vaccine recipients," *Journal of Virology*, vol. 73, no. 7, pp. 5843–5851, 1999.

[13] E. S. Svarovskaia, S. R. Cheslock, W.-H. Zhang, W.-S. Hu, and V. K. Pathak, "Retroviral mutation rates and reverse transcriptase fidelity," *Frontiers in Bioscience*, vol. 8, pp. d117–d134, 2003.

Permissions

List of Contributors

Melbourne Talactac
College of Veterinary Medicine and Biomedical Sciences, Cavite State University, 4122 Cavite, Philippines
College of Veterinary Medicine, Chungnam National University, Daejeon 305-764, Republic of Korea

Jong-Soo Lee, Hojin Moon and Chul Joong Kim
College of Veterinary Medicine, Chungnam National University, Daejeon 305-764, Republic of Korea

Mohammed Y. E. Chowdhury
College of Veterinary Medicine, Chungnam National University, Daejeon 305-764, Republic of Korea
Chittagong Veterinary and Animal Sciences University, Chittagong 4202, Bangladesh

Joseph Erume and Frank N. Mwiine
Department of Biomolecular Resources and Biolab Sciences, College of Veterinary Medicine, Animal Resources and Biosecurity, Makerere University, Kampala, Uganda

Pam D. Luka
Department of Biomolecular Resources and Biolab Sciences, College of Veterinary Medicine, Animal Resources and Biosecurity, Makerere University, Kampala, Uganda
Biotechnology Division, National Veterinary Research Institute, Vom, Plateau State, Nigeria

Bitrus Yakubu and Olajide A. Owolodun
Biotechnology Division, National Veterinary Research Institute, Vom, Plateau State, Nigeria

David Shamaki
Virology Division, National Veterinary Research Institute, Vom, Plateau State, Nigeria

K. H. Chan, P. T. W. Li, T. L. Wong, R. Zhang, K. K. H. Chik and G. Chan
Department of Microbiology, The University of Hong Kong, Pokfulam, Hong Kong

K. K. W. To, H. L. Chen and J. F. W. Chan
Department of Microbiology, The University of Hong Kong, Pokfulam, Hong Kong
State Key Laboratory for Emerging Infectious Diseases, The University of Hong Kong, Pokfulam, Hong Kong
Carol Yu Centre for Infection, The University of Hong Kong, Pokfulam, Hong Kong

K. Y. Yuen
Department of Microbiology, The University of Hong Kong, Pokfulam, Hong Kong
State Key Laboratory for Emerging Infectious Diseases, The University of Hong Kong, Pokfulam, Hong Kong
Carol Yu Centre for Infection, The University of Hong Kong, Pokfulam, Hong Kong
The Collaborative Innovation Center for Diagnosis and Treatment of Infectious Diseases, The University of Hong Kong, Pokfulam, Hong Kong

C. C. Y. Yip
Department of Microbiology, Queen Mary Hospital, Pokfulam, Hong Kong

I. F. N. Hung
Department of Medicine, The University of Hong Kong, Pokfulam, Hong Kong

Ekaterina V. Pimkina, Marina V. Safonova, Ekaterina A. Blinova and German A. Shipulin
Central Research Institute of Epidemiology, Moscow 111123, Russia

Andrey A. Ayginin, Alina D. Matsvay and Kamil Khafizov
Central Research Institute of Epidemiology, Moscow 111123, Russia
Moscow Institute of Physics and Technology, Dolgoprudny 141700, Russia

Anna S. Speranskaya
Central Research Institute of Epidemiology, Moscow 111123, Russia
Lomonosov Moscow State University, Moscow 119991, Russia

Vladimir G. Dedkov
Central Research Institute of Epidemiology, Moscow 111123, Russia
Saint-Petersburg Pasteur Institute, Saint Petersburg 197101, Russia

Ilya V. Artyushin
Lomonosov Moscow State University, Moscow 119991, Russia

R. Eberle
Department of Veterinary Pathobiology, Center for Veterinary Health Sciences, Oklahoma State University, Stillwater, OK 74078, USA

L. Jones-Engel
Department of Anthropology and Center for Studies in Ecology and Demography, University ofWashington, Seattle, WA 98195, USA

Mohammed Abo Elkhair
Department of Virology, Faculty of Veterinary Medicine, University of Sadat City, Sadat City 32897, Minoufiya, Egypt
Research Center for Animal Hygiene and Food Safety, Obihiro University of Agriculture and Veterinary Medicine, Inada 2-11, Hokkaido, Obihiro 080-8555, Japan

Alaa G. Abd El-Razak
Department of Bird and Rabbits Medicine, Faculty of Veterinary Medicine, University of Sadat City, Sadat City 32897, Minoufiya, Egypt

Abd Elnaby Y. Metwally
Animal Health Research Institute, Kafr El Sheikh Provincial Laboratory, Kafr El Sheikh, Egypt

Kayode O. Afolabi, Benson C. Iweriebor and Anthony I. Okoh
SAMRC MicrobialWater Quality Monitoring Centre, University of Fort Hare, Private Bag X1314, Alice 5700, Eastern Cape, South Africa
Applied and Environmental Microbiology Research Group (AEMREG), Department of Biochemistry and Microbiology, University of Fort Hare, Private Bag X1314, Alice 5700, Eastern Cape, South Africa

Larry C. Obi
SAMRC MicrobialWater Quality Monitoring Centre, University of Fort Hare, Private Bag X1314, Alice 5700, Eastern Cape, South Africa
Applied and Environmental Microbiology Research Group (AEMREG), Department of Biochemistry and Microbiology, University of Fort Hare, Private Bag X1314, Alice 5700, Eastern Cape, South Africa
Academic and Research Division, University of FortHare, Private Bag X1314, Alice, Eastern Cape, South Africa

Siti Suri Arshad, Muhammad Salisu Abubakar and Yusuf Abba
Department of Veterinary Pathology and Microbiology, Faculty of Veterinary Medicine, Universiti Putra Malaysia (UPM), 43400 Serdang, Selangor, Malaysia

Faruku Bande
Department of Veterinary Pathology and Microbiology, Faculty of Veterinary Medicine, Universiti Putra Malaysia (UPM), 43400 Serdang, Selangor, Malaysia

Department of Veterinary Services, Ministry of Animal Health and Fisheries Development, PMB 2109, Usman Faruk Secretariat, Sokoto 840221, Sokoto State, Nigeria

Abdul Rahman Omar and Mohd Hair Bejo
Department of Veterinary Pathology and Microbiology, Faculty of Veterinary Medicine, Universiti Putra Malaysia (UPM), 43400 Serdang, Selangor, Malaysia
Laboratory of Vaccine and Immunotherapeutics, Institute of Bioscience, Universiti Putra Malaysia (UPM), 43400 Serdang, Selangor, Malaysia

S. V. Cheresiz and E. A. Semenova
Department of Medicine, Novosibirsk State University, Pirogova Street 2, 630090 Novosibirsk-90, Russia
Institute of Internal and Preventive Medicine, Bogatkova Street 175/1, 630089 Novosibirsk-89, Russia

A. A. Chepurnov
Institute of Clinical Immunology, Yadrincevskaya Street 14, 630047 Novosibirsk-47, Russia

Mohammed A. Hamad
College of Veterinary Medicine, Al-Fallujah University, Al-Anbar 31002, Iraq

Ahmed M. Al-Shammari and and Nahi Y. Yaseen
Iraqi Center for Cancer and Medical Genetic Research, Al-Mustansiriya University, Al-Qadisiyah, Baghdad 1001, Iraq

Shoni M. Odisho
College of Veterinary Medicine, Baghdad University, Baghdad 1001, Iraq

Heidi E. M. Smuts
Division Medical Virology/National Health Laboratory Service, Department of Clinical Sciences, Faculty of Health Sciences, University of Cape Town, Observatory 7925, South Africa

Siti Suri Arshad
Department of Veterinary Pathology and Microbiology, Faculty of Veterinary Medicine, Universiti Putra Malaysia (UPM), 43400 Serdang, Selangor, Malaysia

Nafi'u Lawal
Department of Veterinary Pathology and Microbiology, Faculty of Veterinary Medicine, Universiti Putra Malaysia (UPM), 43400 Serdang, Selangor, Malaysia
Department of Veterinary Microbiology, Faculty of Veterinary Medicine, Usmanu Danfodiyo University, Sokoto (UDUS), 2346 Sokoto, Nigeria

Mohd Hair-Bejo and Abdul Rahman Omar
Department of Veterinary Pathology and Microbiology, Faculty of Veterinary Medicine, Universiti Putra Malaysia (UPM), 43400 Serdang, Selangor, Malaysia
Laboratory of Vaccine and Immunotherapeutics, Institute of Bioscience, Universiti Putra Malaysia (UPM), 43400 Serdang, Selangor, Malaysia

Aini Ideris
Laboratory of Vaccine and Immunotherapeutics, Institute of Bioscience, Universiti Putra Malaysia (UPM), 43400 Serdang, Selangor, Malaysia
Department of Veterinary Clinical Studies, Faculty of Veterinary Medicine, Universiti Putra Malaysia (UPM), 43400 Serdang, Selangor, Malaysia

Daniel Oladimeji Oluwayelu, Comfort Oluladun Aiki-Raji, Emmanuel Chibuzor Umeh, Samat Odunayo Mustapha and Adebowale Idris Adebiyi
Department of Veterinary Microbiology and Parasitology, University of Ibadan, Ibadan 20005, Nigeria

Pit Sze Liew and Mohd Hair-Bejo
Department of Veterinary Pathology and Microbiology, Faculty of Veterinary Medicine, Universiti Putra Malaysia, 43400 Serdang, Malaysia

Abdurrahman Hassan Jibril and Farouk Muhammad Tambuwal
Faculty of Veterinary Medicine, Usmanu Danfodiyo University, PMB 2346, Sokoto, Nigeria

Muhammad Bashir Bello
Faculty of Veterinary Medicine, Usmanu Danfodiyo University, PMB 2346, Sokoto, Nigeria
Laboratory of Vaccines and Immunotherapeutics, Institute of Bioscience, Universiti Putra Malaysia, 43400 Serdang, Selangor, Malaysia

KhatijahMohd Yusoff
Laboratory of Vaccines and Immunotherapeutics, Institute of Bioscience, Universiti Putra Malaysia, 43400 Serdang, Selangor, Malaysia
Faculty of Biotechnology and Biomolecular Sciences, Universiti Putra Malaysia, 43400, Selangor, Malaysia

Aini Ideris, Mohd Hair-Bejo and Abdul Rahman Omar
Laboratory of Vaccines and Immunotherapeutics, Institute of Bioscience, Universiti Putra Malaysia, 43400 Serdang, Selangor, Malaysia

Faculty of Veterinary Medicine, Universiti Putra Malaysia, 43400 Serdang, Selangor, Malaysia

Ben P. H. Peeters
Division of Virology, Central Veterinary Institute, Wageningen University, NL8200 Lelystad, Netherlands

Olusesan Adeyemi Adelabu, Benson Chuks Iweriebor, U. U. Nwodo and Anthony Ifeanyi Okoh
SAMRC Microbial Water Quality Monitoring Centre, University of Fort Hare, Private Bag X1314, Alice, Eastern Cape Province 5700, South Africa
Applied and Environmental Microbiology Research Group (AEMREG), Department of Biochemistry and Microbiology, University of Fort Hare, Private Bag X1314, Alice, Eastern Cape Province 5700, South Africa

Larry Chikwelu Obi
Academic and Research Division, University of FortHare, Private Bag X1314, Alice, Eastern Cape Province, South Africa

Siti Suri Arshad
Department of Veterinary Pathology and Microbiology, Faculty of Veterinary Medicine, Universiti Putra Malaysia (UPM), 43400 Serdang, Selangor Darul Ehsan, Malaysia

Faruku Bande
Department of Veterinary Pathology and Microbiology, Faculty of Veterinary Medicine, Universiti Putra Malaysia (UPM), 43400 Serdang, Selangor Darul Ehsan, Malaysia
Department of Veterinary Services, Ministry of Animal Health and Fisheries Development, PMB 2109, Usman Faruk Secretariat, Sokoto 840221, Sokoto State, Nigeria

Abdul Rahman Omar
Department of Veterinary Pathology and Microbiology, Faculty of Veterinary Medicine, Universiti Putra Malaysia (UPM), 43400 Serdang, Selangor Darul Ehsan, Malaysia
Laboratory of Vaccine and Immunotherapeutic, Institute of Bioscience, Universiti Putra Malaysia (UPM), 43400 Serdang, Selangor Darul Ehsan, Malaysia

Index

www.ingramcontent.com/pod-product-compliance
Lightning Source LLC
Chambersburg PA
CBHW050459200326
41458CB00014B/5233